Second Edition

PHARMACEUTICAL CALCULATIONS

for Pharmacy Technicians

A Worktext

Jahangir Moini, MD, MPH, CPhT

Professor and Former Director, Allied Health Sciences,
including the Pharmacy Technician Program,
Everest University - Melbourne, Florida

CENGAGE

Australia · Brazil · Mexico · Singapore · United Kingdom · United States

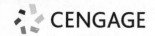

Pharmaceutical Calculations for Pharmacy Technicians: A Worktext, **Second Edition**
Jahangir Moini

Vice President, Editorial: Dave Garza

Director of Learning Solutions: Matthew Kane

Senior Acquisitions Editor: Tari Broderick

Managing Editor: Marah Bellegarde

Associate Product Manager: Meghan E. Orvis

Editorial Assistant: Nicole Manikas

Vice President, Marketing: Jennifer Baker

Marketing Director: Wendy Mapstone

Associate Marketing Manager: Jonathan Sheehan

Senior Director, Education Production:
Wendy A. Troeger

Production Manager: Andrew Crouth

Senior Content Project Manager:
Kara A. DiCaterino

Senior Art Director: Jack Pendleton

For product information and technology assistance, contact us at
Cengage Customer & Sales Support, 1-800-354-9706
or support.cengage.com.

For permission to use material from this text or product, submit all requests online at **www.cengage.com/permissions.**

Library of Congress Control Number: 2011942790

ISBN-13: 978-1-133-13134-2
ISBN-10: 1-133-13134-4

Cengage
20 Channel Street
Boston, MA 02210
USA

Cengage is a leading provider of customized learning solutions with employees residing in nearly 40 different countries and sales in more than 125 countries around the world. Find your local representative at: **www.cengage.com.**

Cengage products are represented in Canada by Nelson Education, Ltd.

To learn more about Cengage platforms and services, register or access your online learning solution, or purchase materials for your course, visit **www.cengage.com.**

Notice to the Reader

Publisher does not warrant or guarantee any of the products described herein or perform any independent analysis in connection with any of the product information contained herein. Publisher does not assume, and expressly disclaims, any obligation to obtain and include information other than that provided to it by the manufacturer. The reader is expressly warned to consider and adopt all safety precautions that might be indicated by the activities described herein and to avoid all potential hazards. By following the instructions contained herein, the reader willingly assumes all risks in connection with such instructions. The publisher makes no representations or warranties of any kind, including but not limited to, the warranties of fitness for particular purpose or merchantability, nor are any such representations implied with respect to the material set forth herein, and the publisher takes no responsibility with respect to such material. The publisher shall not be liable for any special, consequential, or exemplary damages resulting, in whole or part, from the readers' use of, or reliance upon, this material.

Printed at CLDPC, USA, 08-21

PART I

INTRODUCTION

CHAPTER 1

Fundamentals of Math

OBJECTIVES

Upon completion of this chapter, you should be able to:

1. Describe Arabic numbers.
2. Describe Roman numerals.
3. Recognize the symbols used to represent numbers in the Roman numeral system.
4. Convert and correctly write Arabic numbers as Roman numerals and Roman numerals as Arabic numbers.
5. Describe the system of measurement accepted worldwide as well as the household system.
6. List the basic units of weight, volume, and length of the metric system.
7. Explain the rules for changing grams to milligrams and milliliters to liters.
8. Calculate equivalent measurements within the metric system.
9. Summarize metric notation.
10. Recognize the symbols for dram, ounce, grain, and drop.
11. Describe the international unit.
12. Compare apothecary and household equivalents.
13. Explain the use of milliequivalents (mEq) and units in dosage calculations.
14. Describe the use of international units and milliunits (mU) in dosage calculation.

GLOSSARY

apothecary system – A system of measurement that was used in pharmacies until the early twentieth century; it has been replaced by the metric system.

Arabic numbers – The numerical system commonly used, based on the digits 0, 1, 2, 3, 4, 5, 6, 7, 8, and 9.

exponent – A method of expressing a number that is multiplied by itself.

gram – The basic unit of weight in the metric system.

household system – A system of measurement primarily used by patients at home; it is less accurate than the metric system. Its most common units of measure include drops, teaspoons, and tablespoons.

international unit – A measurement used to describe potency of vitamins and chemicals. The quantity that measures biological activity, or effect, of substances, developed from the French "Système Internationale."

liter – The basic unit of volume in the metric system.

meter – The basic unit of length in the metric system.

metric system – The most commonly used system of measurement; it is simple to use because it is based on parts and multiples of 10.

milliequivalent – One-thousandth of an equivalent, the mass of a chemical ion that will combine with 1 gram of hydrogen or 8 grams of oxygen.

milliunit – One-thousandth of a unit.

Roman numerals – The numerical system in which symbols (letters) are used to represent Arabic numbers.

scientific notation – A shorthand method of expressing large numbers that are a product of a number between 1 and 10 and a power of 10.

Système International (SI) – A complete metric system of measurement for scientists; it includes measurements for length, weight, electric current, temperature, matter, and luminous intensity.

unit – A standard of measurement based on the biological activity of a drug rather than its weight; used to express measurement quantities of vitamins, some antibiotics, and certain biologics such as vaccines.

OVERVIEW

To prevent medication errors, the pharmacy technician must master the ability to add, subtract, multiply, and divide whole numbers, fractions, and decimals. Anyone prone to errors in these basic skills will have difficulty computing proper dosages. Pharmacy technicians must master basic mathematics to calculate the dosage of drugs by weight and measures of volume. The technician must be able to solve various types of mathematical problems. Therefore, it is essential for the pharmacy technician to have a sound knowledge of basic mathematical skills.

It also is necessary for pharmacy technicians to understand the systems of measurement and how to convert (change) from one system to another in order to reduce the risk of medication errors. Three systems are used for measuring drugs and solutions: the metric, apothecary, and household systems. The weight of the patient and correct amount of the medication prescribed to the patient are essential factors to performing calculations in the various systems of measurement. Dosage calculations are most concerned with the measurement of weight and volume.

Number Systems

The two systems of numbers currently used in pharmacy are Arabic and Roman. Both systems are used in drug administration. The most common types of numbers used throughout the world today are Arabic. However, the pharmacy technician must also be able to interpret Roman numerals because they are still in use.

Arabic Numbers

Arabic numbers make up a system that is based on the digits 0, 1, 2, 3, 4, 5, 6, 7, 8, and 9. Any number can be represented by combining these digits. Arabic numbers can be written as whole numbers, fractions (e.g., $\frac{1}{3}$), and decimals (e.g., 0.6). The Arabic system is commonly used for counting.

Roman Numerals

Roman numerals consist of letters used to represent number values. The building blocks of the Roman system include the letters I, V, X, L, C, D, and M (**Table 1-1**).

Roman numerals are written as either uppercase or lowercase letters. For example, "iv" represents the number 4, and it is generally written in lowercase to distinguish it from "IV," which is the abbreviation for "intravenous." Sometimes a horizontal line is written above lowercase letters. When the letter "i" is written with this line, the dot of the "i" appears above the line.

TABLE 1-1 Roman Numerals

Roman Numeral	Arabic Equivalent
$\overline{SS}$ or $\overline{ss}$	$\frac{1}{2}$
I or i	1
V or v	5
X or x	10
L or l	50
C or c	100
D or d	500
M or m	1000

Reading Roman Numerals

Roman numerals are read by adding or subtracting the value of the letters. When a letter appears twice in a row, the value of the letter is counted twice. When it appears three times in a row, the value is counted three times. Letters are never used more than three times in a row. If a lower-valued letter follows a larger-valued letter, the letter values should be added. The letter with the largest number equivalent possible should be used to represent a value. If a lower-valued letter is placed before a higher-valued letter, the lower-valued letter is subtracted from the higher-valued letter.

■ EXAMPLE 1:

a. $ii = 1 + 1 = 2$

b. $vi = 5 + 1 = 6$

c. $vii = 5 + 1 + 1 = 7$

d. $xii = 10 + 1 + 1 = 12$

e. $xxv = 10 + 10 + 5 = 25$

f. $xxvii = 10 + 10 + 5 + 1 + 1 = 27$

g. $xxx = 10 + 10 + 10 = 30$

■ EXAMPLE 2:

a. $iv = 5 - 1 = 4$

b. $ix = 10 - 1 = 9$

c. $XL = 50 - 10 = 40$

When a Roman numeral of smaller value comes between two other Roman numerals with larger values, subtract the smaller numeral from the one to its right. Then add the remaining values.

■ EXAMPLE 3:

Calculate the Arabic number for xiv. In xiv, the numeral "i" is located between two numerals with larger values. Subtract i from v first, and then add.

$$xiv = x + iv = x + (v - i) = 10 + (5 - 1)$$
$$= 10 + 4 = 14$$

■ EXAMPLE 4:

Calculate the Arabic for LXIX.

First, subtract I from X, and then add the remaining values.

$$LXIX = L + X + IX = L + X + (X - 1)$$
$$= 50 + 10 + (10 - 1) = 50 + 10 + 9 = 69$$

■ EXAMPLE 5:

a. $vi + xiii = 6 + 13 = 19$

b. $XII + VI = 12 + 6 = 18$

c. $XXIV - IX = 24 - 9 = 15$

d. $XLIX - XXXI = 49 - 31 = 18$

⫸ Remember

- If a letter with a smaller value immediately follows a letter with a larger value, add their values.

- If a letter with a smaller value appears immediately before a letter with a larger value, subtract the smaller value from the larger one. The letters V, L, and D cannot be subtracted from another number.

- When a smaller-valued letter falls between two larger-valued letters, subtract the smaller value from the letter on the right, and then add that value to the letter on the left.

Use of Roman Numerals

Unlike the Arabic system used in everyday counting, the Roman system has no symbol for zero. Roman numerals are used less frequently in dosage calculations. In pharmacy practice, Roman numerals may be used to denote quantities on prescriptions (**Figure 1-1**). The use of this system is restricted because mathematical procedures would become extremely complicated if one were to attempt using these numerals in calculations. The technician needs to understand Roman numerals to interpret prescriptions and drug dosages correctly.

Mary Roberts, M.D.
8264 Palm Tree Way, Melbourne, FL 32101
328-555-9898

Name   Phil Jones

Allegra 180 mg

 # XXX

Sig: one daily

Refills 5

Dr. Mary Roberts

Figure 1-1 Roman numerals may be used on prescriptions.
© *Cengage Learning 2013*

CONVERSION BETWEEN SYSTEMS

To convert Roman numerals to Arabic numbers, convert the Roman symbols to Arabic symbols and add or subtract as described previously. See **Table 1-2** for a list of Roman numerals and their Arabic equivalents.

■ **EXAMPLE 1:**

   a. xv = 10 + 5 = 15

   b. xxviii = 10 + 10 + 5 + 1 + 1 + 1 = 28

   c. xix = 10 + (10 − 1) = 10 + 9 = 19

   d. xxx = 10 + 10 + 10 = 30

TABLE 1-2 Converting the Roman System to Arabic

Roman Numeral	Arabic Number
I, i	1
II, ii	2
III, iii	3
IV, iv	4
V, v	5
VI, vi	6
VII, vii	7
VIII, viii	8
IX, ix	9
X, x	10
XI, xi	11
XII, xii	12
XIII, xiii	13
XIV, xiv	14
XV, xv	15
XVI, xvi	16
XVII, xvii	17
XVIII, xviii	18
XIX, xix	19
XX, xx	20
XXI, xxi	21
XXII, xxii	22
XXIII, xxiii	23
XXIV, xxiv	24
XXV, xxv	25
XXVI, xxvi	26
XXVII, xxvii	27
XXVIII, xxviii	28
XXIX, xxix	29
XXX, xxx	30

METRIC SYSTEM

The **metric system** was developed in France in the eighteenth century for scientific studies and calculations. In the United States, most people use the English system, which utilizes inches, feet, miles, pounds, and tons to describe length and weight. These units are hard to calculate because of how the units relate to each other. For example, 12 inches are in a foot, 5280 feet make up a mile, 16 ounces equal 1 pound, 2000 pounds make up a ton, and so on.

Today, the metric system is the official system of weight and measures used for weighing and calculating pharmaceutical preparations. The metric system is becoming the accepted system throughout the world. This system is sometimes referred to as the *International System of Units* (derived from the French, Système International [SI]). The SI metric system is the most widely accepted system. The basic units that make up the metric system are summarized in **Table 1-3**. Pharmacy technicians need to be concerned primarily with the divisions of weight, volume, and linear measurement of the metric system. Each of these divisions has a primary or basic unit.

TABLE 1-3　SI Metric System

System	Unit	Symbol	Equivalents
Weight	**gram (base unit)**	g	1 g = 1000 mg
	milligram	mg	1 mg = 1000 mcg = 0.001 g
	microgram	mcg	1 mcg = 0.001 mg = 0.00001 g
	kilogram	kg	1 kg = 1000 g
Volume	**liter (base unit)**	L (or l)	1 L = 1000 mL
	milliliter	mL	1 mL = 1 cc = 0.001 L
	cubic centimeter	cc	1 cc = 1 mL = 0.001 L
Length	**meter (base unit)**	m	1 m = 100 cm = 1000 mm
	centimeter	cm	1 cm = 0.01 m = 10 mm
	millimeter	mm	1 mm = 0.001 m = 0.1 cm

Units of Measure

The metric system has three basic units of measurements. Each of these divisions has a primary or basic unit as follows:

- Basic unit of weight is the gram, abbreviated "g"
- Basic unit of volume is the liter, abbreviated "l" or "L"
- Basic unit of length is the meter, abbreviated "m"

Terminology and Abbreviations

The metric system is a decimal system based on multiples of 10 and fractions of 10. It is important to learn the most commonly used prefixes and abbreviations of the metric system. The metric system uses prefixes with all measures. These prefixes indicate the size of the unit (root) being measured in multiples of 10. **Figure 1-2** details the use of prefixes as applied to the appropriate basic unit of measure. It is easily seen that 10 g equals 1 dekagram, 100 g equals 1 hectogram, and 1000 g is referred to as 1 kilogram. Conversely, going down the scale, 0.1 g is referred to as 1 decigram, 0.01 g is called 1 centigram, and 0.001 g is known as a milligram.

1000	100	10	1	0.1	0.01	0.001
Kilo	Hecto	Deka	One	Deci	Centi	Milli
				$\frac{1}{10}$	$\frac{1}{100}$	$\frac{1}{1000}$

Figure 1-2 Metric systems prefixes and their decimal and fractional equivalents.
© Cengage Learning 2013

The basic structure of the metric system's prefixes is shown in **Table 1-4**. **Table 1-5** illustrates examples of common metric abbreviations.

TABLE 1-4 Prefixes

Prefixes for Larger Units	Prefixes for Smaller Units
giga (G) 1,000,000,000 (one billion) m = 1 Gm	deci (d) 0.1 (one-tenth) m = 1 dm
mega (M) 1,000,000 (one million) m = 1 Mm	centi (c) 0.01 (one-hundredth) m = 1 cm
kilo (k) 1,000 (one thousand) m = 1 km	milli (m) 0.001 (one-thousandth) m = 1 mm
hecto (h) 100 (one hundred) m = 1 hm	micro (μ) 0.000001 (one-millionth) m = 1 μm
deka (D) 10 (ten) m = 1 Dm	nano 0.000000001 (one billionth) m = 1 nm

TABLE 1-5 Common Metric Abbreviations

Measure	Abbreviations
nanogram	ng
microgram	mcg
milligram	mg
gram	g
kilogram	kg
milliliter	mL

(Continues)

TABLE 1-5 (Continued)

Measure	Abbreviations
deciliter	dL
liter	L
millimeter	mm
centimeter	cm
meter	m
kilometer	km
kiloliter	kl

Metric Notation

The metric system uses decimals to express units of weight, volume, and length. From these units, temperature, speed, force, and other properties of the physical universe can be measured.

Recall that in the metric system, weight is described in grams, length is described in meters, and volume is described in liters. Each unit can increase or decrease by factors of 10, making calculations easier than in the English system. Note that prefixes like kilo (thousand), mega (million), centi (hundredth), and milli (thousandth) can be used to modify the units. For example, a kilometer is 1000 meters and a centimeter is 0.01 meter.

For writing and interpreting metric notation accurately, remember the following rules:

- Do not guess about the true meaning. When in doubt, ask the writer for clarification.

- The abbreviation always follows the amount (i.e., 25 g, not g 25).

- Decimals are used to designate fractional metric units (i.e., 7.5 mL, not $7\frac{1}{2}$ mL).

- Use a leading zero to emphasize the decimal point for fractional metric units of less than 1 (i.e., 0.75 mg, not .75 mg).

- Omit unnecessary zeros (i.e., 6.5 g, not 6.50 g).

- Write the prefix before the basic unit of measure.

■ **EXAMPLE 1:**

To represent micrograms, write mcg, not gmc or microg.

- Use lowercase letters for metric abbreviations. However, use an uppercase "L" to represent liters.

■ EXAMPLE 2:

Write mg, not MG. Write mL, not ml. Although ml is technically correct, errors can be avoided by using an uppercase L.

- Insert a space between the quantity and the unit.

■ EXAMPLE 3:

Write 15 L, not 15L; write 75 kg, not 75kg.

Exponents and Scientific Notation

An **exponent** is a way of expressing a number that is multiplied by itself (e.g., $5 \times 5 \times 5 \times 5 = 5^4$; this is expressed as 5 to the 4th power). **Scientific notation** is a shorthand method for expressing large numbers that are a product of a number between 1 and 10 and a power of 10 (e.g., 7,000,000 can be expressed as 7×10^6; 7 is multiplied by 1,000,000). Because the metric system uses factors of 10, the use of exponents and scientific notation is an easy way to express large metric units. An easy way to determine the power of 10 is to count the number of zeros in the number or the number of places after the decimal point (e.g., 10^5 means "10 to the 5th power," which is expressed as: $10 \times 10 \times 10 \times 10 \times 10$, equating to 100,000).

■ EXAMPLE 4:

If you are given a value of 5.5×10^5, the number is equivalent to 550,000; 5.5 is multiplied by 100,000.

Stop and Review

Convert the following metric measures.

1. 2500 mL = _____ L

2. 630 mg = _____ g

3. 1600 mcg = _____ mg

4. 1300 mg = _____ g

5. 500 mL = _____ L

6. 150 mg = _____ g

7. 850 cc = _____ L

8. 250 mcg = _____ mg

9. 5500 mcg = _____ mg

10. 100 mg = _____ g

⬭⬭⬭⬭ Remember

- **The basic unit of weight is the gram (g).**

- **The basic unit of volume is the liter (L).**

- **The basic unit of length is the meter (m).**

- **Prefixes accompany the basic units to denote the unit in multiples of 10.**

- **Numbers in the metric system can be presented in scientific notation as a number × 10 to a particular power. To determine the power of 10, count the places from the decimal point in the number.**

Stop and Review

Write the following measures by using official abbreviations and notation rules.

1. five grams = _____

2. two hundred milliliters = _____

3. five-tenths of a liter = _____

4. three-hundredths of a gram = _____

5. four hundred micrograms = _____

6. two-tenths of a milligram = _____

7. four-tenths of a milligram = _____

8. nine hundred micrograms = _____

9. ten and three-tenths micrograms = _____

10. two and seven-tenths kilograms = _____

11. five-hundredths of a gram = _____

12. six and four-tenths kilograms = _____

 Stop and Review

Abbreviate the following metric units.

1. milligram = _____

2. millimeter = _____

3. gram = _____

4. microgram = _____

5. kilogram = _____

6. meter = _____

7. milliliter = _____

8. liter = _____

9. centimeter = _____

10. kiloliter = _____

APOTHECARY SYSTEM

The apothecary system is an old system of measurement. This system is not widely used today because it has been replaced by the metric system. The measures used in the apothecary system are approximate instead of exact. Pharmacy technicians must still be familiar with the apothecary system. Certain medications, especially older ones such as aspirin, quinine, and nitroglycerin, are still measured in apothecary units (**Figure 1-3**).

Figure 1-3 Some medications, such as nitroglycerin, still use apothecary systems of measurement.
Label reproduced with permission of Pfizer, Inc.

The basic unit of weight in the apothecary system is the grain (gr). The apothecary system utilizes Roman numerals. The letters I, V, and X are the basic symbols of this system that pharmacy technicians use in dosage calculations. In medical notation, lowercase letters are typically used to designate Roman numerals such as i, v, and x.

Besides Roman numerals, apothecary notation also uses common fractions, special symbols, and units of measure that precede numeric values. The common units are the grain (gr) and ounce (oz or ℥). **Table 1-6** lists commonly used apothecary system units of measure.

TABLE 1-6 Apothecary System Units of Measure

Solid Weight	Liquid Volume
60 grains = 1 dram	60 minims = 1 fluidram
8 drams = 1 ounce	8 fluidrams = 1 fluid ounce
12 ounces = 1 pound	

In the apothecary system, the symbol or abbreviation comes first, followed by the quantity, which is expressed in lowercase Roman numerals, for example, gr vi, which means 6 grains. Usually only the digits 1 through 10, 20, and 30 are expressed in Roman numerals. Most other quantities are expressed in Arabic numbers. However, numerals from 1 through 10, 20, and 30 are written in Arabic if the entire unit measurement is written in full. For example, 18 grains would not be written xviii grains because the word *grains* is written out; it is either "18 grains" or "gr xviii."

Remember

- Apothecary measures are approximate, not exact.
- The basic unit of apothecary weight is the grain (gr).
- The apothecary system uses Roman numerals and fractions.
- The symbol or abbreviation comes first, followed by the quantity expressed in Roman numerals.

Another difference between the metric system and the apothecary system is that fractions are used in the apothecary system when necessary. (Remember that metric quantities are expressed in decimals.) For example, the fraction "three-quarters" is notated as $\frac{3}{4}$ in the apothecary system but as 0.75 in the metric system. The exception to this rule is the fraction "$\frac{1}{2}$." In apothecary notation, $\frac{1}{2}$ is expressed by the Roman numeral "ss" written below a straight line ($\overline{ss}$). Table 1-7 shows the notations used in the apothecary system.

TABLE 1-7 Apothecary System Abbreviations

Term	Abbreviation	Symbol
Minim	min	ꬆ
Dram	dr	ʒ
Ounce	oz	℥
Grain	gr	(none)
Pound	lb	(none)

Stop and Review

Write the following measurements using apothecary symbols.

1. 3 grains _____

2. $\frac{2}{3}$ dram _____

3. 8 ounces _____

4. 4 pounds _____

5. $\frac{1}{200}$ of a grain _____

6. $\frac{1}{2}$ dram _____

7. 3 ounces _____

8. 2 pounds _____

9. 2 pounds and 11 ounces _____

10. $\frac{1}{2}$ grain _____

HOUSEHOLD SYSTEM

The **household system** of measurement is still commonly used today. It was developed so that patients could measure out dosages at home using ordinary containers found in the kitchen. For example, cups and spoons are simple containers that anyone can use to administer or take medicine. Many over-the-counter medications provide guidelines for patients who depend on household measures. Pharmacy technicians should be familiar with the household system of measurement so that they can explain take-home prescriptions to their patients at the time of discharge. As **Table 1-8** shows, when dispensing medications, the four smallest measures are most frequently used. Household notation places the quantity in Arabic numerals (numbers and common fractions) before the abbreviation for the unit. This system has no standardized system of notation.

TABLE 1-8 Household Abbreviations

Unit	Abbreviation	Equivalents
Drop	gtt	60 drops = 1 tsp
Teaspoon	t (or tsp)	6 tsp = 1 oz
Tablespoon	T (or tbsp)	1 T = 3 t
Ounce (fluid)	oz (℥)	2 T = 1 oz
Ounce (weight)	oz	1 pound (lb) = 16 oz
Cup	cup	1 cup = 8 oz
Pint	pt	1 pt = 2 cups
Quart	qt	1 qt = 4 cups = 2 pt
Gallon	gal	4 qt = 1 gal

Household measurements are inaccurate, with wide variations in the size of teaspoons, tablespoons, and so forth. The generally accepted household measures are the following:

- 60 drops (gtt) = 1 teaspoon (tsp or t)
- 3 tsp = 1 tablespoon (tbsp or T)
- 16 tbsp = 1 glass (or a standard measuring cup)

Household measurements can be equated to apothecary units using the following:

- 1 drop = 1 minim
- 1 tsp = 1 dr
- 1 tbsp = $\frac{1}{2}$ oz

 Remember

- The household system is a common system of measurement used by the lay public in their homes.
- It is very inaccurate due to variations in sizes of household measuring devices.
- It is written in Arabic numbers, with abbreviations used for units of measure following the numbers.

- 2 tbsp = 1 oz

- 1 cup = 6 oz

- 1 glass = 8 oz

- 2 measuring cups = 1 pt

 ## Stop and Review

Convert the following to the equivalent unit indicated using the household system.

1. 75 drops = _____ tsp

2. 24 oz = _____ cups

3. 3 tbsp = _____ oz

4. 4 cups = _____ oz

5. 8 tsp = _____ tbsp

MILLIEQUIVALENTS AND UNITS

Some other measurements can be used for the quantity of medicine ordered. They include: units (formerly abbreviated as U,), milliunits (formerly abbreviated as mU), international units (no longer abbreviated as IU to avoid confusion with IV), and milliequivalents (mEq). The quantity is shown in Arabic numbers with the symbol following. The unit is a standardized amount required to provide a desired effect. Medications such as insulin, heparin, and penicillin have their own meaning and numeric value related to the type of unit. One-thousandth of a unit is a milliunit. The equivalent of one unit is 1000 milliunits. Pitocin is one example of a medication measured in milliunits. The international unit is a unit of potency used to calculate vitamins and chemicals. The milliequivalent (mEq) is one-thousandth of an equivalent weight of a chemical substance. The mEq is the unit used to describe the concentration of serum electrolytes such as sodium, potassium, and calcium.

Medications that are measured in units, international units, and milliequivalents are prepared and administered in the same system. Therefore, there is no need to learn conversions for these systems.

▦ EXAMPLE 1:

Heparin 800 units is ordered, and heparin 1000 units/1 mL is the stock drug.

Heparin.
Courtesy of ESI Lederle, a Business Unit of Wyeth Pharmaceuticals, Philadelphia, PA

▦ EXAMPLE 2:

Potassium chloride 5 mEq is ordered, and potassium chloride 20 mEq per 15 mL is the stock drug.

Potassium Chloride.
Courtesy of Pharmaceutical Associates, Inc.

▦ EXAMPLE 3:

Oxytocin 2 milliunits (0.002 international unit) intravenous per minute is ordered and Oxytocin 10 international units/1 mL to be added to 1000 mL intravenous solution is available.

Oxytocin injection, USP 1 mL contains 10 USP or international units for I.M. or I.V. use.
© *Cengage Learning 2013*

◖▤▥▦▶ *Remember*

- A unit is a standard of measurement based on the biological activity of a drug.

- A milliunit is one-thousandth of a unit.

- A milliequivalent is one-thousandth of a comparable substance whose chemical mass will combine with 1 gram of hydrogen or 8 grams of oxygen.

- An international unit is a measurement of the potency of a vitamin or chemical.

Test Your Knowledge

Convert the following Arabic numbers to Roman numerals.

1. 5 _____
2. 18 _____
3. 9 _____
4. 16 _____
5. 19 _____
6. 22 _____
7. 24 _____
8. 27 _____
9. 29 _____
10. 30 _____
11. 45 _____
12. 89 _____
13. 112 _____
14. 155 _____
15. 198 _____
16. 202 _____
17. 506 _____
18. 534 _____
19. 1000 _____
20. 1025 _____

Convert the following Roman numerals to Arabic numbers.

21. IV _____
22. VII _____
23. IX _____

24. XIII _____

25. XIV _____

26. XVIII _____

27. XIX _____

28. XXIV _____

29. XXVII _____

30. XXIX _____

Calculate the following problems as Arabic numbers.

31. VII + XI _____

32. VIII + IV _____

33. V + VI _____

34. xiv + xvii _____

35. xvi + v _____

36. XIX – xiii _____

37. xxvi – viii _____

38. XV – V _____

39. xiii – iv _____

40. ix – vi _____

Abbreviate the following units of measure.

41. minim _____

42. pint _____

43. grain _____

44. fluid ounce _____

45. dram _____

46. drop _____

47. fluid dram _____

48. quart _____

49. kilogram _____

50. liter _____

51. milligram _____

52. gram _____

53. milliliter _____

54. microgram _____

55. meter _____

56. centimeter _____

57. tablespoon _____

58. cup _____

59. teaspoon _____

60. gallon _____

61. ounce _____

Write the following metric measures using abbreviations and notation rules.

62. four-hundredths of a gram = _____

63. seventeen and five-tenths kilograms = _____

64. three and five-tenths kilograms = _____

65. five and three-tenths milliliters = _____

66. ten and four-tenths micrograms = _____

67. two hundred micrograms = _____

68. fifteen and two-tenths micrograms = _____

69. six-tenths of a liter = _____

70. eight grams = _____

71. four-tenths of a milliliter = _____

72. nine-hundredths of a milligram = _____

Write the amounts using either apothecary or household notation when appropriate.

73. five grains _____

74. one-half teaspoon _____

75. nine ounces _____

76. seven and one-half ounces _____

77. sixteen grains _____

78. one-half grain _____

79. four drams _____

80. twenty-five milliequivalents _____

81. ten thousand units _____

82. one-half tablespoon _____

83. three and one-half ounces _____

84. one-half ounce _____

Give the equivalents to each measurement.

85. 5 tablespoons = _____ t

86. 3 ounces = _____ T

87. 4 cups = _____ oz

88. 5 cups = _____ oz

89. 1 teaspoon = _____ gtt

90. 24 ounces = _____ cups

91. 90 drops = _____ t

92. 6 teaspoons = _____ T

Interpret the following symbols.

93. m = _____

94. 3 = _____ 3

95. ɱ = _____

96. gr = _____

97. qt = _____

98. oz = _____

99. ℥ = _____

100. (s̅s̅) = _____

101. mm = _____

102. g = _____

Write the symbols or abbreviations for the following measurements.

103. drop _____

104. grain _____

105. teaspoon _____

106. minim _____

107. tablespoon _____

108. dram _____

109. milliequivalent _____

110. pint _____

111. ounce _____

Complete the following statements with the correct words.

112. Meters and millimeters are metric units that measure _____.

113. Liters and milliliters are metric units that measure _____.

114. Grams and milligrams are metric units that measure _____.

Fill in the blanks with the correct equivalents to each measurement.

115. 1 kg = _____ g

116. 1000 mcg = _____ mg

117. 1 cm = _____ mm

118. 1 liter = _____ cc

119. 10 mL = _____ cc

120. 1 km = _____ m

121. 1 mm = _____ cm

Circle the correct metric notation.

122. mg10, 10 mG, 10.0 mg, 10 mg, 10 MG

123. 4.5 mL, 4.50 mL, 4.50 ML, $4\frac{1}{2}$ ML, 4.500 mL

124. 7 kg, 7.0 kg, 7-kg, 7 KG, kg 07

125. 2.5 mm, $2\frac{1}{2}$ mm, 2.5 Mm, 2.50 MM, $2\frac{1}{2}$ MM

126. 8.5 mcg, 8.50 mcg, $8\frac{1}{2}$ Mcg, 8.5 MCG, 8.5 mCG

Critical Thinking

1. A pharmacy technician is dispensing a prescription for a patient that reads: 15 mL of cough suppressant three times per day (tid) for 10 days. The technician must answer the following questions:

    a. Which household equipment should the patient use?

    _____

    b. How much medication should the patient take, given the device he was recommended to use? _____

    c. If the medication is supplied in half-pint bottles, how many bottles will the patient need during the 10 days? _____

2. A pharmacy technician is reading a prescription:

    Achromycin 250 mg
    # LXIV

    The technician cannot remember the abbreviation for "L" to dispense the physician's orders. What is the next step that he should take?

    _____

Fractions and Decimals

OBJECTIVES

Upon completion of this chapter, you should be able to:

1. Distinguish the various types of fractions.
2. Compare fractions.
3. Add, subtract, multiply, and divide fractions accurately.
4. Recognize the format of decimals.
5. Convert fractions to mixed numbers and decimals.
6. Add, subtract, multiply, and divide decimals accurately.
7. Round decimals to the nearest tenth, hundredth, and thousandth.

GLOSSARY

common fraction – A fraction in which both the numerator and denominator are whole numbers as opposed to fractions themselves.

complex fraction – A fraction in which the numerator or the denominator, or both, may be a whole number, proper fraction, or mixed number.

decimal fraction – A fraction with a denominator of 10, 100, 1000, or any multiple or power of 10; also known as a decimal.

denominator – The number the whole is divided into.

dividend – The number that is being divided.

divisor – The number performing the division.

fraction – An expression of division with a number that is the portion or part of a whole.

improper fraction – A fraction with the numerator larger than or equal to the denominator.

mixed fraction – A fraction consisting of a whole number and a proper fraction combined.

multiplicand – A number to be multiplied by another.

multiplier – A number by which another is multiplied.

numerator – The portion of the whole being considered.

proper fraction – A fraction with the numerator smaller than the denominator.

quotient – The answer to a division problem.

OVERVIEW

Correct dosage calculations play a large role in ensuring that medications are administered accurately and safely. Pharmacy technicians must learn fractions and decimals to be able to calculate the dosage of drugs by weight and measures of volume. The pharmacy technician must also be able to convert from fractions to decimals as well as from decimals to fractions. Fractions and decimals provide a way to express the relationship of parts to a whole. Fractions measure a portion or part of a whole amount. The decimal system provides another way to represent whole numbers and their fractional parts. Pharmacy technicians use fractions and decimals in their daily work and must be able to work with decimals and fractions proficiently.

FRACTIONS

Fractions can help pharmacy technicians interpret and act on physicians' orders, read prescriptions, and understand patient records and information in the pharmacy literature. Fractions are used in household and apothecary measures for dosage calculations. A **fraction** is a portion of a whole number and represents parts of the whole. The top number is called the **numerator**. The bottom number is called the **denominator**, which represents the whole. Therefore, a fraction has two parts. It can never equal zero. The diagram in **Figure 2-1** represents fractions of a whole.

$$\frac{\text{Numerator (3 parts)}}{\text{Denominator (4 parts)}} = \frac{3}{4}$$

The fraction $\frac{3}{4}$ is used to represent "three-fourths." It means three parts out of a total four parts that make up the whole. The fraction bar also means "divided by." Thus, $\frac{3}{4}$ can be read as "three divided by four," or $3 \div 4$. This definition is important when one changes fractions into decimals.

Distinguishing Types of Fractions

The two types of fractions are common and decimal. A **common fraction** usually is represented as equal parts of a whole. A **decimal fraction** is commonly referred to simply as a decimal. Decimals are covered later in this chapter. The four types of common fractions are proper, improper, mixed, and complex.

Figure 2-1 The fraction 3/4 means three parts out of a total of four parts that make up the whole.
© *Cengage Learning 2013*

Figure 2-2 The value of a proper fraction is always less than 1.
© *Cengage Learning 2013*

Proper Fractions

A **proper fraction** has a numerator that is smaller than the denominator. When the numerator is smaller than the denominator, the value of the fraction is always less than 1 (**Figure 2-2**).

■ **EXAMPLE 1:**

$$\frac{3}{5} = \frac{numerator}{denominator} = \ < 1$$

Other examples of proper fractions are $\frac{2}{5}$, $\frac{1}{10}$, $\frac{26}{47}$, and $\frac{125}{1000}$.

Improper Fractions

An **improper fraction** has a numerator that is equal to or greater than the denominator. The symbol < means "is less than," and > means "is greater than." When the numerator is larger than the denominator, the value of the fraction is always greater than 1 (**Figure 2-3**).

$$\frac{numerator}{denominator} > 1 \ or \ \frac{6}{4} = \ > 1$$

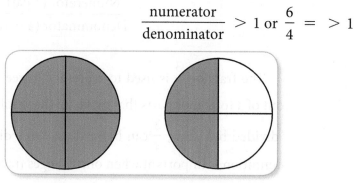

Figure 2-3 The value of an improper fraction is always greater than 1.
© *Cengage Learning 2013*

When the numerator is equal to the denominator, the value of the fraction is always exactly 1 (**Figure 2-4**). If the numerator = the denominator, then:

$$\frac{numerator}{denominator} = 1 \ or \ \frac{6}{6} = 1$$

Figure 2-4 The value of an improper fraction when the numerator and the denominator are equal is always 1.
© Cengage Learning 2013

■ EXAMPLE 2:

Examples of improper fractions include:

$$\frac{7}{5}, \frac{19}{13}, \frac{153}{18}, \text{ and } \frac{1200}{100}$$

■ EXAMPLE 3:

Examples of improper fractions that equal 1 include:

$$\frac{7}{7}, \frac{16}{16}, \frac{111}{111}, \text{ and } \frac{1333}{1333}$$

Mixed Fractions

A **mixed fraction** has a whole number and a proper fraction that are combined. The value of the mixed fraction is always greater than 1 (**Figure 2-5**).

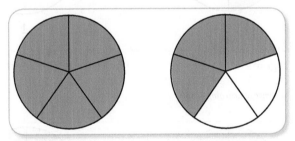

Figure 2-5 The value of a mixed fraction is always greater than 1.
© Cengage Learning 2013

■ EXAMPLE 4:

$$1\frac{3}{5} = 1 + \frac{3}{5} \text{ or } 1\frac{3}{5} > 1$$

Complex Fractions

A **complex fraction** is a fraction in which the numerator or the denominator, or both, may be a whole number, proper fraction, or mixed fraction. The value may be less than, greater than, or equal to 1.

■ EXAMPLE 5:

$$\frac{\frac{4}{9}}{\frac{1}{3}} > 1, \frac{\frac{4}{9}}{2} < 1, \frac{1\frac{4}{9}}{\frac{1}{3}} > 1, \frac{\frac{1}{2}}{\frac{2}{4}} = 1$$

Comparing Fractions

When calculating some drug dosages, it is helpful for the pharmacy technician to know whether the value of one fraction is greater than or less than the value of another fraction. The size of fractions can be determined by comparing the numerators when the denominators are the same, or comparing the denominators when the numerators are the same. If the numerators are the same, the fraction with the smaller denominator has the greater value (**Figure 2-6**).

■ **EXAMPLE 6:**

Compare $\frac{1}{2}$ and $\frac{1}{3}$.

Numerators are both 1.

Denominator 2 is less than 3.

Therefore, $\frac{1}{2}$ has the greater value.

On the contrary, if both the denominators are the same, the fraction with the smaller numerator has the lesser value (**Figure 2-7**).

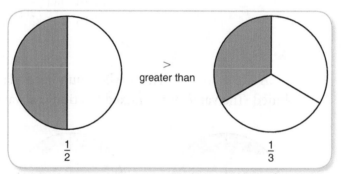

$$\frac{1}{2} \quad > \quad \frac{1}{3}$$
greater than

Figure 2-6 If the numerators are the same, the fraction with the smaller denominator has the greater value.
© Cengage Learning 2013

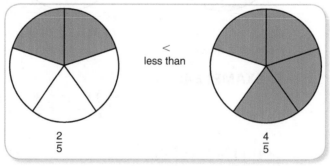

$$\frac{2}{5} \quad < \quad \frac{4}{5}$$
less than

Figure 2-7 If the denominators are the same, the fraction with the smaller numerator has the lesser value.
© Cengage Learning 2013

■ **EXAMPLE 7:**

Compare $\frac{2}{5}$ and $\frac{4}{5}$.

Denominators are both 5.

Numerator 2 is less than 4.

Therefore, $\frac{2}{5}$ has a lesser value.

Converting Improper Fractions to Mixed or Whole Numbers

To convert an improper fraction to an equivalent mixed number or whole number, divide the numerator by the denominator.

■ **EXAMPLE 8:**

$$\frac{6}{3} = 6 \div 3 = 2 \text{ (whole number)}$$

However, in some cases, the numbers do not divide equally. Therefore, a mixed number is the result.

■ **EXAMPLE 9:**

$$\frac{15}{4} = 15 \div 4 = 3\frac{3}{4} \text{ (mixed number)}$$

Because the closest whole number less than 15 that 4 will divide into is 12, 3 is the whole number (4 multiplied by 3 equals 12). Now 15 minus 12 is the remainder, which equals 3. Therefore, 3 out of 4 is the remainder. This fraction is already expressed in the lowest terms, which means that a number can be reduced no further.

■ **EXAMPLE 10:**

$$\frac{9}{4} = 9 \div 4 = 2\frac{1}{4}$$

$$\frac{11}{4} = 11 \div 4 = 2\frac{3}{4}$$

Converting Mixed or Whole Numbers to Improper Fractions

To convert a mixed number to an improper fraction with the same denominator, multiply the whole number by the denominator and add the numerator. Place that value in the numerator, and use the denominator of the fraction part of the mixed number.

■ **EXAMPLE 11:**

Convert $1\frac{3}{7}$ to an improper fraction.

The whole number is 1. The denominator of the fraction is 7. The numerator of the fraction is 3.

Step 1. Multiply the whole number by the denominator of the fraction.

$$1 \times 7 = 7$$

Step 2. Add the product from step 1 to the numerator of the fraction.

$$7 + 3 = 10$$

Step 3. Write the sum from step 2 over the original denominator. Therefore, the answer is $\dfrac{10}{7}$.

Thus,

$$1\dfrac{3}{7} = \dfrac{10}{7}$$

Adding Fractions

If fractions have the same denominator, simply add the numerators and keep the value of the common denominator the same. Then, reduce to the lowest terms.

■ **EXAMPLE 12:**

$$\dfrac{1}{10} + \dfrac{3}{10} = \dfrac{4}{10}$$

■ **EXAMPLE 13:**

$$\dfrac{4}{18} + \dfrac{3}{18} + \dfrac{6}{18} = \dfrac{13}{18}$$

The preceding final fraction is already expressed in the lowest terms.

If you gave an infant $\dfrac{1}{2}$ tablespoon of medication before breakfast, $\dfrac{3}{8}$ tablespoon before lunch, $\dfrac{3}{4}$ tablespoon with dinner, and $\dfrac{3}{8}$ tablespoon at bedtime, you must add the fractions to determine the total amount of medication you have given the infant.

To add the fractions, you must first find the common denominator in all the fractions. Next add the numerators together and keep the value of the common denominator the same. This number is the numerator of the sum of the fractions. The common denominator is the denominator of the sum of the fractions. At the end, reduce the numerator and denominator to the lowest terms.

■ **EXAMPLE 14:**

Add $\dfrac{1}{6}$ and $\dfrac{4}{12}$. To obtain a common denominator of 12, it is necessary to multiply the numerator and denominator of $\dfrac{1}{6}$ by 2. (Note: Both the numerator and denominator must be multiplied so that the value of the fraction remains constant.)

$$\dfrac{1}{6} \times 2 = \dfrac{2}{12}$$

Now we have a common denominator and are able to simply add the numerators.

$$\dfrac{2}{12} + \dfrac{4}{12} = \dfrac{6}{12}$$

Remember

> • To add fractions:
>
> Step 1: Find the least common denominator.
>
> Step 2: Add the numerators together; keep the denominators the same.
>
> Step 3: Reduce the answer to the lowest terms.

Be sure to reduce the final answer.

$$\frac{2}{12} + \frac{4}{12} = \frac{6}{12} = \frac{1}{2}$$

When reduced to the lowest terms, $\frac{6}{12}$ is $\frac{1}{2}$. (The largest number that may be divided into both the numerator and denominator is 6.) So $\frac{6}{12}$ (after both the numerator and denominator are divided by 6) becomes $\frac{1}{2}$.

Subtracting Fractions

If fractions have the same denominator, subtract the smaller numerator from the larger numerator. Keep the denominator the same, and then reduce to the lowest terms to obtain the final answer.

■ **EXAMPLE 15:**

$$\frac{6}{8} - \frac{2}{8} = \frac{4}{8} = \frac{1}{2}$$

If fractions do not have the same denominator, you must change the fractions so that they have the smallest common denominator. Then they can be subtracted as in the preceding example.

■ **EXAMPLE 16:**

$$\frac{13}{24} - \frac{2}{12} =$$

Because 24 is the smallest common denominator for the two denominators shown, you must convert the second fraction by multiplying its numerator and denominator by the number 2.

■ **EXAMPLE 17:**

$$\frac{2}{12} \times \frac{2}{2} = \frac{4}{24}$$

Now that the second fraction has been converted, you may continue with the subtraction as follows:

■ **EXAMPLE 18:**

$$\frac{13}{24} - \frac{4}{24} = \frac{9}{24}$$

■ **EXAMPLE 19:**

$$\frac{9}{24} = \frac{3}{8}$$

Subtracting fractions is similar to adding fractions. To subtract fractions, you must write equivalent fractions with a common denominator. Then subtract the numerators (the difference is the new numerator). Keep the common denominator and reduce your answer to its lowest terms.

■ **EXAMPLE 20:**

Subtract: $\dfrac{2}{6} - \dfrac{3}{12}$

Find a common denominator.

Multiplying the numerator and denominator by 2 produces 12 as the lowest common denominator:

$$\frac{2}{6} - \frac{3}{12} = \frac{4}{12} - \frac{3}{12}$$

Subtract the numerators: $4 - 3 = 1$

Keep the common denominator: $\dfrac{1}{12}$

Multiplying Fractions

To multiply fractions, first multiply the numerators. Second, multiply the denominators, then place the product of the numerators over the product of the denominators, and, finally, reduce to the lowest terms.

■ **EXAMPLE 21:**

$$\frac{3}{5} \times \frac{2}{4} = \frac{6}{20} = \frac{3}{10}$$

In the case of having two fractions that you need to multiply, which could be reduced before multiplying, you may do so as follows:

■ **EXAMPLE 22:**

$$\frac{3}{6} \times \frac{4}{6}$$

Reduce $\dfrac{3}{6}$ to $\dfrac{1}{2}$, then reduce $\dfrac{4}{6}$ to $\dfrac{2}{3}$, and then multiply:

$$\frac{1}{2} \times \frac{2}{3} = \frac{2}{6} = \frac{1}{3}$$

To multiply fractions, first multiply the numerators. Second, multiply the denominators and place the product of the numerators over the product of the denominators. Finally, the resulting value is reduced to its lowest terms.

■ **EXAMPLE 23:**

Multiply $\dfrac{2}{6} \times \dfrac{3}{4}$.

The product of the numerators is $2 \times 3 = 6$. The product of the denominators is $6 \times 4 = 24$. Thus, $\dfrac{2}{6} \times \dfrac{3}{4} = \dfrac{6}{24}$. If $\dfrac{6}{24}$ is reduced, the result is $\dfrac{1}{4}$.

$$\frac{2}{6} \times \frac{3}{4} = \frac{6}{24} = \frac{1}{4}$$

■ **EXAMPLE 24:**

Multiply $4 \times \dfrac{2}{4}$.

First, convert 4 to the improper fraction $\dfrac{4}{1}$.

Now solve.

$$4 \times \frac{2}{4} = \frac{4}{1} \times \frac{2}{4} =$$

$$\frac{4 \times 2}{1 \times 4} = \frac{8}{4} = 2$$

■ **EXAMPLE 25:**

Multiply: $1\frac{4}{7} \times 2\frac{3}{5}$

First, convert the mixed fractions to improper fractions.

$$1\frac{4}{7} = \frac{11}{7} \text{ and } 2\frac{3}{5} = \frac{13}{5}$$

Now multiply the numerators and denominators.

$$1\frac{4}{7} \times 2\frac{3}{5} = \frac{11}{7} \times \frac{13}{5} =$$

$$\frac{11 \times 13}{7 \times 5} = \frac{143}{35}$$

$$\frac{143}{35} \text{ converts to } 4\frac{3}{35}$$

> **Remember**
>
> • **To multiply fractions:**
>
> **Step 1: Reduce all fractions to the lowest terms.**
>
> **Step 2: Multiply the numerators.**
>
> **Step 3: Multiply the denominators.**
>
> **Step 4: Reduce to the lowest terms.**

Dividing Fractions

To divide fractions, first invert (or turn upside down) the divisor, and then multiply.

■ **EXAMPLE 26:**

$$\frac{4}{8} \div \frac{2}{8} = ?$$

Invert the divisor:

$$\frac{4}{8} \times \frac{8}{2} = \frac{32}{16}$$

Reduce, and then multiply the numerators and then the denominators:

$$\frac{32}{16} = \frac{2}{1} = 2$$

■ **EXAMPLE 27:**

$$\frac{32}{12} \div \frac{2}{3} = ?$$

Invert the divisor:

$$\frac{32}{12} \times \frac{3}{2} = \frac{96}{24}$$

Simplify:

$$\frac{16}{4} \times \frac{1}{1} = 4$$

■ **EXAMPLE 28:**

$$3\frac{2}{5} = \frac{5 \times 3 + 2}{5} = \frac{17}{5}$$

■ **EXAMPLE 29:**

$$6\frac{3}{7} = \frac{7 \times 6 + 3}{7} = \frac{45}{7}$$

To divide fractions, multiply the **dividend** (the fraction being divided) by the reciprocal of the **divisor** (the fraction performing the division). First, reduce all fractions to the lowest terms. Next invert (turn upside down) the divisor. Then multiply the two fractions and reduce to the lowest terms.

■ **EXAMPLE 30:**

Suppose you have $\frac{3}{4}$ bottle of liquid medication available. The usual dose you would give a patient is $\frac{1}{16}$ bottle, and you want to know how many doses remain in the bottle. You solve this problem by dividing fractions. To solve $\frac{3}{4} \div \frac{1}{16}$, $\frac{3}{4}$ is the dividend and $\frac{1}{16}$ is the divisor. Therefore, multiply the dividend $\frac{3}{4}$ by the reciprocal of the divisor $\frac{1}{16}$. To determine the reciprocal, the divisor is inverted (or turned upside down).

$$\frac{3}{4} \div \frac{1}{16} = \frac{3}{4} \times \frac{16}{1}$$

You now solve this as a multiplication problem:

$$\frac{3}{4} \times \frac{16}{1} = \frac{48}{4} = \frac{12}{1} = 12$$

The bottle has 12 doses remaining.

■ **EXAMPLE 31:**

Divide $\frac{1}{2}$ by $\frac{1}{4}$.

The problem has no mixed or whole numbers. Invert (flip) the divisor of $\frac{1}{4}$ to find its reciprocal, $\frac{4}{1}$. Then multiply the dividend by the reciprocal of the divisor:

$$\frac{1}{2} \div \frac{1}{4} = \frac{1}{2} \times \frac{4}{1} = \frac{4}{2} = \frac{2}{1} = 2$$

■ **EXAMPLE 32:**

Divide $\frac{1}{75}$ by $\frac{1}{150}$:

The problem has no mixed or whole numbers. Invert the divisor of $\frac{1}{150}$ to find its reciprocal, $\frac{150}{1}$.

Then multiply the dividend by the reciprocal of the divisor:

$$\frac{1}{75} \div \frac{1}{150} = \frac{1}{75} \times \frac{150}{1} = \frac{150}{75} = 2$$

■ **EXAMPLE 33:**

Simplify the following:

$$\frac{\frac{3}{4}}{\frac{1}{16}}$$

The numerator is $\frac{3}{4}$ and the denominator is $\frac{1}{16}$. Rewrite the complex fraction as a regular division problem and then solve it.

$$\frac{3}{4} \div \frac{1}{16} = \frac{3}{4} \times \frac{16}{1}$$

Now solve it as a multiplication problem:

$$\frac{3}{4} \div \frac{1}{16} = \frac{3}{4} \times \frac{16}{1} = \frac{48}{4} = 12$$

> ◁)))) *Remember*
>
> • **To divide fractions:**
>
> Step 1: Reduce all fractions to the lowest terms.
>
> Step 2: Invert the divisor.
>
> Step 3: Multiply the fractions.
>
> Step 4: Reduce to the lowest terms.

⬢ Stop and Review

Answer the following questions relating to common fractions.

1. What is the denominator in $\frac{15}{80}$? _____

2. What is the denominator in $\frac{75}{5}$? _____

3. What is the denominator in $\frac{60}{60}$? _____

4. What is the numerator in $\frac{25}{100}$? _____

5. What is the numerator in $\frac{9}{6}$? _____

6. What is the numerator in $\frac{82}{82}$? _____

7. Which of the following fractions is a proper fraction? _____

   a. $\dfrac{27}{26}$ c. $\dfrac{43}{63}$

   b. $\dfrac{7}{7}$ d. $\dfrac{95}{90}$

8. Which of the following fractions is an improper fraction? _____

   a. $\dfrac{39}{38}$ c. $\dfrac{19}{92}$

   b. $\dfrac{39}{48}$ d. $\dfrac{45}{102}$

Convert the following improper fractions to mixed or whole numbers.

9. $\dfrac{60}{20}$ _____

10. $\dfrac{72}{72}$ _____

11. $\dfrac{26}{4}$ _____

12. $\dfrac{9}{5}$ _____

13. $\dfrac{146}{30}$ _____

14. $\dfrac{200}{8}$ _____

15. $\dfrac{160}{80}$ _____

16. $\dfrac{93}{9}$ _____

Convert the following mixed numbers to improper fractions.

17. $6\dfrac{12}{18}$ _____

18. $19\dfrac{9}{19}$ _____

19. $5\dfrac{1}{10}$ _____

20. $2\dfrac{1}{4}$ _____

21. $3\dfrac{8}{9}$ _____

22. $56\dfrac{4}{8}$ _____

23. $150\dfrac{2}{3}$ _____

24. $192\dfrac{4}{6}$ _____

Finding the Least Common Denominator

It is frequently necessary to find a least common denominator (LCD) for a group of fractions. The least common denominator is the smallest number into which each of the denominators of each of the fractions in the group will divide exactly.

For example, 12 is the least common denominator for the fractions $\dfrac{1}{4}$ and $\dfrac{1}{3}$ because it is the smallest number that both 4 and 3 divide into exactly. For the fractions $\dfrac{1}{4}, \dfrac{1}{6},$ and $\dfrac{1}{8}$, the least common denominator is 24.

The number 48 could have been selected because 4, 6, and 8 also divide exactly into this number, but the least common denominator is the smallest number that all the denominators divide into exactly.

If the least common denominator for a group of fractions cannot be determined by looking, use the following procedure.

> **Remember**
>
> • The least common denominator is the smallest number into which all of the denominators will divide equally.

■ EXAMPLE 34:

Find the least common denominator of $\dfrac{1}{5}, \dfrac{1}{6}, \dfrac{2}{9}, \dfrac{5}{12},$ and $\dfrac{3}{24}$.

SOLUTION:

Write all the denominators in a horizontal row:

5 6 9 12 24

Starting with the number 2, find the smallest whole number that divides exactly into two or more of the denominators. (If two or more of the denominators cannot be exactly divided by the number 2, try the number 3, and so on.)

Write the results of the division directly under the denominators, and bring down all the denominators that cannot be divided, thus completing a totally new row of numbers.

2	5	6	9	12	24
	5	3	9	6	12

Repeat the process until the final row of numbers contains no numbers that can be exactly divided by any whole number other than 1.

2	5	6	9	12	24
2	5	3	9	6	12
3	5	3	9	3	6
	5	1	3	1	2

The least common denominator can then be determined by multiplying each divisor (vertical numbers) and each number in the last row (horizontal numbers).

LCD $= 2 \times 2 \times 3 \times 5 \times 1 \times 3 \times 1 \times 2$

LCD $= 2 \times 2 \times 3 \times 5 \times 3 \times 2$ (the 1s can be dropped)

LCD $= 360$

When the least common denominator is obvious, this procedure is unnecessary.

■ **EXAMPLE 35:**

Find the least common denominator of $\dfrac{1}{4}, \dfrac{3}{12}, \dfrac{3}{20}$, and $\dfrac{7}{40}$.

SOLUTION:

Write the row of denominators:

	4	12	20	40	divide this row by 2
2	2	6	10	20	divide this row by 2
2	1	3	5	10	divide this row by 5
5	1	3	1	2	which is only divisible
	1	3	1	2	by 1

Therefore, the least common denominator is determined by multiplying $2 \times 2 \times 5 \times 1 \times 3 \times 1 \times 2 = 120$.

Reducing Fractions to the Lowest Terms

When calculating dosages, it is usually easier to work with fractions using the smallest numbers possible. Finding these equivalent fractions is called *reducing the fraction to the lowest terms* or *simplifying the fraction*. To reduce a fraction to the lowest terms, *divide* both the numerator and denominator by the *largest nonzero whole number* that will go evenly into both the numerator and the denominator.

■ **EXAMPLE 36:**

Reduce $\dfrac{6}{12}$ to the lowest terms.

The largest number that will divide evenly into both 6 (numerator) and 12 (denominator) is 6.

$$\frac{6}{12} = \frac{6 \div 6}{12 \div 6} = \frac{1}{2} \text{ in lowest terms}$$

Stop and Review

Find the lowest common denominator for these fractions.

1. $\frac{1}{4}, \frac{1}{3}, \frac{1}{6}$ _____

2. $\frac{2}{3}, \frac{5}{6}$ _____

3. $\frac{2}{3}, \frac{3}{4}, \frac{4}{5}$ _____

4. $\frac{8}{10}, \frac{12}{20}$ _____

5. $\frac{7}{8}, \frac{7}{16}$ _____

6. $\frac{3}{4}, \frac{1}{3}$ _____

7. $\frac{7}{8}, \frac{1}{4}, \frac{2}{3}$ _____

8. $\frac{1}{2}, \frac{1}{16}$ _____

9. $\frac{17}{4}, \frac{18}{8}$ _____

10. $\frac{1}{2}, \frac{3}{4}$ _____

Reduce these fractions.

11. $\frac{6}{12}$ _____

12. $\frac{4}{6}$ _____

13. $\frac{6}{8}$ _____

14. $\frac{9}{81}$ _____

15. $\frac{3}{6}$ _____

16. $\frac{10}{20}$ _____

17. $\frac{3}{9}$ _____

18. $\frac{56}{64}$ _____

19. $\frac{18}{24}$ _____

20. $\frac{105}{135}$ _____

Stop and Review

Add the following fractions.

1. $\dfrac{1}{6} + \dfrac{3}{8} = $ _____

2. $\dfrac{1}{9} + \dfrac{7}{8} = $ _____

3. $4 + \dfrac{3}{5} = $ _____

4. $\dfrac{3}{8} + \dfrac{3}{4} + \dfrac{7}{12} = $ _____

5. $\dfrac{1}{6} + \dfrac{3}{6} = $ _____

6. $\dfrac{2}{10} + \dfrac{4}{20} = $ _____

7. $3 + \dfrac{8}{11} = $ _____

8. $\dfrac{1}{7} + \dfrac{2}{12} = $ _____

9. $\dfrac{1}{3} + \dfrac{1}{5} + \dfrac{1}{7} = $ _____

10. $\dfrac{2}{5} + \dfrac{4}{15} = $ _____

11. $\dfrac{1}{5} + \dfrac{1}{4} + \dfrac{1}{3} = $ _____

12. $\dfrac{5}{6} + \dfrac{7}{9} = $ _____

13. $2\dfrac{3}{6} + \dfrac{1}{5} = $ _____

14. $\dfrac{3}{5} + \dfrac{4}{15} = $ _____

15. $3\dfrac{1}{2} + 2\dfrac{1}{2} = $ _____

Subtract the following fractions.

16. $7\dfrac{7}{15} - 4\dfrac{4}{15} = $ _____

17. $\dfrac{7}{25} - \dfrac{2}{25} = $ _____

18. $\dfrac{11}{3} - \dfrac{2}{6} = $ _____

19. $6\dfrac{1}{3} - \dfrac{5}{6} = $ _____

20. $6\dfrac{7}{7} - 2\dfrac{21}{5} = $ _____

21. $7 - \dfrac{3}{7} =$ _____

22. $\dfrac{4}{7} - \dfrac{3}{21} =$ _____

23. $\dfrac{3}{4} - \dfrac{1}{6} =$ _____

24. $1\dfrac{7}{8} - \dfrac{1}{4} =$ _____

25. $2\dfrac{5}{8} - \dfrac{1}{2} =$ _____

26. $14\dfrac{9}{10} - 3\dfrac{1}{2} =$ _____

27. $14 - \dfrac{3}{7} =$ _____

28. $8\dfrac{1}{12} - 3\dfrac{1}{4} =$ _____

29. $25 - 17\dfrac{7}{9} =$ _____

30. $1\dfrac{2}{3} - 1\dfrac{1}{12} =$ _____

 ## Stop and Review
Multiply these fractions.

1. $\dfrac{1}{3} \times \dfrac{1}{5} =$ _____

2. $\dfrac{2}{7} \times \dfrac{4}{5} =$ _____

3. $\dfrac{2}{5} \times \dfrac{6}{8} =$ _____

4. $\dfrac{5}{3} \times \dfrac{8}{10} =$ _____

5. $\dfrac{6}{9} \times \dfrac{2}{6} =$ _____

6. $\dfrac{9}{7} \times \dfrac{7}{2} =$ _____

7. $\dfrac{10}{16} \times \dfrac{5}{9} =$ _____

8. $\dfrac{3}{8} \times \dfrac{4}{9} =$ _____

9. $\dfrac{12}{9} \times \dfrac{2}{2} =$ _____

10. $\dfrac{14}{12} \times \dfrac{4}{5} =$ _____

11. $3\dfrac{1}{3} \times \dfrac{9}{15} =$ _____

12. $1\dfrac{5}{6} \times 7\dfrac{4}{5} =$ _____

13. $3\dfrac{6}{8} \times 7\dfrac{2}{9} =$ _____

14. $1\dfrac{7}{8} \times \dfrac{4}{5} =$ _____

15. $\dfrac{3}{6} \times \dfrac{7}{16} \times \dfrac{3}{4} =$ _____

16. $\dfrac{8}{5} \times \dfrac{3}{10} \times \dfrac{4}{5} =$ _____

17. $\dfrac{14}{36} \times \dfrac{2}{24} \times 14 =$ _____

18. $7 \times \dfrac{5}{15} \times \dfrac{5}{14} =$ _____

19. $\dfrac{45}{22} \times \dfrac{14}{7} \times \dfrac{7}{24} =$ _____

20. $\dfrac{12}{24} \times \dfrac{7}{8} \times \dfrac{15}{18} =$ _____

Stop and Review
Solve the following problems.

1. $\dfrac{4}{8} \div \dfrac{6}{9} =$ _____

2. $\dfrac{5}{11} \div \dfrac{3}{4} =$ _____

3. $\dfrac{4}{9} \div \dfrac{1}{2} =$ _____

4. $\dfrac{1}{5} \div \dfrac{3}{4} =$ _____

5. $\dfrac{5}{7} \div \dfrac{2}{6} =$ _____

6. $\dfrac{6}{9} \div \dfrac{3}{7} =$ _____

7. $\dfrac{9}{10} \div \dfrac{3}{5} =$ _____

8. $\dfrac{5}{14} \div \dfrac{23}{36} =$ _____

9. $1\dfrac{5}{7} \div \dfrac{4}{5} =$ _____

10. $\dfrac{5}{8} \div 1\dfrac{3}{4} =$ _____

11. $6\dfrac{2}{9} \div 2\dfrac{3}{8} = $ _____

12. $5\dfrac{1}{2} \div 1\dfrac{1}{6} = $ _____

13. $1\dfrac{5}{6} \div 7 = $ _____

14. $8 \div \dfrac{3}{6} = $ _____

15. $\dfrac{\frac{9}{12}}{\frac{4}{6}} = $ _____

16. $\dfrac{\frac{2}{7}}{\frac{3}{8}} = $ _____

DECIMALS

Generally, decimal fractions and decimal numbers are referred to simply as *decimals*. Decimal fractions are used with the metric system, which is the system most often used in the calculation of drug dosages. The pharmacy technician must be able to manipulate decimals easily and accurately. Each decimal fraction consists of a numerator that is expressed in numerals, a decimal point placed so that it designates the value of the denominator, and the denominator that is understood to be 10, or some power of 10. In writing a decimal fraction, always place a zero to the left of the decimal point so that the decimal point can readily be seen. This also ensures that the decimal will not be mistaken for the whole number 1. Table 2-1 shows some examples.

Remember

- Whole numbers are to the left of the decimal point.
- Fractions are to the right of the decimal point.
- Always write a zero to the left of the decimal point when the decimal number has no whole number part. Using the zero makes the decimal point more noticeable. It also helps prevent errors caused by illegible handwriting.

TABLE 2-1 Equivalent Mixed Fractions and Decimals

Mixed Fraction	Decimal	Description
$15\dfrac{3}{10}$	15.3	Fifteen and three-tenths
$85\dfrac{7}{10}$	85.7	Eighty-five and seven-tenths
$172\dfrac{25}{100}$	172.25	One hundred seventy-two and twenty-five hundredths
$\dfrac{42}{100}$	0.42	Forty-two hundredths
$2\dfrac{355}{1000}$	2.355	Two and three hundred fifty-five thousandths

Figure 2-8
© Cengage Learning 2013

To understand how to read and write decimals, examine **Figure 2-8**, which shows that all whole numbers are to the left of the decimal point and all fractions are to the right.

Converting Fractions to Decimals and Decimals to Fractions

Recognizing that there is a relationship between fractions and decimals is useful when it becomes necessary to convert a fraction to its decimal equivalent. To accomplish this task, simply divide the numerator of the fraction (the top of the fraction) by the denominator of the fraction (the bottom number of the fraction).

■ **EXAMPLE 1:**

Convert $\frac{3}{4}$ to a decimal.

SOLUTION:

Divide the numerator of the fraction by the denominator.

$$
\begin{array}{r}
0.75 \\
4\overline{)3.00} \\
2.8 \\
\hline
20 \\
20 \\
\hline
\end{array}
$$

Therefore, $\frac{3}{4} = 0.75$

■ **EXAMPLE 2:**

Convert $\frac{1}{100}$ to a decimal.

SOLUTION:

Divide the numerator of the fraction by the denominator.

$$
\begin{array}{r}
0.01 \\
100\overline{)1.00} \\
1.00 \\
\hline
\end{array}
$$

Therefore, $\frac{1}{100} = 0.01$

))))) Remember

- All decimal fractions and decimal numbers are referred to simply as *decimals*.

- To convert fractions to decimals, divide the numerator by the denominator.

- To convert decimals to fractions, make the number without the decimal point the numerator. The number 1 followed by as many zeros as decimal places becomes the denominator. Then reduce to the lowest terms.

■ **EXAMPLE 3:**

Convert 0.75 to a fraction.

SOLUTION:

Make the decimal number without the decimal point the numerator of the fraction. The number 1 followed by as many zeros as there are digits to the right of the decimal point is the denominator.

$$\frac{75}{100} = \frac{3}{4}$$

Therefore, $0.75 = \frac{3}{4}$

 Stop and Review

Change the following fractions into decimals.

1. $\frac{1}{2}$ _____

2. $\frac{2}{5}$ _____

3. $\frac{1}{6}$ _____

4. $\frac{5}{8}$ _____

5. $\frac{2}{15}$ _____

6. $\frac{1}{158}$ _____

7. $\frac{3}{200}$ _____

8. $\frac{1}{12}$ _____

9. $\frac{1}{500}$ _____

10. $\frac{1}{3000}$ _____

Change the following decimals to fractions.

11. 0.005 _____

12. 0.009 _____

13. 0.0033 _____

14. 0.05 _____

15. 0.25 _____

16. 0.0002 _____

17. 0.075 _____

18. 0.15 _____

19. 0.84 _____

20. 2.75 _____

Adding Decimals

To add decimals, write the decimals in a column, with the decimal points placed directly under each other. Then add the numbers, as in the addition of whole numbers, and place the decimal point in the sum directly under the decimal points in the column.

■ **EXAMPLE 4:**

Add 4.27 and 0.51.

To perform the operation, write it as follows:

$$\begin{array}{r} 4.27 \\ + 0.51 \\ \hline \end{array}$$

Then add vertically to keep the decimal points aligned:

$$\begin{array}{r} 4.27 \\ + 0.51 \\ \hline 4.78 \end{array}$$

■ **EXAMPLE 5:**

Add $18.4 + 7.52 + 8 + 0.631$.

To perform the operation, write it as follows:

$$\begin{array}{r} 18.4 \\ 7.52 \\ 8 \\ + 0.631 \\ \hline \end{array}$$

Then add:

$$\begin{array}{r} 18.4 \\ 7.52 \\ 8.0 \\ + 0.631 \\ \hline 34.551 \end{array}$$

Subtracting Decimals

To subtract decimals, write the decimals in columns, keeping the decimal points under each other. Then subtract the decimals, as with whole numbers. A zero may be added after the decimal without changing the value.

 Remember

- **To add decimals:**

  Step 1: Write the decimals in a column, aligning the decimal points.

  Step 2: Add the columns vertically right to left, carrying numbers over as necessary.

  Step 3: Place the decimal point in the answer directly under the decimal point in the column.

Then place the decimal point in the remainder, directly under the decimal point in the column. Remember to carry numbers over as necessary when subtracting.

■ **EXAMPLE 6:**

Subtract $68.07 - 17.44$.

To perform the operation, write it as follows:

$$\begin{array}{r} 68.07 \\ -\ 17.44 \\ \hline 50.63 \end{array}$$

■ **EXAMPLE 7:**

Subtract $9.5 - 3.008$.

To perform the operation, write it as follows:

$$\begin{array}{r} 9.5 \\ -\ 3.008 \end{array}$$

Or

$$\begin{array}{r} 9.500 \\ -\ 3.008 \\ \hline 6.492 \end{array}$$

Stop and Review

Add or subtract the following numbers.

1. $9.32 + 4.92 = $ _____

2. $155.07 + 31.02 = $ _____

3. $17.435 + 0.034 = $ _____

4. $72.308 + 4.916 = $ _____

5. $4.06 + 0.8 = $ _____

6. $5.45 + 0.009 = $ _____

7. $0.025 + 0.68 = $ _____

8. $8 + 0.033 = $ _____

9. $53.62 - 0.07 = $ _____

10. $18.36 - 1.225 = $ _____

11. $7.88 - 0.08 = $ _____

12. $16.5 - 0.9 = $ _____

Remember

- To subtract decimals:

Step 1: Write the decimals in a column, aligning the decimal points.

Step 2: Subtract the columns vertically right to left, borrowing numbers as necessary.

Step 3: Place the decimal point in the answer directly under the decimal point in the column.

13. $5.22 - 0.6 = $ _____

14. $12.8 - 0.777 = $ _____

15. $9 - 0.023 = $ _____

16. $17 - 0.07 = $ _____

Multiplying Decimals

To multiply decimals, first find the product as usual. Second, count the number of decimal places in both the **multiplicand** (the number being multiplied) and the **multiplier** (the number doing the multiplying). Finally, mark the total number of decimal places in the product and insert a decimal point.

■ EXAMPLE 8:

Step 1: Multiply 3.07×0.8.

3.07 (multiplicand)

$\underline{\times 0.8}$ (multiplier)

2456 (product)

Step 2:

Count the number of decimal places in the multiplicand and multiplier.

 3.07

$\underline{\times 0.8 =}$ Total of three decimal places

Step 3:

Mark off three decimal places in the product.

New decimal $= 2.456$

■ EXAMPLE 9:

Step 1: Multiply 3.85×2.2.

3.85 (multiplicand)

$\underline{\times 2.2}$ (multiplier)

 8470 (product)

Step 2:

Count the number of decimal places in the multiplicand and multiplier.

3.85

$\underline{\times 2.2 =}$ Total of three decimal places

Step 3:

Mark off three decimal places in the product.

New decimal $= 8.47$

Remember

- To multiply decimals:

Step 1: Multiply the whole numbers.

Step 2: Add the number of decimal places in the numbers being multiplied.

Step 3: Place the decimal point in the answer the number of spaces to the left equal to the number of decimal places in the numbers being multiplied.

Stop and Review
Multiply the following numbers.

1. $9.7 \times 8.6 =$ _____

2. $4.9 \times 0.7 =$ _____

3. $6.28 \times 3.3 =$ _____

4. $7.06 \times 0.08 =$ _____

5. $0.77 \times 0.7 =$ _____

6. $0.082 \times 0.6 =$ _____

7. $0.009 \times 0.03 =$ _____

8. $0.25 \times 0.85 =$ _____

9. $5.04 \times 18 =$ _____

10. $17 \times 0.08 =$ _____

11. $0.003 \times 19.7 =$ _____

12. $0.007 \times 55.05 =$ _____

Dividing Decimals

To divide a decimal by a whole number, first write the problem as usual. Second, place a decimal point in the quotient line directly above the decimal in the dividend, and then find the **quotient** (the answer). Division is written using several symbols, such as $1 \div 2$, or $\frac{1}{2}$. The divisor (the number performing the division) is on the right of the symbol in the first example and on the bottom of the symbol in the second example. The divisor must be a whole number (a number with no decimal point), and the decimal point must be correctly placed in the answer. When a decimal number is being divided by a whole number, the decimal point is placed directly above the decimal point in the dividend (number being divided). When a number is being divided by a decimal number, the decimal point in the divisor must be moved to the right as many places as needed to make the divisor a whole number. The decimal point in the dividend must be moved the same number of places to the right. The decimal point in the quotient is placed directly above the new position of the decimal point in the dividend.

■ EXAMPLE 10:

Divide $0.6 \div 0.02$.

First, write the problem as a fraction:

$$\frac{0.6}{0.02}$$

Second, move the decimal point two places to the right in both the numerator and the denominator. The denominator is now a whole number:

$$\frac{0.6}{0.02} = \frac{60}{2}$$

This step is equivalent to multiplying:

$$\frac{0.6}{0.02} \times \frac{100}{100}$$

Third, complete the division:

$$\frac{0.6}{0.02} = \frac{60}{2} = 30$$

so that $0.6 \div 0.02 = 30$

■ EXAMPLE 11:

Divide $0.088 \div 0.11$.

First:

$$\frac{0.088}{0.11}$$

Second:

$$\frac{0.088}{0.11} = \frac{8.8}{11} = 0.8$$

Move the decimal point two places to the right, in both the numerator and denominator, so that the denominator (divisor) is a whole number.

Third, complete the division:

$$0.088 \div 0.11 = 0.8$$

> **⟨⟨⟨⟩ Remember**
>
> • **To divide decimals:**
>
> **Step 1: Write the division problem as a fraction.**
>
> **Step 2: Move the decimal point so that the denominator is a whole number.**
>
> **Step 3: Move the decimal point in the numerator the same number of places to the right.**
>
> **Step 4: Complete the division.**

Stop and Review

Divide the following numbers.

1. $6.2 \div 1.4 = $ _____

2. $36.8 \div 0.6 = $ _____

3. $84.6 \div 1.8 = $ _____

4. $0.004 \div 0.002 = $ _____

5. $1.5 \div 0.5 =$ _____

6. $0.62 \div 0.4 =$ _____

7. $0.08 \div 0.02 =$ _____

8. $14.6 \div 2 =$ _____

9. $60 \div 0.6 =$ _____

10. $0.88 \div 8.8 =$ _____

11. $39.06 \div 100 =$ _____

12. $4.44 \div 1000 =$ _____

13. $66.666 \div 0.03 =$ _____

14. $82.82 \div 0.004 =$ _____

15. $126.26 \div 2000 =$ _____

16. $38.42 \div 2.1 =$ _____

17. $6.6 \div 0.11 =$ _____

18. $77.7 \div 3.3 =$ _____

19. $0.888 \div 1000 =$ _____

20. $8.875 \div 3.25 =$ _____

Rounding Decimals

To round a decimal, it is necessary to obtain an answer one decimal place after the desired place. Therefore, if the last digit is less than 5, the last digit is simply dropped. However, if the last digit is 5 or greater, the prior digit must increase by one number.

■ EXAMPLE 12:

Round 3.3 to the nearest whole number.

Consider the tenths column. Because 3 is less than 5, the answer is 3, and 0.3 is discarded. Round 3.57 to the nearest tenth. Because the hundredths column includes 7, and this number is greater than 5, the answer is 3.6 and the 7 is dropped.

Round 2.896 to the nearest hundredth. Because the last digit is 6, and this number is greater than 5, the answer is 2.90 and the 6 is dropped.

> **))))) Remember**
>
> • **To round decimals:**
>
> Step 1: If the last digit is less than 5, the last digit is simply dropped.
>
> Step 2: If the last digit is greater than 5, the number is increased by one, and the last digit is dropped.

Test Your Knowledge

Calculate the following numbers and give the answer in the lowest terms.

1. $\dfrac{8}{4} + \dfrac{2}{6} =$ _____

2. $\dfrac{3}{5} + 1\dfrac{2}{5} =$ _____

3. $\dfrac{4}{10} + \dfrac{2}{20} + \dfrac{1}{50} =$ _____

4. $8 + \dfrac{5}{8} + \dfrac{1}{4} + \dfrac{6}{12} =$ _____

5. $\dfrac{18}{9} - \dfrac{4}{6} =$ _____

6. $\dfrac{4}{5} - \dfrac{3}{4} =$ _____

7. $6\dfrac{1}{2} - 2\dfrac{7}{8} =$ _____

8. $3 - \dfrac{2}{7} =$ _____

9. $\dfrac{8}{6} \times \dfrac{2}{4} =$ _____

10. $\dfrac{7}{7} \times \dfrac{3}{14} =$ _____

11. $4\dfrac{6}{3} \times \dfrac{10}{5} =$ _____

12. $\dfrac{6}{8} \times 11 =$ _____

13. $\dfrac{2}{8} \div \dfrac{4}{6} =$ _____

14. $\dfrac{17}{13} \div \dfrac{3}{56} =$ _____

15. $2\dfrac{7}{8} \div \dfrac{2}{6} =$ _____

16. $\dfrac{1}{4} \div 1\dfrac{1}{4} =$ _____

Convert the following mixed numbers to improper fractions.

17. $1\dfrac{2}{7} = $ _____

18. $21\dfrac{3}{8} = $ _____

19. $8\dfrac{6}{10} = $ _____

20. $6\dfrac{4}{8} = $ _____

21. $4\dfrac{3}{6} = $ _____

22. $11\dfrac{2}{6} = $ _____

Reduce the following fractions to their lowest terms.

23. $\dfrac{12}{48} = $ _____

24. $\dfrac{66}{92} = $ _____

25. $\dfrac{48}{8} = $ _____

26. $\dfrac{92}{8} = $ _____

27. $\dfrac{112}{62} = $ _____

28. $\dfrac{186}{93} = $ _____

Find the least common denominator, and then write an equivalent fraction for each.

29. $\dfrac{5}{10}$ and $\dfrac{3}{5} = $ _____

30. $\dfrac{3}{6}$ and $\dfrac{4}{9} = $ _____

31. $\dfrac{7}{10}, \dfrac{1}{4},$ and $\dfrac{2}{3} = $ _____

32. $\dfrac{3}{5}, \dfrac{3}{2},$ and $\dfrac{1}{6} = $ _____

Round to the nearest tenth.

33. 4.62 = _____

34. 7.75 = _____

35. 8.991 = _____

36. 0.053 = _____

Round to the nearest hundredth.

37. 8.091 = _____

38. 0.444 = _____

39. 64.004 = _____

40. 9.882 = _____

Round to the nearest whole number.

41. 20.4 = _____

42. 6.86 = _____

43. 0.821 = _____

44. 12.668 = _____

Calculate the following numbers.

45. $0.021 + 0.88 =$ _____

46. $7.18 + 14.38 =$ _____

47. $4.69 + 0.7 =$ _____

48. $16 + 0.008 + 1.3 =$ _____

49. $5.47 - 0.39 =$ _____

50. $6.26 - 3.31 =$ _____

51. $0.684 - 0.89$ (Note: The answer to this problem will be a negative decimal.)

_____

52. $19.02 - 0.647 =$ _____

53. $5.3 \times 7.9 =$ _____

54. $0.67 \times 0.004 =$ _____

55. $9 \times 0.992 =$ _____

56. $12.09 \times 1.009 =$ _____

57. $48.62 \div 2.1 =$ _____

58. $6.876 \div 3.36 =$ _____

59. $4.4 \div 0.11 =$ _____

60. $1.6 \div 0.08 =$ _____

Circle the correct answer.

61. Which is the largest number?   0.015   0.15   0.024

62. Which is the smallest number? 0.325   0.6   0.073

63. True or false? $0.465 = 0.0465$

64. True or false? 4.6 grams $= 4.06$ grams

65. True or false? 8.8 ounces $= 8.800$ ounces

Critical Thinking

A pharmacy technician is opening a box of instruments in various sizes. The technician is asked to arrange a set of instruments on the shelf in order, from smallest to largest on the basis of the instruments' diameters. The diameters are marked $\frac{1}{4}, \frac{1}{16}, \frac{1}{2}, \frac{7}{16}, \frac{3}{16}$, and $\frac{5}{16}$.

1. How should the technician arrange the instruments?

   _____

2. Look at the pattern of increase in these measurements. Are any instruments missing in the sequence? If so, which ones?

   _____

Ratios, Proportions, and Percents

OBJECTIVES

Upon completion of this chapter, you should be able to:

1. Distinguish the numerical relationships represented by ratios.
2. Describe the concept of proportions.
3. Explain the relationship between percents and ratios.
4. Solve for x using proportions.
5. Convert percentages into ratios and fractions, and convert ratios and fractions into percentages.

GLOSSARY

extremes – The two outside terms in a ratio.

means – The two inside terms in a ratio.

percent – A fraction whose numerator is expressed and whose denominator is understood to be 100.

proportion – A statement of two equal ratios.

OVERVIEW

Pharmacy technicians must understand percents, ratios, and proportions to deal with a variety of medications and treatments and to ensure accuracy in preparing and calculating these medications. The ability to express percents and ratios, and how they are related to fractions and decimals, is a skill that is essential to correctly measuring and calculating medications. The pharmacy technician needs to practice using percents, ratios, and proportions to become skilled in this area of mathematics.

RATIOS

A ratio is the relation between two numbers. Ratios may be used to relate a quantity of liquid medication to a quantity of intravenous solution. Pharmacy technicians can also use ratios to calculate dosages of dry medication such as caplets or tablets. Ratios are written either as fractions or linearly. The two numbers in a ratio (or "quantities") are separated by a colon (:). The use of the colon is a traditional way to write the division sign within a ratio, which is expressed as "4 is to 9" in the following example.

■ EXAMPLE 1:

$\frac{4}{9}$ may be expressed as a ratio: 4:9.

A ratio also can be expressed as a fraction. The first number of the ratio becomes the numerator and the second number becomes the denominator. When expressed as a fraction, a ratio can be reduced to its lowest terms.

■ EXAMPLE 2:

5:250 may be expressed as a fraction:

$$\frac{5}{250} = \frac{1}{50}$$

■ EXAMPLE 3:

$$7:21 = \frac{7}{21} = \frac{1}{3}$$

■ EXAMPLE 4:

4:8 can be expressed as $\frac{4}{8}$ and can be reduced to $\frac{1}{2}$.

Ratios should generally be expressed in lowest terms, such as the following: $\frac{5}{25}$, which reduces to $\frac{1}{5}$. Therefore, the ratio 5:25 should be written as 1:5. Another example would be $\frac{25}{100}$, which can be reduced to $\frac{1}{4}$, or 1:4.

> **)))) Remember**
>
> - Ratios express a relationship.
> - The quantities in a ratio are separated by a colon.
> - To change a ratio into a fraction, the first number in the ratio becomes the numerator and the second number becomes the denominator.
> - Ratios should be expressed in lowest terms.

Stop and Review
Convert the following fractions into ratios.

1. $\dfrac{250}{1000} =$ _____

2. $\dfrac{20}{100} =$ _____

3. $\dfrac{40}{60} =$ _____

4. $\dfrac{6}{8} =$ _____

5. $\dfrac{300}{900} =$ _____

6. $\dfrac{25}{200} =$ _____

7. $\dfrac{60}{1200} =$ _____

8. $\dfrac{75}{1500} =$ _____

9. $\dfrac{3}{9} =$ _____

10. $\dfrac{25}{50} =$ _____

11. $\dfrac{40}{100} =$ _____

12. $\dfrac{17}{170} =$ _____

13. $\dfrac{50}{1000} =$ _____

14. $\dfrac{8}{100} =$ _____

15. $\dfrac{20}{4000} =$ _____

16. $\dfrac{150}{3000} =$ _____

17. $\dfrac{500}{2000} =$ _____

18. $\dfrac{32}{160} =$ _____

19. $\dfrac{10}{40} = $ _____

20. $\dfrac{12}{120} = $ _____

PROPORTIONS

A **proportion** is the relationship between two equal ratios. Because ratios are usually written as fractions, a proportion is also expressed as two equal fractions. The proportion (equation) uses an equal sign or double colon to demonstrate that the ratios on both sides of the equal sign (=) or double colon (::) are equal. Therefore, a proportion can be shown in two ways:

As two equal fractions,

$$\frac{A}{B} = \frac{C}{D}$$

or using a colon,

$$A{:}B = C{:}D$$

When two ratios are equal, the cross products of the ratios are equal. Using cross products tests whether the two ratios are equal. To find the cross products of a proportion, multiply the outer terms, called the **extremes**, and the middle terms, called the **means**. This relationship is shown in **Figure 3-1**. In a proportion, the product of means is equal to the product of extremes.

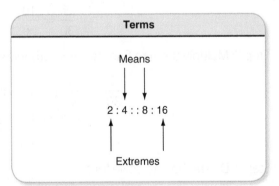

Figure 3-1 The means and the extremes.
© Cengage Learning 2013

Remember

- A proportion is the relationship between two equal ratios.

- An equal sign or double colon represents the relationship between the two parts.

- Both sides of the proportion must be the same. This can be verified by multiplying the means and the extremes.

■ **EXAMPLE 1:**

$$A{:}B = C{:}D \text{ or } A \times D = B \times C$$

$$\frac{5}{10} = \frac{13}{26}$$

or, $5 \times 26 = 10 \times 13$, $130 = 130$

■ **EXAMPLE 2:**

$$20:25 = 4:5$$

In this example, 20 and 5 are the extremes, and 25 and 4 are the means. Because the cross products are both equal to 100, these ratios are equal and this proportion is true ($20 \times 5 = 25 \times 4$ or $100 = 100$).

To write a ratio proportion as a fraction proportion, use the following rule:

1. Change the double colon to an equal sign.

2. Convert both ratios to fractions.

■ **EXAMPLE 3:**

$$3:5 :: 9:15 \text{ or}$$

$$3:5 = 9:15 \text{ or}$$

$$\frac{3}{5} = \frac{9}{15}$$

■ **EXAMPLE 4:**

$$5:100 :: 50:1000 \text{ or}$$

$$5:100 = 50:1000 \text{ or}$$

$$\frac{5}{100} = \frac{50}{1000}$$

In a case when one quantity is missing from the proportion, substitute the letter "x" for the missing term. You must take three steps:

Step 1: Write the proportion as a fraction:

$$\frac{5}{30} = \frac{10}{x}$$

Step 2: Multiply them to find the cross products:

$$\frac{5}{30} = \frac{10}{X} \text{ (cross multiply)}$$
$$5 \times X = 10 \times 30$$
$$5X = 300$$

Step 3: Divide them to solve for X:

$$X = \frac{300}{5} = 60$$

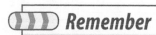 **Remember**

- **To solve for X:**
  Write the proportion.
  Cross multiply.
  Divide to solve for X.

 Stop and Review

Solve for X in the following proportions.

1. $6:30 = 15:X$ _____

2. $2:10 = 3:X$ _____

3. $5:20 = 3:X$ _____

4. $50:250 = 10:X$ _____

5. 21:63 = 45:X _____

6. 32:128 = 4:X _____

7. 8:72 :: 5:X _____

8. 0.4:0.8 = X:80 _____

9. 30:120 = X:12 _____

10. 128:1 = X:5 _____

11. X:625 = 1:5 _____

12. 20:40 = X:100 _____

PERCENTS

Percent (denoted by the symbol "%") stands for "hundredths." A percent is a ratio of a number to 100. It can be written in the form of "x" with the symbol %, or "X%." Think of the symbol % to be a distortion of the 100 in a ratio of X:100. The ratio of 30 to 100 is 30 percent, or 30%; this is the same as 30 hundredths, or 0.30. A percent may be expressed as a fraction, a decimal, or a ratio, each of which provides a way to express the relationship of parts to a whole.

■ EXAMPLE 1:

Percent	Fraction	Decimal	Ratio
30%	$= \dfrac{30}{100}$	= 0.30	= 30:100

Percents are frequently used to show the strength of intravenous (IV) solutions. They are also used to indicate the strength of medications such as ointments; for example, two percent (2%) of an ointment means 2 parts of 100, and 0.9% of a solution means 0.9 part (less than 1 part) of 100.

Changing Percents to Decimals

To change a percent to a decimal, move the decimal point two places to the left to signify hundredths; add zeros as necessary. This also can be done by removing the percent sign and dividing by 100.

■ EXAMPLE 2:

Convert 38% to a decimal.

$$38\% = 38.\% = .38. = 0.38$$

■ EXAMPLE 3:

Convert 125% to a decimal.

$$125\% = 125.\% = 1.25. = 1.25$$

■ **EXAMPLE 4:**

Convert $15\frac{1}{2}$% to a decimal.

$$15\frac{1}{2} = 15\frac{5}{10}\% = 15.5\% = 015.5\% = 0.15.5 = 0.155$$

Changing Decimals to Percents

To change a decimal to a percent, move the decimal point two places to the right to signify hundredths; add zeros as necessary. This also can be done by multiplying by 100 and adding the percent sign.

■ **EXAMPLE 5:**

Convert 0.22 to a percent.

$$0.22 \times 100 = 22\%$$

$$0.22 = 0.22. = 22\%$$

Changing Percents to Fractions

To convert a percentage to a fraction, convert the percent to a decimal, and then convert the decimal to a fraction. Another way is to put the percent over 100 and reduce.

■ **EXAMPLE 6:**

Change 30% to a fraction.

$$30 \div 100 = 0.30$$

$$\frac{3}{10}$$

■ **EXAMPLE 7:**

Change 0.1% to a fraction.

$$0.1 \div 100 = 0.001$$

$$\frac{1}{1000}$$

Changing Fractions to Percents

To change a fraction to a percent, convert the fraction to a decimal, and then convert the decimal to a percent by multiplying by 100 and adding a percent sign.

■ **EXAMPLE 8:**

Convert $\frac{3}{5}$ to a percent.

$$\frac{3}{5} = 0.6 = 60\%$$

◖▮▮▯ Remember

- **Percents stand for hundredths.**

- **Percents can be expressed as ratios, decimals, or fractions.**

- **To change a percent to a decimal, move the decimal point two places to the left or divide by 100.**

- **To change a decimal to a percent, move the decimal point two places to the right or multiply by 100.**

- **To change a percent to a fraction, convert the percent to a decimal and then the decimal to the fraction.**

- **To change a fraction to a percent, convert the fraction to a decimal and then the decimal to a percent.**

- **To determine a specific percentage, change the percent to a decimal or fraction and then multiply by the number.**

■ **EXAMPLE 9:**

Convert $\frac{1}{4}$ to a percent.

$$\frac{1}{4} = 0.25 = 25\%$$

Determining Percents

To determine the percentage of a given number, first convert the percentage to a decimal or fraction. Next multiply the decimal or fraction by the number.

■ **EXAMPLE 10:**

What percent of 10 ounces is 3 ounces? You are looking for a percentage in this case.

Convert the percentage to a decimal or fraction.

$$10\% = 0.1 = \frac{1}{10}$$

Next multiply the decimal or fraction by the number.

$$0.1 \times 3 = 0.3 = 30\%$$

$$\frac{1}{10} = \frac{X}{3}$$

$$3 = 10X \text{ or } 10X = 3$$

X divided by 10 = 3 divided by 10

$$X = \frac{3}{10} \text{ or } X = 0.30 = 30\%$$

Stop and Review

Solve the following problems on determining percents.

1. 60% of 20 = _____

2. 50% of 1000 = _____

3. 0.02% of 100 = _____

4. $\frac{1}{2}$ % of 2000 = _____

5. 25% of 1000 = _____

6. 10% of 75 = _____

7. $\frac{8}{10}$ % of 1000 = _____

8. 75% of 250 = _____

9. $\frac{1}{4}$ % of 1200 = _____

10. 7% of 500 = _____

11. 0.9% of 1200 = _____

12. 5% of 5000 = _____

13. $\frac{1}{2}$ % of 250 = _____

14. 15% of 400 = _____

15. 20% of 150 = _____

 Test Your Knowledge

Express the following percents as decimals.

1. 6%   _____

2. 35%   _____

3. 0.3%   _____

4. 0.01%   _____

5. 0.004%   _____

Express the following percents as fractions and reduce the answers to the lowest terms.

6. 5%   _____

7. 20%   _____

8. 0.3%   _____

9. .25%   _____

10. 0.05%   _____

Express the following as ratios.

11. $\frac{1}{3}$ _____

12. $\frac{1}{500}$ _____

13. $\frac{\frac{2}{3}}{\frac{3}{4}}$ _____

14. $\dfrac{2}{150}$ _____

15. $\dfrac{\frac{1}{500}}{\frac{1}{1000}}$ _____

Express the following percents as ratios.

16. 1% _____

17. 50% _____

18. 12.5% _____

19. 0.25% _____

20. 0.33% _____

Solve for X in the following proportions.

21. 1:5 = X:20 _____

22. X:3 = 7:21 _____

23. $\dfrac{1}{2}$: X = 3:12 _____

24. $\dfrac{1}{3}:\dfrac{2}{3}=\dfrac{1}{6}$:X _____

25. 25:X = 75:1500 _____

26. $\dfrac{1}{6}:\dfrac{1}{8}$ = X:3 _____

27. 0.3:0.4 = X:0.5 _____

28. 0.5:0.125 = 2:X _____

29. 0.25:3 = 0.75:X _____

30. $\dfrac{1}{150}:\dfrac{1}{100}$ = X:1 _____

Are the following statements true or false?   True   False

31. 3:5 and 12:20 are equal ratios.   _____   _____

32. If cross products are equal, the ratios are equal.   _____   _____

33. A proportion is the relationship between two equal quotients.   _____   _____

34. 7 miles in 10 minutes = 3.5 miles in 5 minutes.   _____   _____

35. If $\dfrac{x}{15}=\dfrac{2}{36}$, then x = 3   _____   _____

36. If $\dfrac{3}{5} = \dfrac{6}{10}$, then $3 \times 6 = 5 \times 10$ _____ _____

37. 6 for $0.85 is better than 8 for $1.00. _____ _____

38. $\dfrac{4}{5} = \dfrac{16}{18}$ _____ _____

39. 18 for $0.56 is better than 9 for $1.50. _____ _____

40. $\dfrac{25}{55} = \dfrac{4}{8}$ _____ _____

Critical Thinking

A pharmacy technician received a prescription for 125 mcg of a medication. The pharmacy has 0.25 mg scored tablets on hand. The technician calculated that the patient should take two tablets per dose. The drug label indicates that 0.25 mg is equivalent to 250 mcg.

1. Is the pharmacy technician performing the calculation correctly?

   _____

2. If not, how many tablets should the patient take?

   _____

Celsius and Fahrenheit Temperature Conversions

OBJECTIVES

Upon completion of this chapter, you should be able to:

1. Describe the Fahrenheit and Celsius temperature scales.

2. Convert between Celsius and Fahrenheit temperatures.

3. Explain the formula used to convert between Fahrenheit and Celsius temperatures.

GLOSSARY

Celsius scale – A temperature measurement scale wherein water freezes at 0 degrees and boils at 100 degrees; Celsius was the last name of the scale's inventor.

centigrade – Identical to the Celsius scale and used interchangeably.

Fahrenheit scale – A temperature measurement scale wherein water freezes at 32 degrees and boils at 212 degrees; Fahrenheit was the last name of the scale's inventor.

temperature – The measure of heat associated with metabolism of the body, or from any heat source.

OVERVIEW

Pharmacy technicians should be familiar with measurements of temperature and also be able to convert them. Correct temperatures are essential for the proper storage of drugs and vaccines. Many different medications and substances must be kept refrigerated until use. The temperature of the pharmacy refrigerator must be kept constant and requires regular monitoring by the pharmacy technician. Many medications list storage temperatures in either Celsius or Fahrenheit. Also, because body temperature is measured as part of diagnosing medical conditions, the ability to convert between Celsius and Fahrenheit temperatures is essential for pharmacy technicians.

TEMPERATURE

Temperature is defined as a relative measure of sensible heat or cold. Normally, the human body is maintained at a constant level of 98.6° Fahrenheit (F) (or 37° Celsius [C]) by the body's thermotaxic nerve mechanism that balances heat gains and heat losses.

Temperature scales have two basic points: from when water starts to freeze and when it starts to boil. Between these two temperatures, a scale is made. The most popular scales are the Celsius (created by Anders Celsius) and Fahrenheit (made by Gabriel Fahrenheit) scales. The Fahrenheit scale is defined so that the freezing point of water occurs at 32 degrees and the boiling point occurs at 212 degrees. This means that there are 180 divisions between the freezing point and boiling point.

The Celsius scale differs in that the freezing point of water occurs at 0 degrees and the boiling point occurs at 100 degrees. This scale (also referred to as "centigrade") exists on 100-unit divisions and is also known as a "centiscale." In 1948, the "centidegrees" (centigrade scale) was replaced by "degrees Celsius" (°C).

Converting between the Celsius and Fahrenheit Scales

Temperatures are most often reported in Fahrenheit and, occasionally, also in Celsius. A formula has been developed to compute conversions between the two scales based on the differences between the freezing and boiling points of each scale (**Figure 4-1**). Recall that there are 100 degrees between the boiling and freezing points on the Celsius thermometer, and 180 degrees between the boiling and freezing points on the Fahrenheit thermometer. The ratio of the difference between the Fahrenheit and Celsius scales can be expressed as 180:100, or:

$$\frac{180}{100}$$

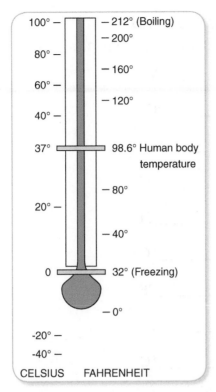

100° — — 212° (Boiling)
— 200°

80° — — 160°

60° —
— 120°

40° —

37° — 98.6° Human body
temperature

— 80°

20° —

— 40°

0 — 32° (Freezing)

— 0°

-20° —
-40° —

CELSIUS   FAHRENHEIT

Figure 4-1 Comparison of Celsius and Fahrenheit scales.
© *Cengage Learning 2013*

When reduced, this ratio is equivalent to 1.8.

This equivalent of 1.8 is constantly used in temperature conversions between Fahrenheit and Celsius via the following formula:

$$°C = \frac{°F - 32}{1.8}$$

■ EXAMPLE 1:

Convert: 99.4°F to °C.

Substituting 99.4 for °F in the conversion formula, 99.4°F = °C

$$\frac{99.4 - 32}{1.8} = \frac{67.4}{1.8} = 37.4°C$$

Use the following formula to convert a temperature from Celsius to Fahrenheit.

$$°F = (1.8 \times °C) + 32$$

■ EXAMPLE 2:

Convert: 20°C to °F.

Substituting 20 for °C in the conversion formula,

$$(1.8 \times 20) + 32 = 36 + 32 = 68$$

Thus, 20°C = 68°F

Remember

• To convert Fahrenheit to Celsius, use the following formula:

$$°C = \frac{°F - 32}{1.8}$$

• To convert Celsius to Fahrenheit, use the following formula:

$$°F = (1.8 \times °C) + 32$$

Stop and Review

Convert the following temperatures.

1. 37°C = _____ °F

2. 93°F = _____ °C

3. 62°F = _____ °C

4. 104°F = _____ °C

5. 42.7°C = _____ °F

6. 188°F = _____ °C

7. 100°C = _____ °F

8. 87°C = _____ °F

9. 109°F = _____ °C

10. 22°C = _____ °F

Convert the following statements of temperature to Celsius or Fahrenheit.

11. Normal body temperature is 98.6°F. _____

12. Medication must not be exposed to a temperature > 88°F. _____

13. A patient has a fever of 102.8°F. _____

14. You need to keep a vaccine at the temperature of 6°C. _____

15. A physician orders antipyretic medication and adds a note that the patient should stop taking it if his body temperature lowers to 38.5°C. _____

Another method can be used to convert Fahrenheit to Celsius: subtract 32 and then multiply the result by $\frac{5}{9}$.

1. To begin, subtract 32 from the Fahrenheit number.

2. Divide the answer by 9.

3. Multiply the answer by 5.

■ **EXAMPLE 3:**

Convert: 95°F to Celsius.

$$95 - 32 = 63 \quad 63 \div 9 = 7 \quad 7 \times 5 = 35°C$$

Table 4-1 lists a few common temperatures with approximate descriptions.

TABLE 4-1 Common Temperatures

°F	°C	Description
212	100	Boiling point of water
98.6	37	Normal body temperature
86	30	Very hot summer day
72	22	Room temperature
68	20	Mild spring day
50	10	Warm winter day
32	0	Freezing point of water
20	−7	Very cold winter day

Test Your Knowledge

Give the following temperature equivalents as indicated. Those temperatures given in °F should be converted to °C and vice versa.

1. 63.4°F _____

2. 99.5°F _____

3. 87.2°F _____

4. 178°F _____

5. 132°F _____

6. 32°F _____

7. 112°F _____

8. 212°F _____

9. 44°F _____

10. 97.8°F _____

11. 164°F _____

12. 48°F _____

13. 0°C _____

14. 6.8°C _____

15. 2.4°C _____

16. 37.4°C _____

17. 100°C _____

18. 43.6°C _____

19. 32°C _____

20. 8.4°C _____

21. 55°C _____

22. 17°C _____

23. 0.12°C _____

24. 27°C _____

Critical Thinking

1. A prescription is written for a child who has a fever of more than 101°F. She is to be given acetaminophen every 4 hours. Her mother asks a pharmacy technician to tell her the Celsius temperature equivalent of 101°F. _____

2. A vaccine must be kept in the pharmacy refrigerator at 8°C. What is the equivalent Fahrenheit temperature? _____

PART II

DOSAGE CALCULATIONS

Ratio and Proportion Method

OBJECTIVES

Upon completion of this chapter, you should be able to:

1. Use common fractions to express ratio and proportion in dosage calculations.
2. Use colons to express ratio and proportion in dosage calculations.
3. Perform calculations using different units of measure.
4. Define the terms *ratio* and *proportion*.

GLOSSARY

ratio – A statement of the relation of one quantity to another.

true proportion – A proportion in which the ratios have been proven to be equal by multiplying the means and extremes.

OVERVIEW

Ratio and proportion form the basis for nearly all calculations. The ratio and proportion method is a concept that is widely understood and used. Even so, many pharmacy technicians have difficulty interpreting such calculations and identifying a place to start. A ratio states the relation of one quantity to another. Ratios may be written as common fractions (implying division) or with a colon between the two numbers.

In previous chapters, this book discussed how to read the dosage on drug labels. Each of these dosages was expressed as a ratio: a specific weight (strength of a drug in forms such as tablets, capsules, or certain volumes of solution). Liquid solutions are commonly measured in mL. Common dosages are expressed as follows: 50 mg per mL, 100 mcg per tablet, and 1000 units per mL.

RATIO AND PROPORTION EXPRESSED USING COMMON FRACTIONS

A **ratio** is made up of two numbers or quantities that have a significant relationship. They can be expressed (written) as either common fractions or separated by a colon (:). A proportion is used to show the relationship between two ratios. The ratios in a proportion are separated by an equal (=) sign. Conversions may be made by setting up a proportion of two ratios expressed as fractions. A **true proportion** contains two ratios that are equal (for example, $\frac{1}{50} = \frac{2}{100}$). In a true proportion, the cross-multiplied products will be identical.

The pharmacy technician must make sure that the units in the numerators match and the units in the denominators match. The units in each ratio must then be labeled.

■ EXAMPLE 1:

Convert: 1.5 g to grains (gr).

Known approximate equivalent: 1 g = gr 15.

This proportion in fractional form looks like this:

$$\frac{\text{gr } 15}{1 \text{ g}} = \frac{\text{gr x}}{1.5 \text{ g}} \quad \text{(Cross multiply.)} \quad 22.5 = 1x$$

Therefore, x = 22.5.

In the preceding equation, the unknown "x" is the numerator. It is important that the sequence is the same (the numerator units match and the denominator units match). Remember, a proportion must compare "like things" to "like things."

> ⬤⬤⬤⬤ **Remember**
>
> In a proportion, the ratio for a known equivalent equals the ratio for an unknown equivalent. The following two steps are involved in this method:
>
> 1. Set up a proportion of two equivalent ratios.
>
> 2. Cross-multiply to solve for an unknown quantity (X).

EXAMPLE 2:

Convert: 10 grains to milligrams.

$$\frac{gr\ i}{60\ mg} = \frac{gr\ 10}{x\ mg} \quad x = 60 \times 10 = 600\ mg$$

EXAMPLE 3:

Convert: 75 mL to tsp.

Known approximate equivalent: 1 tsp = 5 mL.

$$\frac{1\ t}{5\ mL} = \frac{xt}{75\ mL} \quad 5x = 75$$

$$\frac{5x}{5} = \frac{75}{5} \quad x = \frac{75}{5}t = 15\ t$$

EXAMPLE 4:

Convert: 176 lb to kg.

Known approximate equivalent: 1 kg = 2.2 lb.

$$\frac{1\ kg}{2.2\ lb} = \frac{x\ kg}{176\ lb} \text{ (Cross multiply.) } 2.2x = 176$$

$$\frac{2.2\ x}{2.2} = \frac{176}{2.2} \quad x = \frac{176}{2.2} = kg = 80\ kg$$

EXAMPLE 5:

How many tablets will contain 100 mg if 1 tablet contains 50 mg?

$$\frac{1\ tablet}{50\ mg} = \frac{X\ tablets}{100\ mg}$$

Therefore,

$$50X = 100\ mg,\ so\ X = 2\ tablets$$

EXAMPLE 6:

Cross-multiply this proportion to determine if it is a true proportion.

$$\frac{1\ mL}{10\ units} = \frac{2\ mL}{20\ units}$$

Therefore,

$$1 \times 20 = 10 \times 2$$

$$20 = 20$$

Yes, this is a true proportion because the products of cross-multiplying—20—are equal.

Dosage Calculations

In dosage calculations, ratio and proportion are important because they can be used when only one ratio is known (or complete), and the second ratio is incomplete.

■ EXAMPLE 7:

A solution strength of 8 mg per mL is needed to prepare a dosage of 10 mg. The solution strength available (8 mg per mL) provides the *known ratio*. The dosage to be given is the *incomplete ratio* (10 mg). The letter "X" is used to represent the mL that will contain 10 mg. Notice that both numerators are expressed as milligrams while both denominators are expressed as milliliters. The ratios in a proportion must be written in the same sequence of measurement units.

$$\frac{8\,mg}{1\,mL} = \frac{10\,mg}{X\,mL}$$

The first fraction is a complete ratio that expresses the drug strength. The second fraction is an incomplete ratio that expresses the dosage to give. By cross-multiplying, it is easy to see that:

$$8X = 10, \text{ therefore, the answer is } 1.25\,mL$$

The ordered dosage of 10 mg is contained in 1.25 mL.

It is important to double-check your calculations and to assess that each answer is logical. In the preceding example, because 1 mL contains 8 mg, you will need a larger volume than 1 mL to obtain 10 mg. The answer, 1.25 mL, is larger, so it is logical. While this does not verify that the calculation is correct, at least it shows you that you set up the proportion correctly and cross-multiplied sufficiently.

■ EXAMPLE 8:

A dosage of 20 mg has been ordered. The strength available is 25 mg in 1.5 mL.

$$\frac{25\,mg}{1.5\,mL} = \frac{20\,mg}{X\,mL}$$

When you cross-multiply,

$$25X = 1.5 \times 20$$

Therefore, X = 1.2 mL.

Because the dosage ordered (20 mg) is smaller than the strength available (25 mg in 1.5 mL), the answer should be smaller than 1.5 mL, and it is. Therefore, it is logical.

■ EXAMPLE 9:

The solution strength on hand is 80 mg per mL. A dosage of 200 mg is ordered.

$$\frac{80\,mg}{1\,mL} = \frac{200\,mg}{X\,mL}$$

Therefore,

$$80X = 200$$

$$\text{So, } X = 2.5 \text{ mL}$$

This answer is logical because 2.5 mL is larger, and the dosage ordered (200 mg) is larger than the solution on hand (80 mg per mL) and must be contained in more than 1 mL.

■ EXAMPLE 10:

Shortcuts can be used to simplify the math in these problems. To do so, after cross-multiplying, immediately divide by the number in front of X. You can also reduce numbers to their lowest common terms whenever possible. For example, if you have a 300 mg per 1.2 mL solution and need to prepare a dosage of 120 mg:

$$\frac{300 \text{ mg}}{1.2 \text{ mL}} = \frac{120 \text{ mg}}{X \text{ mL}}$$

Cross-multiply and immediately divide by the number in front of X:

$$X = \frac{1.2 \times 120}{300}$$

Reduce the 120 and 300 numbers by 60. Do the final division, and, depending on the medication you are using, round to the nearest tenth:

$$X = \frac{1.2 \times 2}{5} = \frac{2.4}{5} = 0.48 = 0.5 \text{mL}$$

A dosage of 120 mg requires fewer mL than the 300 mg per 1.2 mL strength available. Therefore, the smaller 0.5 mL answer is logical.

■ EXAMPLE 11:

You have on hand a 1.5 mg in 0.5 mL solution. You must prepare a 2 mg dosage.

$$\frac{1.5 \text{ mg}}{0.5 \text{ mL}} = \frac{2 \text{ mg}}{X \text{ mL}}$$

Therefore,

$$X = \frac{1 \times 2}{3} = \frac{2}{3} = 0.66 = 0.7 \text{ mL}$$

Because the 0.7 mL answer is a larger volume than the 1.5 mg in 0.5 mL dosage strength, it is logical for this 2 mg dosage.

■ EXAMPLE 12:

The solution available is 80 mg per mL. A 120 mg dosage is ordered.

$$\frac{80 \text{ mg}}{1 \text{ mL}} = \frac{120 \text{ mg}}{X \text{ mL}}$$

Therefore,

$$X = \frac{120}{80} = \frac{3}{2} = 1.5 \text{ mL}$$

Because the 120 mg dosage ordered requires a volume larger than the 80 mg per mL available dosage strength, the answer (1.5 mL) is larger, and therefore, logical.

Stop and Review

Use the ratio-proportion method to convert each of the following amounts to the unit indicated. Indicate the approximate equivalent used in the conversion.

1. 160 ml = _____ L

2. 84 lb = _____ kg

3. 30 mg = _____ gr

4. 625 mcg = _____ mg

5. 2 qt = _____ L

6. 32 g = _____ mg

7. 18.5 cm = _____ in

8. gr $\overline{ss}$ = _____ mg

9. gr $\dfrac{1}{8}$ = _____ mg

10. 250 mL = _____ L

Determine if these proportions are true by cross-multiplying.

11. $\dfrac{34 \text{ mg}}{2 \text{ mL}} = \dfrac{51 \text{ mg}}{3 \text{ mL}}$ _____

12. $\dfrac{15 \text{ mg}}{4 \text{ mL}} = \dfrac{45 \text{ mg}}{12 \text{ mL}}$ _____

13. $\dfrac{1.3 \text{ mL}}{46 \text{ mg}} = \dfrac{0.65 \text{ mL}}{23 \text{ mg}}$ _____

14. $\dfrac{2.3 \text{ mL}}{150 \text{ units}} = \dfrac{1.9 \text{ mL}}{130 \text{ units}}$ _____

15. $\dfrac{40 \text{ mg}}{1.1 \text{ mL}} = \dfrac{80 \text{ mg}}{2.2 \text{ mL}}$ _____

Calculate the following dosages and express the answers to the nearest tenth. Assess your answers to determine if they are logical. Make sure to include the units of measure in your answers.

16. Ordered:	24 mg
Solution strength available:	12.5 mg in 1.5 mL
Give:	_____
17. Ordered:	30 mg
Solution strength available:	40 mg in 2.5 mL
Give:	_____
18. Ordered:	0.3 mg
Solution strength available:	0.6 mg in 0.8 mL
Give:	_____
19. Ordered:	24 mg
Solution strength available:	36 mg per 2 mL
Give:	_____
20. Ordered:	52 mg
Solution strength available:	78 mg in 0.9 mL
Give:	_____
21. Ordered:	150 mg
Solution strength available:	100 mg per mL
Give:	_____

22. Ordered:	600 mcg
Solution strength available:	750 mcg in 3 mL
Give:	_____
23. Ordered:	4 g
Solution strength available:	1.5 g per mL
Give:	_____
24. Ordered:	0.25 mg
Solution strength available:	0.5 mg per mL
Give:	_____
25. Ordered:	3 g
Solution strength available:	4 g in 2.7 mL
Give:	_____

RATIO AND PROPORTION EXPRESSED USING COLONS

Ratios and proportions may also be expressed using colons. For example,

$$\frac{3}{4} = \frac{15}{20}$$

$$3 : 4 :: 15 : 20$$

Remember

It is easy to remember which numbers are the means and which are the extremes in a proportion. The means begin with the letter "m", as does the *middle* of the equation. The extremes begin with the letter "e", as do the *ends* of the equation.

In a proportion, the ratios also may be separated by an equal sign. When using colons instead of fractions for ratio and proportion, the numbers on the ends of the proportion (3 and 20 in the preceding example) are called the *extremes*. The numbers in the middle (4 and 15) are called the *means*. If you multiply the means and then the extremes, their products (answer) will be equal. However, you must never mix up the means and extremes in proportions or the answer you obtain will be incorrect.

Dosage Calculations

■ EXAMPLE 1:

Ordered: Biaxin® 0.5 g p.o. q8h

On hand: Biaxin® 250 mg

Desired dose = X

Biaxin 250 mg.
Courtesy of Abbott Laboratories

■ EXAMPLE 2:

1 tablet : 50 mg = 2 tablets : 100 mg

The means are 50 and 2, while the extremes are 1 and 100.

Therefore: $50 \times 2 = 100 \times 1$

$$100 = 100$$

meaning the ratios are equal and the proportion is true.

Remember

- **To find the desired dose:**

  Use the conversion factor formula, or

  Use the ration and proportion method

■ EXAMPLE 3:

2 mL : 500 mg = 1 mL : 250 mg

Therefore: $500 \times 1 = 2 \times 250$

$$500 = 500$$

meaning the ratios are equal and the proportion is true.

■ EXAMPLE 4:

1 mL : 10 units = 2 mL : 20 units

Therefore: $10 \times 2 = 20$

$$20 = 20$$

This is a true proportion.

 Stop and Review

Use mathematics to determine if these proportions are true.

1. 34 mg : 2 mL = 51 mg : 3 mL _____

2. 15 mg : 4 mL = 45 mg : 12 mL _____

3. 1.3 mL : 46 mg = 0.65 mL : 23 mg _____

4. 2.3 mL : 150 units = 1.9 mL : 130 units _____

5. 40 mg : 1.1 mL = 80 mg : 2.2 mL _____

CALCULATIONS USING DIFFERENT UNITS OF MEASURE

When units of measure are different, the ratio and proportion method may still be used. For example, a common situation is when the medication order is in grams and the dosage strength is available in milligrams per milliliter.

■ EXAMPLE 1:

The order is for 0.15 g of medication. The dosage strength available is 200 mg per mL. Because the order and the dosage are different, conversion is required. Also, it is safer to use smaller units of measure to eliminate or avoid decimal points. Therefore, convert the 0.15 grams to milligrams (150 milligrams). To better show the math in this example, the ratios and proportions are shown as common fractions.

$$\frac{200 \text{ mg}}{1 \text{ mL}} = \frac{0.15 \text{ g}}{X \text{ mL}}$$

Change grams to milligrams.

$$\frac{200 \text{ mg}}{1 \text{ mL}} = \frac{150 \text{ mg}}{X \text{ mL}}$$

Therefore,

$$200X = 1 \times 150$$

So,

$$X = \frac{150}{200} = 0.75 \text{ or } 0.8 \text{ mL}$$

To check, because 150 mg is smaller than 200 mg, it must be contained in a smaller volume than 1 mL. Therefore, the answer, 0.8 mL, is logical.

■ EXAMPLE 2:

The dosage ordered is 0.5 mg. You have a dosage strength of 200 mcg per mL.

$$\frac{200 \text{ mcg}}{1 \text{ mL}} = \frac{0.5 \text{ mg}}{X \text{ mL}}$$

Change mg to micrograms (mcg).

$$\frac{200 \text{ mcg}}{1 \text{ mL}} = \frac{500 \text{ mcg}}{X \text{ mL}}$$

Therefore,

$$200X = 500$$

So,

$$X = 2.5 \text{ mL}$$

Because 500 mcg is larger than 200 mcg, it must be contained in a larger quantity than 1 mL. Therefore, the answer, 2.5 mL, is logical.

■ EXAMPLE 3:

In this example, ratio and proportion are used to solve a calculation for unit and mEq dosages. The order is for 1200 units. The available dosage strength is 1000 units per 1.5 mL.

$$\frac{1000 \text{ units}}{1.5 \text{ mL}} = \frac{1200 \text{ units}}{X \text{ mL}}$$

Therefore,

$$1000X = 1.5 \times 1200$$

So,

$$X = \frac{1.5 \times 1200}{1000}$$

The answer is 1.8 mL. Because 1200 units is a larger dosage than 1000 units, the answer (in mL) should be larger than 1.5 mL, which is logical.

■ EXAMPLE 4:

A drug has a dosage strength of 2 mEq per mL. You are to give 10 mEq.

$$\frac{2 \text{ mEq}}{1 \text{ mL}} = \frac{10 \text{ mEq}}{X \text{ mL}}$$

Therefore,

$$2X = 10$$

So,

$$X = 5 \text{ mL}$$

Because 10 mEq is larger than 2 mEq, the answer should also be significantly larger, and, therefore, it is logical.

Stop and Review

Solve the following dosage problems and express answers to the nearest tenth. Make sure to include the units of measure.

1. Ordered:	0.4 mg
Drug label reads:	1000 mcg in 2 mL
Give:	_____

2. Ordered:	275 mg
Drug label reads:	0.5 g per 2 mL
Give:	_____
3. Ordered:	0.15 mg
Drug label reads:	0.2 mg in 1.5 mL
Give:	_____
4. Ordered:	600 mg
Drug label reads:	1 g in 3.6 mL
Give:	_____
5. Ordered:	10,000 units
Drug label reads:	8000 units in 1 mL
Give:	_____
6. Ordered:	15 mEq
Drug label reads:	20 mEq per 20 mL
Give:	_____
7. Ordered:	200,000 units
Drug label reads:	150,000 units per 2 mL
Give:	_____

Test Your Knowledge

Use the ratio and proportion method to calculate the following parenteral dosages. Answers should be in milliliters and expressed to the nearest tenth or hundredth as needed. Check each answer to make sure it is logical. Measure the dosages on the syringes provided.

Dosage Ordered   **mL required**

1. Depo-Provera® 0.3 g   _____

Depo-Provera 400 mg/mL.
Used with permission from Pharmacia Corporation, Peapack, NJ.

2. furosemide 15 mg   _____

Furosemide 20 mg/Ml.
Used with permission of American Regent, Inc.

3. heparin sodium 2000 units   _____

Heparin Sodium Injection, USP.
© *Cengage Learning 2013*

Dosage Ordered	**mL required**

4. Cleocin® 0.75 g for an IV additive _____

Cleocin Phosphate 900 mg.
Used with permission from Pharmacia Corporation, Peapack, NJ.

5. naloxone 350 mcg _____

Narcan®
Used with permission from Endo Pharmaceuticals Inc.

6. clindamycin 225 mg _____

Clindamycin 150 mg/mL.
Used with permission from Bedford Laboratories.

7. Robinul® 75 mcg (calculate to the nearest hundredth) _____

Robinul® 75 mcg.
Copyright Baxter International Inc. Robinul is a trademark of Wyeth Pharmaceuticals Division of Wyeth.

Dosage Ordered   **mL required**

8.   midazolam HCl 4 mg   _____

Midazolam 25 mg/5 mL.
Used with permission from Bedford Laboratories.

9.   benztropine mesylate 2.4 mg   _____

Benztropine mesylate 2 mg per 2 mL.
© Cengage Learning 2013

10.   cyanocobalamin 800 mcg   _____

Cyanocobalamin 1000 mcg/mL.
Used with permission of American Regent, Inc.

11.   potassium chloride 16 mEq for IV additive   _____

Potassium Chloride 40 mEq.
Used with permission from Abraxis BioScience, Inc.

Dosage Ordered	**mL required**

12. calcium gluconate 0.93 mEq for an IV additive   _____

Calcium Gluconate 10 mL.
Used with permission of American Regent, Inc.

13. morphine sulfate 1.5 mg   _____

Duramoprh 10 mg/10 mL.
Copyright Baxter International Inc. Duramorph is a trademark of Baxter International Inc. or its subsidiaries

14. heparin 450 units (calculate to the nearest hundredth)   _____

Heparin Sodium 1000 USP.
© Cengage Learning 2013

15. Dilantin® 0.1 g   _____

Dilantin 250 mg/5 mL.
Labels reproduced with permission of Pfizer, Inc.

Dosage Ordered	**mL required**

16. gentamicin 70 mg   _____

Gentamicin 40 mg/mL.
Uses with permission from Abraxis BioScience, Inc.

17. sodium chloride 60 mEq for an IV additive   _____

Sodium Chloride.
© Cengage Learning 2013

18. meperidine 75 mg   _____

Meperidine 100 mg/mL.
Copyright Baxter International Inc.

19. Betamethasone sodium phosphate and
Betamethasone acetate 10 mg   _____

Betamethasone sodium phosphate and Betamethasone acetate, USP 5 mL mutiple-
Dose Vial, 6 mg per mL.
© Cengage Learning 2013

Dosage Ordered	**mL required**

20. gentamicin 0.1 g _____

Gentamicin 40 mg/mL.
Reprinted with permission of Abraxis BioScience, Inc.

21. doxorubicin HCl 16 mg for an IV additive _____

Doxorubicin HCl 20 mg.
Used with permission from Bedford Laboratories, Bedford, Ohio

22. methotrexate 40 mg _____

Methotrexate 200 mg.
© *Cengage Learning 2013*

23. haloperidol decanoate 75 mg _____

Haldol 50 mcg/mL.
Used with permission form Ortho-McNeill Pharmaceuticals, Inc.

Dosage Ordered	**mL required**

24. chlorpromazine HCl 40 mg

_____

Thorazine 25 mg/mL.
Reprinted with permission from GlaxoSmithKline

25. nalbuphine HCl 30 mg

_____

Nubain 20 mg/mL.
Used with permission form Endo Pharmaceuticals, Inc.

26. cyanocobalamin 750 mg

_____

Cyanocobalamin 1000 mcg/mL.
Used with permission of American Regent, Inc.

27. naloxone HCl 0.5 mg

_____

Naloxone 400 mcg/mL.
Copyright Baxter Healthcare Corporation

Dosage Ordered	**mL required**

28. chlorpromazine (Thorazine®) 60 mg   _____

Thorazine 25 mg/mL.
Reprinted with permission from GlaxoSmithKline

29. Robinul® 180 mcg   _____

Robinul 1 mL.
Copyright Baxter International Inc. Robinul is a trademark of Wyeth Pharmaceuticals Division of Wyeth.

30. Penicillian G benzathine/Penicillin G procaine   _____

Penicillian G benzathine/Penicillin G procaine 900/300 1,200 UNITS per 2 mL
NOT FOR INTRAVENOUS USE.
© *Cengage Learning 2013*

Dimensional Analysis

OBJECTIVES

Upon completion of this chapter, you should be able to:

1. Simplify units using dimensional analysis.
2. Use dimensional analysis to calculate dosages.
3. Convert between metric and household systems using dimensional analysis.

GLOSSARY

clinical ratios – Common fractions used in dimensional analysis calculations.

metric conversion – A process of converting between different metric values, such as from milligrams to grams.

unit conversion – Dimensional analysis (also known as "units conversion"). This is the process of mathematically changing or converting units of measure.

OVERVIEW

Dimensional analysis is the process of mathematically changing or converting units of measure. It is also referred to as **unit conversion** or **units conversion**. It utilizes a simplified version of ratio and proportion, reducing multistep calculations to a single equation. In this process, arithmetical terms (quantities and units) are logically sequenced and placed into equations. All units cancel out except for the unit or units of the desired answer. Dimensional analysis consolidates multiple arithmetical steps into a single expression.

To understand dimensional analysis, you must first understand clinical ratios. Dimensional analysis consolidates many steps of arithmetic into a single expression. It is used widely in chemistry, and pharmacists or pharmacy technicians often prefer it to the ratio-proportion method.

CLINICAL RATIOS

In dimensional analysis, clinical ratios are written as common fractions, such as the following:

$$\frac{1 \text{ tablet}}{250 \text{ mg}} \qquad \frac{2 \text{ grams}}{1.5 \text{ mL}} \qquad \frac{1 \text{mL}}{10 \text{ units}}$$

BASIC DIMENSIONAL ANALYSIS

To set up an equation for dimensional analysis, you must follow these steps:

1. Write the unit of measure being calculated, such as milliliters (mL). This eliminates confusion over which measure is being calculated and determines how the first clinical ratio is entered into the equation.

2. Identify the complete clinical ratio that contains the milliliters, as provided by the dosage strength available. This should be entered as a common fraction.

3. All additional ratios are entered so that each denominator matches with its successive numerator. If the first ratio denominator is milligrams, then the next numerator also must be in milligrams.

4. Cancel the alternate denominator/numerator measurement units (but not their quantities). They must match. If so, all clinical ratios were entered correctly. After cancellation, only the unit of measure being calculated may remain in the equation.

5. Calculate the equation now that all components are in place.

> ### Remember
>
> The unit of measure being calculated is written first, followed by an equal sign. It is then matched in the numerator of the first clinical ratio entered. The unit of measure in each denominator is matched in the successive numerator entered.

EXAMPLE 1:

The available drug strength is 500 mg in 2 mL. How many mL are needed to prepare a 300 mg dosage?

$$mL = \frac{2\ mL}{500\ mg}$$

Therefore, based on the desired 300 mg dosage,

$$mL = \frac{2\ mL}{500\ mg} \times \frac{X\ mL}{300\ mg}$$

Therefore, by cross-multiplying, 2 mL × 300 mg = 600 mg. This amount, when divided by 500 mg, gives an answer of 1.2 mL, which contains the desired 300 mg of medication.

This type of equation works the same way for every calculation, no matter how many ratios are entered. There are no complicated rules to remember.

EXAMPLE 2:

Because 1 liter (L) is equal to 1000 milliliters (mL), how many fluidounces (fl oz) are in 2.5 liters? Approximately 30 milliliters are in 1 fluidounce. Use ratio and proportion as follows:

$$\frac{2.5\ L}{1\ L} \times \frac{XmL}{1000\ mL}$$

Therefore, X = 2500 mL. So,

$$\frac{1\ fl\ oz}{X\ fl\ oz} \times \frac{30\ mL}{2500\ mL}$$

Therefore, X = 83.3 fl oz, which may be rounded to 83 fl oz.

EXAMPLE 3:

To solve the same equation by dimensional analysis, you would do the following:

$$\frac{1\ fl\ oz}{30\ mL} \times \frac{1000\ mL}{1\ L} \times 2.5L$$

Therefore, the same answer, 83.3 fl oz., can be easily found.

EXAMPLE 4:

If 1000 mL of dextrose is needed intravenously, to be infused over 8 hours, and an IV set delivering 10 drops per mL is used, how many drops per minute should be delivered to the patient? Using ratio and proportion:

Because 8 hours = 480 minutes:

$$\frac{1000 \text{ mL}}{X \text{ mL}} \times \frac{480 \text{ minutes}}{1 \text{ minute}}$$

Therefore, X = 2.1 mL/minute.

Then

$$\frac{2.1 \text{ mL/minute}}{1 \text{ mL}} \times \frac{X \text{ drops/minute}}{10 \text{ drops}}$$

Therefore, X = 21 drops per minute.

◾ EXAMPLE 5:

To solve the same equation by dimensional analysis, you would do the following (the terms should have "drops" in the numerator and "minutes" in the denominator to give the desired answer in drops per minute):

$$\frac{10 \text{ drops}}{1 \text{ mL}} \times \frac{1}{480 \text{ minutes}} \times 1000 \text{ mL}$$

Therefore, the same answer is easily found: 21 drops per minute.

Stop and Review

Using dimensional analysis, perform the following dosage calculations, expressing answers in mL, rounded to the nearest tenth.

1. A dosage strength of 0.4 mg in 2.5 mL is available. How many milliliters should be administered if a dose of 0.15 mg is required?

   _____

2. A pharmacy technician must prepare a 200,000-unit dosage from an available solution containing 150,000 units in 2 mL. How many milliliters should be administered to contain the correct dosage?

   _____

3. A dosage strength of 0.8 mg in 2 mL must be used to prepare a 0.5 mg dosage.

   _____

4. An IV additive has a dosage strength of 20 mEq per 20 mL. A dosage of 15 mEq has been ordered.

   _____

5. A dosage of 0.3 g has been prescribed. The strength available is 0.4 g in 1.5 mL.

   _____

EQUATIONS REQUIRING METRIC CONVERSIONS

Dimensional analysis allows multiple ratios to be entered into a single equation. It is sometimes easier to do the conversion before the equation is set up. For instance, if a medication is available in milligrams (mg) but is labeled in another amount, such as grams or micrograms, metric conversion must be done.

■ EXAMPLE 1:

The IM dosage ordered is 250 mg. The drug available is labeled 1 g per 2 mL. How many mL must you give?

$$mL = \frac{2\,mL}{1\,g}$$

Because the dosage ordered is in milligrams and the drug available is in grams, a conversion ratio is needed: 1 gram equals 1000 milligrams. Therefore, you can change "1 g" to "1000 mg":

$$mL = \frac{2\,mL}{1000\,mg}$$

Next you must add the dosage ordered into the equation:

$$mL = \frac{2\,mL}{1000\,g} \times \frac{250\,mg}{1}$$

Then remove the "milligrams" and carry out the multiplication:

$$mL = \frac{2 \times 250}{1000}$$

This leaves:

$$mL = \frac{500}{1000}$$

The result is ½ mL. Therefore, ½ mL contains the desired dosage of 250 mg.

■ EXAMPLE 2:

An intramuscular medication order is for 0.5 mg of medication in solution. The drug label reads "750 mcg in 2 mL". Enter the mL to be calculated followed by an equal sign to the left of the equation. Locate the ratio containing mL, 750 mcg in 2 mL. Enter 2 mL as the numerator to match the mL being calculated. The denominator becomes 750 mcg.

$$mL = \frac{2\,mL}{750\,mcg}$$

Because the medication order was for milligrams, a conversion ratio is needed. Enter the 1000 mcg = 1 mg conversion ratio. The numerator is 1000 mcg, matching the mcg of the previous denominator. The denominator becomes 1 mg.

$$mL = \frac{2\ mL}{750\ mcg} \times \frac{1000\ mcg}{1\ mg}$$

The mg denominator is now matched by the 0.5 mg dosage to be administered, completing the equation.

$$mL = \frac{2\ mL}{750\ mcg} \times \frac{1000\ mcg}{1\ mg} \times 0.5\ mg$$

Cancel the alternate denominator-numerator mcg/mcg and mg/mg units of measure, which checks for the correct ratio entry. Only the mL being calculated should remain. Do the math as follows:

$$mL = \frac{2\ mL}{750} \times \frac{1000}{1} \times 0.5 = 1.33$$

To give a dosage of 0.5 mg from the available 2 mL per 750 mcg strength, you must prepare 1.33 mL.

■ **EXAMPLE 3:**

Prepare a 0.5 mg dosage from an available strength of 200 mcg per mL. Enter the mL being calculated to the left of the equation followed by an equal sign. Enter the 1 mL in 200 mcg dosage as the starting ratio, with 1 mL as the numerator to match the mL being calculated; 200 mcg becomes the denominator.

$$mL = \frac{1\ mL}{200\ mcg}$$

A mcg to mcg conversion ratio is needed. Enter 1000 mcg as the numerator to match the mcg in the previous denominator; 1 mg becomes the new denominator.

$$mL = \frac{1\ mL}{200\ mcg} \times \frac{1000\ mcg}{1\ mg}$$

The mg denominator is now matched by the 0.5 mg dosage ordered to complete the equation.

$$mL = \frac{1\ mL}{200\ mcg} \times \frac{1000\ mcg}{1\ mg} \times 0.5\ mg$$

Cancel the alternate mcg/mcg and mg/mg units of measure to double-check for correct ratio entry. Only the mL unit being calculated remains in the equation. Do the math.

$$mL = \frac{1\ mL}{200} \times \frac{1000}{1} \times 0.5 = 2.5\ mL$$

A 0.5 dosage requires a 2.5 mL volume of the 200 mcg per mL strength solution available.

■ EXAMPLE 4:

The medication has a strength of 0.5 mg in 1.5 mL. The order is for 750 micrograms. Therefore, how many mL should be given?

Enter the mL to be calculated to the left of the equation followed by an equal sign. Enter the starting ratio, the 1.5 mL in 0.5 mg dosage available, with 1.5 mL as the numerator, to match the mL being calculated; 0.5 mg becomes the denominator.

$$mL = \frac{1.5\ mL}{0.5\ mg}$$

The problem has no "milligram" dosage, but asks for micrograms, which signals the need for a conversion ratio. Enter the 1 mg = 1000 mcg conversion ratio, with 1 mg as the numerator, to match the milligrams denominator of the starting ratio; 1000 mcg becomes the new denominator.

$$mL = \frac{1.5\ mL}{0.5\ mg} \times \frac{1\ mg}{1000\ mcg}$$

Enter the dosage ordered (750 mcg) as the final numerator to match the mcg in the previous denominator. The equation is complete.

$$mL = \frac{1.5\ mL}{0.5\ mg} \times \frac{1\ mg}{1000\ mcg} \times 750\ mcg$$

Cancel the alternate mg/mg and mcg/mcg units of measure to check the accuracy of ratio entry, and then complete the math.

$$mL = \frac{1.5\ mL}{0.5} \times \frac{1}{1000} \times 750 = 2.25 = 2.3\ mL$$

Therefore, a 750 mcg dosage requires 2.3 mL of the 0.5 mg in 1.5 mL medication.

⫸ Remember

For calculations using dimensional analysis:

- **The unit of measure being calculated is written first to the left of the equation.**

- **The unit of measure is followed by an equal sign.**

- **All ratios entered must include the quantity and the unit of measure.**

- **The numerator in the starting ratio must be in the same measurement unit as the unit of measure being calculated.**

- **The unit of measure in each denominator must be matched in the numerator of each successive ratio entered.**

- **Metric system conversions can be made by incorporating a conversion ratio directly into the dimensional analysis equation.**

- **The unit of measure in each alternate denominator and numerator must cancel. This leaves only the unit of measure being calculated remaining in the equation.**

- **The numerator of the starting ratio is never cancelled.**

Test Your Knowledge

Calculate the following dosages using dimensional analysis.

1. A prescriber ordered 0.2 g tablets. On hand are tablets labeled "80 mg". How many tablets should be given to the patient?

   _____

2. A physician ordered a dosage of 85 mg. The drug on hand is labeled "0.1 g in 1.5 mL". How many mL should be given to the patient?

   _____

3. A pharmacy technician prepares 0.1 g of an IM medication from a strength of 200 mg per mL. How many mL must be administered?

   _____

4. The prescriber ordered 0.5 mg of a medication. The dosage strength on hand is 200 mcg per mL. How many mL should be administered to the patient?

   _____

5. A pharmacy technician is preparing a 0.75 mg dosage. The strength available is 500 mcg in 1.5 mL. How many mL should be given?

   _____

6. If you want to prepare a 130 mg dosage of a drug labeled "0.1 g in 2 mL", how many mL must be given?

   _____

7. A physician ordered a dosage of 1500 mcg. The solution available is 0.5 mg per mL. How many mL should be administered?

   _____

8. A technician prepares 500 mg for IM injection from an available strength of 1 g per 3 mL. How many mL must be administered?

   _____

9. An oral solution has a dosage of 500 mg in 5 mL. If a 0.7 g dosage is required, how many mL must be given?

   _____

10. A technician prepares a 0.75 g dosage from a 250 mg per mL strength solution. How many mL are needed?

    _____

Using dimensional analysis, calculate the dosages from the medication labels provided. Your answers should be in mL, rounded to the nearest tenth or hundredth. Use the syringes that are shown to measure your dosages.

Dosage Ordered   **mL Needed**

11. terbutaline sulfate 800 mcg   _____

Terbutaline 1 mg/mL.

Used with permission from Bedford Laboratories. A Division of Ben Venue Laboratories Inc. A Boehringer Ingelheim Company

12. Vistaril® 70 mg   _____

Vistaril 50 mg/mL.

Used with permission from Pfizer, Inc.

13. fentanyl citrate 0.15 mg   _____

Fentanyl 250 mcg/5 mL.

Copyright Baxter Healthcare Corporation

14. naloxone 350 mcg   _____

Narcan® 1 mL.

Used with permission from Endo Pharmaceuticals, Inc.

Dosage Ordered   **mL Needed**

15. clindamycin 225 mg   _____

Clindamycin 150 mg/mL.
Used with permission from Bedford Laboratories. A Division of Ben Venue Laboratories Inc. A Boehringer Ingelheim Company

16. Robinul® 75 mcg (Calculate to the nearest hundredth.) _____

Robinul Injectable.
Copyright Baxter International Inc. Robinul is a trademark of Wyeth Pharmacueticals Division of Wyeth.

17. midazolam HCl 4 mg   _____

Midazolam 25 mg/mL.
Used with permission from Bedford Laboratories. A Division of Ben Venue Laboratories Inc. A Boehringer Ingelheim Company.

18. Inapsine® 3 mg   _____

Inapsine 5mg/2 mL.
Used with permission from Akorn Inc., and Taylor Pharmaceuticals

Dosage Ordered	**mL Needed**

19. morphine sulfate 1.5 mg   _____

Duramorph 10 mg/10 mL.
Copyright Baxter International Inc. Duramorph is a trademark of Baxter International Inc. or its subsidiaries

20. heparin sodium 450 units (Calculate to the nearest hundredth.)   _____

Heparin Sodium 1000 Units/mL.
© Cengage Learning 2013

21. droperidol 4 mg   _____

Inapsine 5mg/2 mL.
Used with permisison from Akron Inc. and Taylor Pharmaceuticals

22. Dilantin® 0.1 g   _____

Dilantin 250 mg.
Used with permission form Pfizer Inc.

Dosage Ordered	**mL Needed**

23. medroxyprogesterone 0.9 g　　　　　　　　　_____

Depo-Provera® 400 mg.
Used with permission from Pfizer, Inc.

24. Vistaril® 120 mg　　　　　　　　　_____

Vistaril 50 mg/mL.
Used with permission from Pfizer, Inc.

25. sodium chloride 60 mEq for an IV additive　　　　_____

Sodium Chloride 100 mL.
© *Cengage Learning 2013*

26. atropine sulfate 150 mcg　　　　　　　　　_____

Atropine Sulfate 0.1 mg/mL.
1 mg per 10 mL For IV use/Single Dose.
© *Cengage Learning 2013*

Dosage Ordered	**mL Needed**

27. meperidine 75 mg

_____

Meperidine 100 mg/mL.
Copyright Baxter Healthcare Corporation

28. fentanyl citrate 80 mcg

_____

Fentanyl Citrate 250 mcg/5 mL.
Copyright Baxter Healthcare Corporation

29. gentamicin 0.1 g

_____

Gentamicin 40 mg/mL.
Used with permision of Abraxis BioScience, Inc.

30. Dilantin® 0.15 g

_____

Dilantin 250 mg.
Used with permission from Pfizer, Inc.

Dosage Ordered   **mL Needed**

31. doxorubicin HCl 16 mg for an IV additive   _____

Doxorubicin Hydrochloride Injection.
Used with permission from Bedford Laboratories. A Division of Ben Venue Laboratories Inc. A Boehringer Ingelheim Company

32. meperidine HCl 30 mg   _____

Meperidine 25 mg/mL.
Copyright Baxter Healthcare Corporation

33. methotrexate 40 mg   _____

Methotrexate 200 mg.
Copyright Baxter Healthcare Corporation

34. midazolam HCl 3 mg   _____

Midazolam 25 mg/mL.
Used with permission from Bedford Laboratories. A Division of Ben Venue Laboratories Inc. A Boehringer Ingelheim Company

Dosage Ordered	**mL Needed**

35. ondansetron 3 mg   _____

Ondansetron 4 mg/2 mL.
Used with permission from Bedford Laboratories. A Division of Ben Venue Laboratories Inc. A Boehringer Ingelheim Company

36. hydroxyzine HCl 40 mg   _____

Vistaril 25 mg/mL.
Used with permission from Pfizer, Inc.

37. Ketorolac tromethamine 20 mg   _____

Ketorolac 15 mg/mL.
Used with permission from Bedford Laboratories. A Division of Ben Venue Laboratories Inc. A Boehringer Ingelheim Company

38. nalbuphine HCl 30 mg   _____

Nubain 20 mg/mL.
Used with permission from Endo Pharmaceuticals, Inc.

Dosage Ordered	**mL Needed**

39. morphine 15 mg   _____

Morphine 10 mg/mL.
Copyright Baxter Healthcare International Inc.

40. Dilantin® 125 mg   _____

Dilantin 250 mg.
Used with permission from Pfizer Inc.

41. Ketorolac 25 mg   _____

Ketorolac 15 mg/mL.
Used with permission from Bedford Laboratories. A Division of Ben Venue Laboratories Inc. A Boehringer Ingelheim Company

42. Vistaril 50 mg   _____

Vistaril 25 mg/mL.
Used with permission from Pfizer, Inc.

Dosage Ordered	**mL Needed**

43. Robinul® 180 mcg   _____

Robinul Injectable 1 mL.

Copyright Baxter International Inc. Robinul is a trademark of Wyeth Pharmacueticals Division of Wyeth

44. hydroxyzine HCl 70 mg   _____

Vistaril 50 mg/mL.

Used with permissions from Pfizer Inc.

45. potassium chloride 20 mEq for an IV additive   _____

Potassium Chloride 30 mEq.

© Cengage Learning 2013

46. Inapsine® 4.5 mg   _____

Inapsine 5mg/2 mL.

Used with permisison from Akron Inc. and Taylor Pharmaceuticals

Dosage Ordered   **mL Needed**

47. Nubain 15 mg   _____

Nubain 20 mg/mL.
Used with permission from Endo Pharmaceuticals, Inc.

48. phenytoin Na 0.1 g   _____

Dilantin 250 mg.
Used with permission from Pfizer, Inc.

49. lidocaine HCl 15 mg   _____

Lidocaine 20 mg/mL.
Copyright Baxter Healthcare Corporation

Formula Method

OBJECTIVES

Upon completion of this chapter, you should be able to:

1. Explain the basic formula used in the formula method.
2. Use the formula method with metric conversions.
3. Identify the use of the formula method with units and milliequivalent calculations.

GLOSSARY

desired dosage – The amount of a medication that is needed for administration.

dosage ordered – The amount of a medication in milligrams, grams, and so forth from a prescriber for a patient.

dosage strength available – The amount of medication on hand in milligrams, grams, and so forth.

OVERVIEW

The *formula method* is used for simple, one-step dosage calculations. It is a variation of ratio and proportion. Various initials are used to represent the components used in the formula method. In this book, the initials used are "D", "H", "Q", and "X". It is not important which initials are used, as long as the answer achieved is correct.

BASIC FORMULA

The following initials are usually used in the formula method:

$$\frac{D}{H} \times Q = X$$

These initials mean:

D = "desired" (dosage ordered in milligrams, grams, and so forth)

H = "have" (dosage strength available in mg, g, and so forth)

Q = "quantity" (the mL volume that the dosage strength available is contained in)

X = "unknown" (the mL volume that the desired dosage will be contained in)

The "unknown" (X) is always expressed in the same units of measure as the "quantity" (Q), which is the mL volume that the dosage available is contained in.

> ◖▮▮▮◗ **Remember**
>
> You must memorize the formula used in the formula method. Always double-check calculations. Determine if answers are logical. Ask for help if you doubt the accuracy of your calculations.

▮ EXAMPLE 1:

You have on hand a dosage strength of 80 mg in 2 mL. A dosage of 60 mg is ordered. How many mL are necessary to administer this dosage?

Desired dosage (D) = 60 mg

On hand (H) = 80 mg in (Q) 2 mL

Remember that X must be expressed in the same units of measure as Q, which is mL in this example. Always include the units of measure in the formula:

$$\frac{(D)\ 60\ mg}{(H)\ 80\ mg} \times (Q)\ 2\ mL = X\ mL$$

$$\frac{60}{80} \times 2 = X = 1.5\ mL$$

Therefore, to give a dosage of 60 mg, 1.5 mL must be administered.

Because 60 mg is required, which is a smaller dosage than the dosage strength available of 80 mg in 2 mL, the answer, 1.5 mL, is smaller, and because of this, logical.

■ **EXAMPLE 2:**

A dosage of 0.5 mg is ordered. On hand is 0.45 mg in 1.2 mL. So, D = 0.4 mg. H = 0.45 mg in (Q) 1.2 mL.

$$\frac{0.5 \text{ mg}}{0.45 \text{ mg}} \times 1.2 \text{ mL} = X \text{ mL}$$

$$\frac{0.5}{0.45} \times 1.2 = X = 1.33 = 1.3 \text{ mL}$$

Therefore, to give 0.5 mg, you must administer 1.3 mL. Because 0.5 mg ordered is larger than the 0.45 mg strength available and the volume containing it must be larger, 1.3 mL is larger, so it is logical.

■ **EXAMPLE 3:**

The strength available is 1000 mcg per mL. A dosage of 660 mcg has been ordered.

$$\frac{660 \text{ mg}}{1,000 \text{ mcg}} \times 1 \text{mL} = X \text{ mL}$$

$$\frac{660}{1,000} \times 1 = X = 0.66 = 0.7 \text{ mL}$$

Therefore, to give a dosage of 660 mcg, you must administer 0.7 mL. The answer must be a smaller quantity than 1 mL, and it is.

 Stop and Review

Calculate the dosages and express your answers to the nearest tenth.

1. Ordered:	0.6 g
Strength available:	1 g in 2.5 mL
Give:	_____
2. Ordered:	150 mg
Strength available:	250 mg in 1.5 mL
Give:	_____

3. Ordered:	0.4 mg
Strength available:	1 mg in 3 mL
Give:	_____
4. Ordered:	275 mcg
Strength available:	600 mcg in 1.2 mL
Give:	_____

USE WITH METRIC CONVERSIONS

When drug strengths are in different units of measure, one of them must be changed before a dosage can be determined. The drug strengths (D and H) must always be expressed in the same units of measure.

■ EXAMPLE 1:

A dosage (D) of 200 mcg is ordered. However, the strength available (or "dose on hand") is 0.4 mg in 1.5 mL. This is labeled as "H". First, you must convert mg to mcg to eliminate the decimal point:

$$0.4 \text{ mg} = 400 \text{ mcg}$$

Then use the formula for the calculation as follows:

$$\frac{200 \text{ mcg}}{400 \text{ mcg}} \times 1.5 \text{ mL} = X \text{ mL}$$

The result is 0.75 mL.

Therefore, to give 200 mcg, you must administer 0.75 mL of 0.4 mg medication. Remember that your answer must be smaller than 1.5 mL (which it is) because the dosage ordered is smaller than the strength available. Therefore, this example is logical.

■ EXAMPLE 2:

On hand is a strength of 1000 mg in 1.5 mL. A dosage of 0.8 g has been ordered. First, convert g to mg to eliminate the decimal point:

$$0.8 \text{ g} = 800 \text{ mg}$$

Then use the formula for calculation:

$$\frac{800 \text{ mg}}{1,000 \text{ mg}} \times 1.5 \text{ mL} = X \text{ mL}$$

The result is 1.2 mL.

Therefore, to give 0.8 g, you must administer 1.2 mL. The answer must be less than 1.5 mL (which it is) because the 800 mg ordered is less than the 1000 mg strength available.

Stop and Review

Calculate the dosages and express your answers to the nearest tenth.

1. Ordered:	870 mcg
Strength available:	1 mg per mL
Give:	_____
2. Ordered:	450 mg
Strength available:	0.1 g per mL
Give:	_____
3. Ordered:	0.6 mg
Strength available:	1000 mcg per 2 mL
Give:	_____
4. Ordered:	0.4 g
Strength available:	500 mg per 1.3 mL
Give:	_____

USE WITH UNITS AND MILLIEQUIVALENT CALCULATIONS

The same as with metric conversions, it also is easy to convert dosages expressed in units or milliequivalents (mEq).

■ EXAMPLE 1:

If a dosage of 6500 units is ordered, and the available strength is 10,000 units per mL, first do the following:

$$\frac{6500 \text{ units}}{10,000 \text{ units}} \times 1 \text{ mL} = X \text{ mL}$$

Therefore, to give 6500 units, you must administer 0.7 mL (which is rounded to the nearest tenth from the answer of 0.65 mL). Because the dosage ordered (6500 units) is less than the strength available (10,000 units), it must be contained in less solution than 1 mL (which it is).

■ EXAMPLE 2:

If a dosage of 40 mEq is ordered, and the available strength is 70 mEq in 5 mL, first do the following:

$$\frac{40 \text{ mEq}}{70 \text{ mEq}} \times 5 = X \text{ mL}$$

Therefore, to give 40 mEq, you must administer 3.75 mL (which is rounded to the nearest tenth from the answer of 2.86 mL). Because the dosage ordered (40 mEq) is less than the dosage strength available (70 mEq), it must be contained in a smaller volume than 5 mL, and it is.

Stop and Review

Calculate the dosages and express the answers to the nearest tenth.

1. Ordered:	1250 units
Strength available:	1000 units per 1.5 mL
Give:	_____
2. Ordered:	45 units
Strength available:	80 units per mL
Give:	_____
3. Ordered:	50 mEq
Strength available:	200 mEq per 20 mL
Give:	_____

4. Ordered:	30 mEq
Strength available:	80 mEq per 5 mL
Give:	_____

Test Your Knowledge

After calculating the following dosages, express your answers as decimal fractions, rounding to the nearest tenth.

1. A 50 mg dosage is ordered. Strength available is 60 mg in 1.5 mL. _____

2. A 300 mcg dosage is ordered. Strength available is 0.4 mg per mL. _____

3. Prepare a 0.45 g dosage. Strength available is 300 mg per mL. _____

4. An 8 mg dosage has been ordered. The medication is labeled 5 mg per mL. _____

5. A 70 mg dosage must be prepared from a solution labeled 250 mg in 5 mL. _____

6. A dosage of 30 mg has been ordered. The drug is labeled 25 mg per mL. _____

7. Prepare a 60 mg dosage. The label reads 50 mg per mL. _____

8. The vial is labeled 5 mg per mL. The order is for 12 mg. _____

9. The vial label reads 10 mg per mL. A dosage of 7 mg has been ordered. _____

10. A dosage of 8 mg has been ordered. The dosage strength is 10 mg in 1 mL. _____

11. A medication is labeled 900 mg per 6 mL. Prepare a 0.3 g dosage. _____

12. A vial is labeled 0.5 g in 20 mL. Prepare a 300 mg IV dosage. _____

13. A dosage of 750 mg has been ordered. The vial is labeled 0.5 g per 2 mL. _____

14. An available dosage is 250 mcg in 5 mL. Prepare a dosage of 0.2 mg.

    _____

15. A single-use ampule is labeled 0.1 g per 2 mL. The order is for 130 mg.

    _____

16. A vial is labeled 15 mg in 5 mL. Draw up a 12 mg dosage.

    _____

17. Prepare 14 mg. The ampule is labeled 20 mg in 2 mL.

    _____

Using the given information, calculate the milliliters (mL) needed for each question.

18. Draw up an 800 mg dosage for IV administration from a container labeled 1.2 g per 30 mL. _____

19. Prepare an 80 mg dosage of a medication. The container is labeled 100 mg in 2 mL. _____

20. A dosage of 300 mcg is ordered. The solution strength is 0.4 mg per mL.

    _____

21. An available dosage strength is 0.4 g per mL. Prepare a 600 mg dosage.

    _____

22. A solution is labeled 40 mEq per 20 mL. Draw up a 60 mEq dosage for addition to an IV. _____

23. A dosage of 0.6 mg has been ordered. The label reads 400 mcg per mL.

    _____

24. A 60 mg dosage must be prepared from a 75 mg per mL strength.

    _____

25. A vial is labeled 40 mg per mL. Prepare a 0.1 g dosage.

    _____

26. The order is for 8 mg. The drug is labeled 50 mg in 10 mL.

    _____

27. An available strength is 1000 mcg per mL. Measure a 0.8 mg dosage.

    _____

28. A vial is labeled 25 mg per mL. Prepare 40 mg. _____

29. You have an available strength of 4000 mcg per mL. A dosage of 10 mg has been ordered. _____

30. A medication is labeled 0.25 g per 25 mL. Prepare 200 mg for IV use.

    _____

31. A dosage of 10 mg has been ordered. The dosage strength available is 15 mg in 1 mL. _____

32. An available strength is 5 mg per mL. Prepare a 4 mg dosage.
    _____

33. An available strength is 90 units in 1.5 mL. A dosage of 75 units has been ordered. _____

34. The solution available is labeled 80 mEq per 20 mL. You are to prepare 100 mEq for addition to an IV solution. _____

35. The solution is 0.15 g in 1 mL, and you must prepare a dosage of 180 mg.
    _____

36. An available strength is 1000 units per mL. Prepare a 750-unit dosage.
    _____

37. A vial is labeled 40 mEq in 20 mL. Draw up a 60 mEq dosage for addition to an IV solution. _____

38. A dosage of 400,000 units has been ordered. The available strength is 300,000 units in 1 mL. _____

39. Prepare a 250 mcg dosage. A dosage of 0.2 mg per 2 mL is available.
    _____

40. The solution is labeled 50 mEq per 50 mL. A dosage of 35 mEq has been ordered. _____

PART III

PRESCRIPTIONS, DRUG LABELS, AND PERCENTAGE OF ERROR

Interpretation of Prescriptions and Drug Labels

OBJECTIVES

Upon completion of this chapter, you should be able to:

1. List the components of a prescription.
2. Explain the parts of a drug label.
3. List the seven rights of drug administration.
4. Describe types of prescriptions.
5. Explain the role of computer systems in reducing medication errors.
6. Define *verbal orders* versus *stat orders*.

GLOSSARY

bar coding – A system of marking products with printed horizontal bars and spaces (and sometimes numerals) that uniquely reference information; they are read via scanners attached to computers and offer improved timeliness and accuracy in recordkeeping and dispensing of medical products.

dispensing – The preparation and distribution of prescription medications.

expiration date – A specific date when it is determined that a drug product will have lost a significant amount of potency.

inscription – The part of a prescription that lists the names and quantities of the ingredients to be used.

lot number – A number printed by a drug manufacturer on each medicine bottle that identifies the batch that the medication came from.

signa – A Latin term that means "mark" or "label." The signa is the portion of a prescription where the prescriber writes the directions for use.

stat – An abbreviation used on prescriptions and other medical orders; it means "immediately."

subscription – The part of a prescription that includes directions for compounding. Most physicians do not include this information anymore, and pharmacists prepare the compound based on accepted standards.

superscription – The area on a prescription form below the patient's name and address. The superscription usually is designated with the "Rx" symbol and is considered the "body of the prescription."

supply dosage – An amount of a drug's measured units per a specific quantity.

OVERVIEW

The ability to calculate drug dosages is a skill that should not be taken lightly. In fact, pharmacy technicians and nurses who deal with the preparation and administration of medications should aim for 100 percent success in performing this task.

THE PRESCRIPTION

A prescription is an order written by the licensed health care professional for the compounding or dispensing and administering of medications to a particular patient. Pharmacy technicians must be familiar with the commonly used abbreviations, which are listed in **Table 8-1**.

The components of a prescription include the following:

- Name, address, and phone number of the prescriber's office

- Name and address of the patient (Note: The patient's address is often filled in by the pharmacy instead of the physician's office.)

- Date

- Medication prescribed (inscription)

- Rx symbol (superscription) (Note: This is not required by federal law.)

- Dispensing directions to the pharmacist (subscription)

- Directions for the patient (signa)

- Refill and special labeling

- Prescriber's signature

- License number or Drug Enforcement Administration (DEA) number (on controlled substances only) (Note: DEA numbers are often filled in by the pharmacy instead of the physician's office.)

Figure 8-1 is an example of a prescription.

TABLE 8-1 Abbreviations Commonly Used in Prescriptions and Pharmacy

Abbreviation	Meaning
A	Before
ā ā, aa	Of each
ac	Before meals
ad lib	As desired
AM, am	Morning

(Continues)

TABLE 8-1 (Continued)

Abbreviation	Meaning
Amt	Amount
aq	Water
bid, BID	Twice a day
$\overline{C}$	With
cap, caps	Capsule
Comp	Compound
D	Day
dil	Dilute
disp	Dispense
dr	Dram
dx	Diagnosis
elix	Elixir
gr	Grain
gtt	Drop
h, hr	Hour
hs	At bedtime ("hour of sleep")
ID	Intradermally
IM	Intramuscularly
inj	Inject
IV	Intravenously
liq	Liquid
mcg	Microgram
mEq	Milliequivalent
mg	Milligram
mixt	Mixture
mL, ml	Milliliter
non rep	Do not repeat, no refills
NPO	Nothing by mouth
Oint	Ointment
OTC	Over-the-counter
oz	Ounce
pc	After meals

(Continues)

TABLE 8-1 (Continued)

Abbreviation	Meaning
per	Through or by
PM, pm	Afternoon
po	By mouth
pr	Through the rectum
prn, PRN	As needed
pt	Pint
pulv	Powder
q	Every
qam	Every morning
qh	Every hour
q2h	Every 2 hours
qid, QID	Four times a day
QPM, QHS	Every night
qs, qv	Quantity sufficient per directions
qt	Quart
rx, Rx	Prescription
$\bar{S}$	Without
Sig	Write on label
Sol	Solution
Stat	Immediately
Supp	Suppository
T, tbsp	Tablespoon
t, tsp	Teaspoon
Tab	Tablet
tid, TID	Three times a day
TO	Telephone order
Top	Topically
tr, tinct	Tincture
tx	Treatment
ud	As directed
ung	Ointment
vo	Verbal order
x	Times, multiplied by

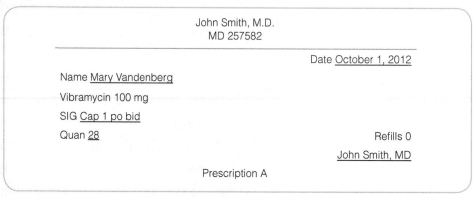

Figure 8-1 The prescription.
© *Cengage Learning 2013*

Stop and Review

Refer to Prescription A to answer the following questions.

1. How often should the patient take Vibramycin?

2. How much Vibramycin should the patient take at one time?

3. What components are missing from Prescription A?

4. How much Vibramycin should the pharmacy technician dispense?

5. How many times can Prescription A be refilled?

John Smith, M.D.
MD 257582

Date June 6, 2012

Name David Fish

Baclofen 20 mg

SIG tab 1 po tid

Quan 90

Refills 5

John Smith, MD

Prescription B

Refer to Prescription B to answer the following questions.

6. What strength tablets should be dispensed?

7. How often should the patient take baclofen?

8. How many baclofen tablets should the pharmacy technician dispense?

9. If the patient receives the original prescription and gets three refills, how many tablets has the patient received in total?

10. What components, if any, are missing from Prescription B?

_____

_____

John Smith, M.D.
MD 257582

Name Alice Harp

SIG tab 1 po tid

Quan 90

Refills 5

John Smith, MD

Prescription C

Refer to Prescription C to answer the following questions.

11. What components, if any, are missing from Prescription C?

12. How many tablets of ampicillin should the pharmacy technician dispense?

13. How often should the patient take the ampicillin?

14. How much ampicillin should the patient take at one time?

15. How many times can this prescription be refilled?

_____

_____

The Medication Order

The term *drug order* (also known as "medication order" or "chart order") is usually used for patients who are in the hospital, nursing homes, or other institutional settings. Drug orders are usually written on physicians' order forms. Orders may also be entered into a computer. Sometimes, the physician's order is called *stat*, meaning this order must be dispensed in less than 15 minutes. Information that is commonly required for completing inpatient medication orders includes the following:

- Patient name and patient identification or medical record number
- Patient room or bed number
- Date and time of order
- Name, quantity, strength of medications ordered, and dosage to be administered
- Route of administration
- Prescriber's name and signature
- Name or initials of the nurse who transcribed the order or called in a verbal order

An example of a drug order for inpatients is shown in **Figure 8-2**.

Stop and Review

Refer to the physician's order in Figure 8-2 to answer the following questions.

1. What is the only medication ordered to be given as needed for intense pain?

    _____

    _____

2. What is the maximum amount of Tylenol that should be given in a 24-hour period if this medication is ordered *as needed*?

    _____

    _____

3. What is the ordered route of administration for insulin?

    _____

    _____

4. What time of day is the insulin to be administered?

    _____

    _____

			ENTERED	FILLED	CHECKED	VERIFIED

NOTE: A NON-PROPRIETARY DRUG OF EQUAL QUALITY MAY BE DISPENSED - IF THIS COLUMN IS NOT CHECKED!

DATE	TIME WRITTEN	PLEASE USE BALL POINT - PRESS FIRMLY	✓	TIME NOTED	NURSES SIGNATURE
11/3/xx	0815	Keflex 250 mg p.o. q.6h	✓		
		Humulin N NPH U-100 Insulin 40 U SC ā breakfast	✓	0830	
		Demerol 75 mg IV q. 3–4 h p.r.n. severe pain	✓		
		Codeine 30 mg p.o. q.4h p.r.n. mild–mod pain	✓		G. Pickar, R.N.
		Tylenol 650 mg p.o. q.4h p.r.n., fever > 101° F	✓		
		Lasix 40 mg p.o. q.d.	✓		
		Slow-K 8 mEq p.o. b.i.d.	✓		
		J. Physician, M.D.			
11/3/xx	2200	Lasix 80 mg IV stat	✓		
		J. Physician, M.D.		2210	M. Smith, R.N.

AUTO STOP ORDERS: UNLESS REORDERED, FOLLOWING WILL BE D/Cᴰ AT 0800 ON:

DATE	ORDER		
		☐ CONT	PHYSICIAN SIGNATURE
		☐ D/C	
		☐ CONT	PHYSICIAN SIGNATURE
		☐ D/C	
		☐ CONT	PHYSICIAN SIGNATURE
		☐ D/C	

CHECK WHEN ANTIBIOTICS ORDERED ☐ Prophylactic ☐ Empiric ☐ Therapeutic

Allergies:
None Known

PATIENT DIAGNOSIS
Diabetes

HEIGHT 5' 5"   WEIGHT 130 lb

FORM 959-706 (8-xx)   **PHYSICIANS ORDER**   Reynolds • Reynolds LITHO IN U.S.A. K41814 (7-xx) D339080

Patient, Mary Q.
#3-11316-7

①

Figure 8-2 The physician's order.
© Cengage Learning 2013

5. How many times a day will Lasix be administered?

_____

_____

6. The patient has hypertension. Which medication will reduce the volume of blood?

_____

_____

7. A dosage of 8 mEq of slow-K is ordered. What does mEq mean?

_____

_____

8. What does a physician's order indicate as the route(s) of administration for Lasix?

_____

_____

9. What is the equivalent of the scheduled administration time(s) for Lasix, as converted to international time?

_____

_____

10. What is the route of administration for codeine?

_____

_____

THE DRUG LABEL

The label of a drug is the information attached to a container that identifies the contents of the container. For example, the label for a bottle of regular-strength aspirin would identify the contents as "aspirin, 325 mg."

The United States Food and Drug Administration (FDA) requires that manufacturers include extensive information as part of a drug product's label, especially for prescription drugs. Because the FDA requires more information than can be printed on a bottle's label, the agency allows drug manufacturers to list this information on papers that are inserted into or attached to the container. These labels, commonly called "package inserts," contain information that includes the drug's chemistry, intended uses, pharmacology, side effects, drug interactions, normal dose, warnings, precautions, contraindications, and how it is supplied. In some cases, a package insert can contain many pages of information.

Drug Name

When a manufacturer assigns a new drug its name, this name is called its *trade name*. This is the same as a product name or a *brand name*. Trade names are a challenge because there may be an unlimited amount of them, all containing similar ingredients. It is often followed by the sign "®," meaning that both the name and formulation are registered.

The *generic name* is given by the United States Adopted Name Council. Generic names are usually preferred and less complicated than any of the other naming methods. By law, the generic name must be identified on all drug labels. Each drug has only one generic name, and students generally must memorize it. For example, ibuprofen is an anti-inflammatory drug. Ibuprofen is the generic name. Brand or trade names for ibuprofen are Advil® and Motrin®. The drug has only one chemical, or "active ingredient," but several trade names. See the following labels (**Figure 8-3a and b**) for examples of a brand name (Carafate) and a generic name (furosemide).

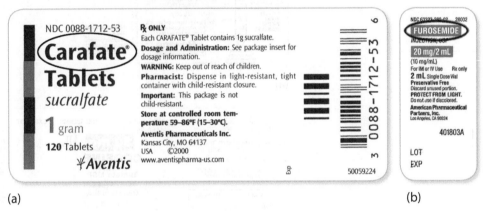

(a)   (b)

Figure 8-3 Circled on these labels are the drug names. (a) Carafate is the brand name (b) Furosemide is the generic drug name.
(a) *Courtesy of Aventis Pharmaceuticals Inc.* (b) *Courtesy of American Pharmaceuticals Partners, Inc.*

Dosage Strength

The dosage strength is the amount of active ingredient(s) found in a drug. Generally, the "weight" of the ingredient(s) in the drug may be measured on drug labels, such as grams (g), milligrams (mg), micrograms (mcg), milliequivalents (mEq), and units (formerly the abbreviation "U"). (Note: Completely avoid the use of the abbreviation U due to its being mistaken for an "O" or zero. Instead, the word *units* should be written out.) Reading the label can help determine the dosage strength (**Figure 8-4**).

Figure 8-4 Circled on this Lipid® label is the dosage strength.
Label reproduced with permission of Pfizer, Inc.

Form of the Drug

Drugs are available in different forms, and, commonly, a single drug may be available in a number of various forms. Drug dosage forms are classified according to their physical state and chemical composition. They may include solids, semisolids, liquids, and gases. Examples of liquid and solid drugs are shown in **Figure 8-5a–d**.

(a)

(b)

(c)   (d)

Figure 8-5 Different drug dosage forms (a) oral (b) tablets (c) capsules, and (d) liquid. (a) Used with permission of Roxane Laboratories, Inc. (b) *Used with permission of Roxane Laboratories, Inc.* (c) © *Cengage Learning 2013* (d) *Courtesy of Akorn, Inc.*

Route of Administration

The pathway by which a drug is given to a patient is known as its "route of administration." Depending on the patient's condition and the characteristics of the drug, the route of administration may include oral, sublingual, rectal, vaginal, topical, intravenous injection, intramuscular injection, subcutaneous injection, transcutaneous patch, inhalation, and many others (**Figure 8-6a–c**).

Figure 8-6 Circled are different routes of administration. (a) sublingual (b) oral, and (c) intramuscular or intravenous.

(a) *Labels reproduced with permission of Pfizer, Inc.* (b) *Used with permission of Roxane Laboratories, Inc.*
(c) *Courtesy of Endo Pharmaceuticals, Inc.*

Supply Dosage

The term **supply dosage** pertains to both *dosage strength* and *form*. It is read as "X measured units per some quantity." For liquid drugs, the supply dosage is the same as the drug's concentration, such as "X measured units per milliliter." For solid-form drugs such as tablets, the supply dosage is X measured units per tablet. Pharmacy technicians should take a minute to read the supply dosage printed on the following labels (**Figure 8-7a and b**).

Figure 8-7 Circled in these labels are supply dosage.

(a) *Courtesy of ESI Lederle, a Business Unit of Wyeth Pharmaceuticals, Philadelphia, PA* (b) *Courtesy of Endo Pharmaceuticals, Inc.*

Total Volume

The full quantity contained in a package, bottle, or vial is called the "total volume" (**Figure 8-8a and b**). For solid drugs, the total number of individual items must be considered. For liquids, it is the total fluid volume.

(a)

(b)

Figure 8-8 Circled in these labels is the total volume.
(a) © Copyright Eli Lilly and Company. Used with permission. (b) Used by permission of Novartis AG.

Warnings and Storage Information

Many environmental factors may influence the effect of medications. These factors include light, temperature, air, and humidity. Environmental factors, human error, or negligence can cause further complications. It is essential for pharmacy technicians to handle and store medications properly to ensure drug quality.

Many drugs require specific storage conditions, and anyone who deals with or handles medications must understand the storage guidelines. The technician must be aware of the temperature guidelines and read the label, which may state some storage directions, such as "Store at controlled room temperature" (**Figure 8-9a and b**). Other label warnings include "Do not freeze," "Protect from extreme heat," "Keep refrigerated," "Protect from high humidity," and "Protect from light."

Information about Mixing or Reconstituting

Reconstitution is the process of adding water or another solvent to a powdered form of a medication in order to make a solution or a suspension (**Figure 8-10a and b**).

(a)

(b)

Figure 8-9 Circled are particular warning and storage information for these drugs.
(a) Storage temperature information for Ciprofloxacin hydrocholoride (b) Several labels for Erythomycin Ethylsuccinate, including proper storage temperature and container type.
(a) © *Cengage Learning 2013* (b) *Courtesy of Mylan Pharmaceuticals, Inc.*

(a)

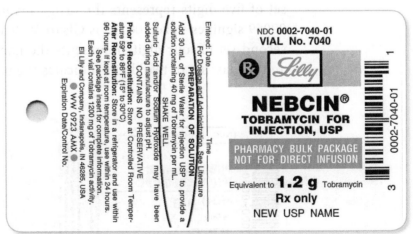

(b)

Figure 8-10 Circled is information regarding how to safely and properly reconstitute or mix these drugs.
(a) © *Copyright Eli Lilly and Company. Used with permission.* (b) © *Copyright Eli Lilly and Company. Used with permission.*

Expiration Date

A specific day or month that has been determined as the time when a drug product has lost a significant amount of its potency is known as its expiration date. For example, many antibiotic oral suspensions lose significant potency within 14 days of the time they are mixed and, therefore, have a 14-day expiration date. In other cases, the assigned expiration date may be arbitrary. Pharmaceutical manufacturers must assign expiration dates to all of their products, even if they do not lose significant potency over many years of storage (**Figure 8-11**). In these cases, a drug company may assign an expiration date that usually varies between three or four years after manufacture. The expiration date is based on how the testing of the drug was conducted. For example, if the manufacturer does not test the drug past two years, the expiration date cannot be longer than two years.

Figure 8-11 Circled is the expiration date for this drug.
Courtesy of Ortho-McNeil Pharmaceuticals Inc.

National Drug Code (NDC)

The American coding system for prescription drugs whereby each drug is individually identified down to its package size is known as the "National Drug Code (NDC)." The NDC usually employs an 11-digit design, formatted as follows: XXXXX-YYYY-ZZ (**Figure 8-12**). In this scheme, the first set of five digits represents the drug's manufacturer or distributor (e.g., 00069 signifies Pfizer, 00173 is Glaxo-Wellcome, and 00002 is Lilly). The second set of four digits represents the name and strength of the drug, and the last set of two digits indicates the package size. Only the first set

Figure 8-12 Circled is the 11-digit National Code.
© Cengage Learning 2013

of digits is standardized. All the other numbers are assigned by the drug companies themselves.

However, the NDC sometimes changes their coding for various drug products. The first set of digits is sometimes only 4 digits long instead of 5. Likewise, the second set of digits is sometimes only 3 digits long instead of 4. The NDC is commonly used to identify the exact drug dispensed to a patient (e.g., NDC-61570-069-60 for Procanbid), as well as its strength and package size.

Lot Number

A lot number is a number printed by the drug manufacturer on each bottle of medicine that identifies the batch that the particular medication came from (**Figure 8-13**). Lot numbers are important in case of a recall of a defective product. The lot number has been invaluable for vaccine and over-the-counter medication recalls.

Figure 8-13 Circled in the label is the lot number.
Reprinted with the permission of Roche Laboratories, Inc. All rights reserved.

Bar Code Symbols

Bar code symbols are commonly used in retail sales. They also document drug dosing for recordkeeping and stock reorders and may soon help in the automation of medication documentation right at the patient's bedside. Overall, the process of bar coding is greatly beneficial, though it has influenced changes in package sizes, production processes, and label designs. The horizontal types of bar codes look like picket fences, and the vertical types look like ladders (**Figure 8-14a and b**).

Combination Drugs

When a medication contains more than one active ingredient, it is known as a "combination drug." The ingredients may be combined in order to treat a wider spectrum of symptoms, to decrease side effects, or to increase the effectiveness of one of the ingredients. Read the following labels and notice the different substances that are combined in each tablet (**Figure 8-15a and b**). Combination drugs are usually prescribed by the number of tablets, capsules, or milliliters to be given rather than by the dosage strength.

(a)

(b)

Figure 8-14 Circled in these labels are bar code symbols, commonly found in retail sales.
(a) *Courtesy of ESI Lederle, a Business Unit of Wyeth Pharmaceuticals, Philadelphia, PA* (b) *Used by permission of Novartis AG.*

(a)   (b)

Figure 8-15 Circled in these labels are combination drugs.
(a) *© Cengage Learning 2013* (b) *© Cengage Learning 2013*

 Stop and Review

Use the following labels A through F to find the information requested in questions 1 through 13. In questions h through m, show your answers by using the letter of the corresponding label.

(a)

Versed 5 mg.
Courtesy of Roche Laboratories, Inc.

(b)

Guaifenesin 1 mg/mL.
© Cengage Learning 2013

(c)

Biaxin 250 mg.
Used with permisson of Abbott Laboratories

(d)

Klonopin .5 mg.
Reprinted with the permission of Roche Laboratories, Inc. All rights reserved.

(e)

Tamoxifen citrate 20 mg 30 tablets.
© Cengage Learning 2013

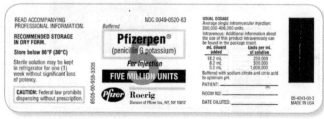

Each CLAFORAN® STERILE vial contains 2g cefotaxime for injection, Dextrose Hydrous, USP to adjust osmolality, sodium citrate hydrous, USP to buffer injection, and hydrochloric acid to adjust pH.
R ONLY   Dosage and Administration: Read package insert for prescribing information and reconstitution. Shake to dissolve. Store dry powder below 30°C. Protect from excessive light.
Mfd for: Hoechst-Roussel Pharmaceuticals
Division of Aventis Pharmaceuticals Inc.
Kansas City, MO 64137   ©2000
Made in United Kingdom   50053567   CND 70100

NDC 0039-0019-01
Claforan® Sterile
cefotaxime for injection, USP
(formerly sterile cefotaxime sodium)
Lot BA799
Exp 8/2008
2g IM/IV   ⨏Aventis

(f)

Claforan Sterile.
Courtesy of Aventis Pharmaceuticals Inc.

1. Determine the route of administration on label A. _____

2. What does the term *Filmtab* mean on label C? _____

3. Determine how much of the supply drug you will administer to the patient per dose for the order *Tamoxifen* 40 mg p.o. q12h on label E. _____

4. Look at label D and determine the supply dosage. _____

5. Indicate which labels have an imprinted bar code symbol. _____

6. Look at label A and list the manufacturer of Versed. _____

7. What is the name of the manufacturer on label E? _____

8. On which label is the lot number circled? _____

9. On which label is the total volume of the liquid bottle circled? _____

10. On which label is the expiration date circled? _____

11. On which label is the brand name of the drug circled? _____

12. On which label is the form of the drug circled? _____

13. On which label is the dosage strength circled? _____

Refer to the following label to identify the specific drug information described in questions 14 through 19.

READ ACCOMPANYING PROFESSIONAL INFORMATION.
RECOMMENDED STORAGE IN DRY FORM.
Store below 86°F (30°C)
Sterile solution may be kept in refrigerator for one (1) week without significant loss of potency.
CAUTION: Federal law prohibits dispensing without prescription.

NDC 0049-0520-83
Buffered
Pfizerpen®
(penicillin G potassium)
For Injection
FIVE MILLION UNITS
Pfizer Roerig
Division of Pfizer Inc, NY, NY 10017

USUAL DOSAGE
Average single intramuscular injection: 200,000-400,000 units.
Intravenous: Additional information about the use of this product intravenously can be found in the package insert.

mL diluent added	Units per mL of solution
18.2 mL	250,000
8.2 mL	500,000
3.2 mL	1,000,000

Buffered with sodium citrate and citric acid to optimum pH.
PATIENT: _____
ROOM NO: _____
DATE DILUTED: _____
05-4243-00-3
MADE IN USA

6505-00-958-3305

Pfizerpen 5 million units.
Label reproduced with permission of Pfizer Inc.

14. Brand name _____

15. Generic name _____

16. Dosage strength _____

17. Route of administration _____

18. National Drug Code _____

19. Manufacturer _____

Refer to the following label to answer questions 20 through 22.

Lidocaine 1 %.
Courtesy of Baxter Healthcare Corporation

20. The supply dosage of the drug is _____ mg per mL.

21. The supply dosage of the drug is _____ %.

22. The dosage of the drug is _____ g per _____ mL.

INTERPRETING AND PROCESSING A DRUG ORDER

The prescription must be read carefully to verify that the ingredients or quantities of medications are correct.

Processing a drug order in most states may follow a specific sequence that technicians should be familiar with. For example, the drug is written first, followed by the dosage, route, and frequency. The brand (or trade) name of the drug begins with an uppercase letter and the generic name begins with a lowercase letter.

■ EXAMPLE 1:

Ziagen 300 mg p.o. b.i.d.

1.   Ziagen is the brand name of the drug.

2.   300 mg is the dosage.

3.   p.o. is the route.

4.   b.i.d. is the frequency.

This order means: "Give 300 milligrams of Ziagen orally twice daily."

■ **EXAMPLE 2:**

Advil 400 mg p.o. b.i.d.

1. Advil is the trade name of the drug.

2. 400 mg is the dosage.

3. p.o. is the route.

4. b.i.d. is the frequency.

This order means: "Give 400 mg of Advil orally twice daily."

If the technician follows the steps of processing a drug order properly, interprets the order correctly, and understands the drug label, then these factors will assist in the accurate calculation of drug dosages. Medication errors can thus be preventable.

■ **EXAMPLE 3:**

Tagamet 300 mg tab 1 p.o. b.i.d.

Reads: "Give 300 milligrams of Tagamet orally 2 times a day."

■ **EXAMPLE 4:**

Humulin N U-100 insulin 30 units SC q.d. 30 min ā breakfast

Reads: "Give 30 units of Humulin N U-100 insulin subcutaneously every day 30 minutes before breakfast."

 Stop and Review

Fill in the blanks regarding drug order processing.

1. Write the first four steps of processing a prescription.

_____

_____

_____

_____

2. What is the last step that pharmacy technicians must take regarding the processing of a prescription?

_____

3. State the reasons that filling a prescription correctly is a very important task for the pharmacy technician.

_____

4. Describe the role of computer systems in the filling of prescriptions.

_____

5. What information is contained on a medication label that helps the pharmacy technician process the prescription?

_____

Interpret the following medication orders.

6. atropine sulfate ophthalmic 1% 2 gtt OU q 15 min x 4

_____

_____

7. Biaxin 250 mg p.o. b.i.d.

_____

_____

8. Lasix 20 mg IM ā breakfast

_____

_____

9. Nitroglycerin gr $\dfrac{1}{400}$ SL stat

_____

_____

10. Solu-Medrol 10 mg IM q6h

_____

_____

11. meperidine 20 mg SC q3-4h p.r.n. pain

_____

_____

12. heparin 750 units SC stat

_____

_____

13. Narcan 0.3 mg IM stat

_____

_____

14. Benadryl 40 mg p.o. stat

_____

_____

15. Valium 3.5 mg IM q6h p.r.n., anxiety

_____

_____

16. Synthroid 150 mcg p.o. q.d.

_____

_____

17. tobramycin sulfate 90 mg IM q8h

_____

_____

18. Cortisporin otic suspension 2 gtt A.S. t.i.d.

_____

_____

19. Fortaz 250 mg IV q12h

_____

_____

20. Elixophyllin liquid 0.24 g p.o. stat

_____

_____

REDUCING MEDICATION ERRORS

One of the best ways to minimize the occurrence of errors is to become familiar with the most common causes of medication errors. Medication errors are often attributed to one or more of the following:

- Calculation errors
- Careless use of zeros and decimal points

- Abbreviations
- Verbal orders
- Drug concentration
- Poor handwriting of prescribers
- Apothecary system
- Manufacturer of drug products
- Look-alike and sound-alike drug names
- Product labeling
- Lack of color coding
- Drug preparation errors
- Labeling
- Outdated medication (very rare)
- Work environment
- Drug interactions

Pharmacy technicians can reduce medication errors by doing the following:

- Recheck calculations
- Verify drug orders
- Check for current allergy history and current medication list
- Confirm the patient's identity

▪ EXAMPLE 1:

A physician wrote "0.5 mg" IV morphine for postoperative pain on a 9-month-old child. An inexperienced pharmacy technician read the prescription as "5 mg every 4 hours." The technician dispenses the drug; fortunately, the pharmacist notices the error and explains the technician's mistake to him.

▪ EXAMPLE 2:

A physician ordered "calcium gluconate 400 mg IV" for a 2-day-old baby. The product label states "0.465 mEq Ca⁺⁺mL" in bold print on the front of the label, but also states "each mL contains calcium gluconate 94 mg" in the fine print on the back. The label further mentions "9.3 mg Ca⁺⁺/mL" in bold in another spot on the label. The pharmacy technician is confused and divides 400 by 9.3 to get 43 mL. A 50 mL vial of calcium gluconate (approximately 1g/10 mL) was removed from a shelf, and 43 mL (approximately 4 g of calcium gluconate, or 20 mEq of calcium ion) was dispensed for the infant, instead of around 4 mL or 400 mg. Fortunately, the pharmacist found the error because he knew that calcium and calcium gluconate are measured differently, and their normal doses are different.

■ EXAMPLE 3:

The elixir sulfanilamide calamity in 1937 is an example of formulation or manufacturing errors. The tragedy occurred shortly after the introduction of sulfanilamide (the first sulfa antimicrobial drug), when diethylene glycol was used as the diluent in the formulation of a liquid preparation of sulfanilamide known as Elixir Sulfanilamide. Because no pharmacological studies had been done on this preparation, it was sold to the public without the knowledge that diethylene glycol was toxic. As a result of this error, 105 patients died from its therapeutic use. Mislabeling, contamination, the wrong drug, the wrong concentration, or the wrong doses of drugs are other causes of medication errors.

■ EXAMPLE 4:

A 260 mg preparation of Taxol was ordered by a physician, but the pharmacist mistakenly prepared 260 mg of Taxotere instead. These drugs are both used as chemotherapy for different cancers. Their recommended dosages differ. The patient died several days later. His death couldn't be connected to the error because he was already severely ill.

■ EXAMPLE 5:

A patient died as a result of 200 units of insulin being accidentally injected. This occurred because 20 units of insulin was abbreviated as "20 U." The health practitioner mistook the "U" for another zero following the number "20." (The abbreviation "U" for units must be avoided, and you must write out the word *units* in its entirety.)

■ EXAMPLE 6:

Methotrexate is typically used in daily doses to treat people with cancer, although low doses of it have been prescribed for other conditions, including arthritis, asthma, and inflammatory bowel disease. One elderly patient with rheumatoid arthritis received a 10 mg daily dose of methotrexate, rather than the intended 10 mg weekly dose, and died as a result.

Computers

Computers can reduce medication errors. Prescription dispensing and associated record maintenance can be done by computer systems more precisely and accurately than by hand, ensuring that fewer medication errors occur. Computer dispensing and record maintenance also provide all kinds of information about potential drug complications that the physician might not have considered.

Bar Coding

Bar coding offers assurance that the identity and dose of the drug are as prescribed for the correct patient, and it improves timeliness and accuracy. The advent of bar coding of pharmaceuticals has required changes in label designs, production processes, and size of packages. Bar coding saves dollars, time, and, most important, lives.

Stop and Review
Answer the following questions.

1. Medication errors during dispensing may be reduced if the pharmacy technician does the following:

   a. _____

   b. _____

   c. _____

   d. _____

2. Describe the effect of bar coding and its reduction of medication errors.

   _____

   _____

3. Give an example of a medication error that resulted in the death of more than 100 patients.

   _____

   _____

4. How can computers reduce medication errors?

   _____

   _____

Test Your Knowledge

Answer questions 1 through 4 regarding the components of prescriptions.

1. Name five components of a prescription.

   _____

   _____

   _____

   _____

   _____

2. Define a "stat" order.

   _____

3. The DEA number always must be shown on a prescription for

   _____

4. Name the terms for the following parts of a prescription.
   - Medication prescribed _____
   - Directions to the patient _____
   - Dispensing directions to the pharmacist _____
   - Rx symbol _____

Mary Keho, M.D.

265 Sunrise Blvd., Fort Lauderdale, FL 33601

954-555-9876

Name	Phil Jones _____
	Allegra 60 mg
Sig	Tab 1 po bid _____
Quan	30
Refills	5

Prescription A

Refer to Prescription A to answer questions 5–7.

5. How many times should the patient take Allegra per day? _____

6. How many times can Prescription A be refilled? _____

7. How much Allegra should you dispense? _____

Mary Keho, M.D.

265 Sunrise Blvd., Fort Lauderdale, FL 33601

954-555-9876

Name	Connie Griffin
	Trycet 100 mg
Sig	Tab 1 q4h po prn pain
Quan	30
Refills	0

Prescription B

Refer to Prescription B to answer questions 8–10.

8. How much Trycet should the patient take at one time? _____

9. What strength tablets should be dispensed? _____

10. How often should the patient take Trycet? _____

Mary Keho, M.D.

265 Sunrise Blvd., Fort Lauderdale, FL 33601

954-555-9876

Name	John Kay
	timolol malente 0.5%
Sig	gtt 1 bid in affected eye
Quan	5 mL
Refills	2

Prescription C

Refer to Prescription C to answer questions 11–13.

11. How much timolol should the patient use at one time? _____

12. What strength drops should be dispensed? _____

13. How many times can this prescription be refilled? _____

Mary Keho, M.D.

265 Sunrise Blvd., Fort Lauderdale, FL 33601

954-555-9876

Name   Nancy Novel

Phenobarbital 15 mg

Sig   tab 1 po tid

Quan   60

Refills   3

Prescription D

Refer to Prescription D to answer questions 14–16.

14. How many times should the patient take phenobarbital each day?
_____

15. How much phenobarbital should the patient take at one time? _____

16. If the patient gets the original prescription and only 2 refills, how many tablets will the patient take in total? _____

Mary Keho, M.D.

265 Sunrise Blvd., Fort Lauderdale, FL 33601

954-555-9876

Name   Terri Perez

guaifenesin 100 mg

Sig   syr ii tsp q4h pm

Quan   100 mL

Refills   0

Prescription E

Refer to Prescription E to answer questions 17–19.

17. How often should the patient take guaifenesin? _____

18. How many teaspoons should the patient take at one time? _____

19. How many times can this prescription be refilled? _____

Write the meaning of the following abbreviations commonly used in prescriptions.

20. Oint _____

21. q _____

22. vo _____

23. Amt. _____

24. ac _____

25. sig _____

26. pc _____

27. hs _____

28. aq _____

29. prn _____

30. gtt _____

31. s̄ _____

32. stat _____

33. c̄ _____

NDC 63323-006-50   0650

SODIUM BICARBONATE

INJECTION, USP, 8.4%

84 mg/mL

50 mEq/50 mL

(1mEq/mL)

For IV Use Only

50 mL   Rx only
Single Dose Vial

Sterile, Nonpyrogenic
Preservative Free
Discard unused portion.
Each mL contains: Sodium bicarbonate 84 mg; Water for Injection q.s. Carbon dioxide is added for pH adjustment.
50 mEq/50 mL
2 mOsmol/mL (calc.)
Usual Dosage: See Insert.
DO NOT USE IF PRECIPITATE IS PRESENT.
Use only if seal is intact.
Store at controlled room temperature 15°–30°C (59°–86°F).

APP
AMERICAN PHARMACEUTICAL PARTNERS, INC.
Los Angeles, CA 90024

3   63323-006-50   1

4017868

Label A

Sodium Bicarbonate 84 mg/mL.
Courtesy of American Pharmaceuticals Partners, Inc.

Refer to Label A to answer questions 34–37.

34. What is the supply dosage of the medication in milliequivalents?

_____

35. What is the supply dosage of the medication in milligrams?

_____

36. What is the National Drug Code number?

_____

37. What is the route of administration?

_____

Label B

Vantin 100 mg.
Courtesy of Pharmacia Corporation Peapack, NJ

Refer to Label B to answer questions 38–41.

38. What is the generic name of the drug?

_____

39. What is the reconstitution instruction to mix a supply dosage of 100 mg per 5 mL for oral suspension?

_____

_____

_____

40. What is the name of the manufacturer of the drug?

_____

41. What is the National Drug Code number?

_____

Label C

Methotrexate 250 mg.
Courtesy of Baxter Healthcare Corporation

Refer to Label C to answer questions 42–44.

42. What is the supply dosage?

_____

43. What is the total volume of the medication container?

_____

44. How much will you administer to the patient per dose for the order *Methotrexate 25 mg IV stat?*

_____

Label D

Nebcin 1.2 g.
© Copyright Eli Lilly and Company. Used with permission.

Refer to Label D to answer questions 45–48.

45. What is the generic name of the drug?

_____

46. What is the brand name of the drug?

_____

47. How many milligrams are in each mL?

_____

48. What is the total volume of the medication container?

_____

FOR INTRAMUSCULAR USE ONLY.
USUAL ADULT DOSE: Intramuscularly: 25 - 100 mg stat; repeat every 4 to 6 hours, as needed.
See accompanying prescribing information.

Each mL contains **50 mg** of hydroxyzine hydrochloride, 0.9% benzyl alcohol and sodium hydroxide to adjust to optimum pH.

To avoid discoloration, protect from prolonged exposure to light.

Rx only

10 mL   NDC 0049-5460-74

Vistaril®
(hydroxyzine hydrochloride)

Intramuscular Solution
50 mg/mL

Pfizer **Roerig**
Division of Pfizer Inc, NY, NY 10017

Store below 86°F (30°C).
PROTECT FROM FREEZING.

PATIENT: _____

ROOM NO.: _____

05-1111-32-4   **9249**
MADE IN USA

Label E

Vistaril 50 mg/mL.
Label reproduced with permission of Pfizer Inc.

Refer to Label E to answer questions 49–53.

49. What is the drug form?

_____

50. What is the administration route?

_____

51. What is the total volume of the drug container?

_____

52. What is the appropriate temperature for storage of the drug?

_____

53. What is the name of the manufacturer of the drug?

_____

Label F

Inderal 20 mg.
Courtesy of Wyeth Pharmaceuticals, Philaelphia, PA

Refer to Label F to answer questions 54–57.

54. What is the generic name of the medication?

_____

55. What is the form of the drug?

_____

56. What is the name of the manufacturer of the drug?

_____

57. What is the NDC number of the drug?

_____

Label G

Potassium Chloride.
Courtesy of American Pharmaceuticals Partners, Inc.

Refer to Label G to answer questions 58–59.

58. What is the dosage strength of the drug?

_____

59. What is the expiration date of the drug?

_____

Interpret the following physician medication orders.

60. Apresoline 30 mg IV q6h

_____

61. neostigmine 0.5 mg IM t.i.d.

_____

62. Novolin N NPH U-100 insulin 25 USC ā breakfast

_____

63. Demerol 50 mg IM q3-4h p.r.n. pain _____

64. Lanoxin 0.25 mg p.o. q.d.

_____

65. Maalox 5 mL p.o. 1h a.c., 1h p.c., h.s.

_____

66. Motrin 600 mg p.o. b.i.d.

_____

67. Cytoxan 50 mg p.o. q.d.

_____

68. Cephalexin 0.5 g p.o. q.i.d.

_____

69. potassium chloride 16 mEq p.o. q.d.

_____

70. Toradol 60 mg IM stat et q6h

_____

71. Decadron 4 mg IV b.i.d.

_____

Label H

Label I

(h) Lortab 5 mg/500 mg (i) Furosemide 20 mg/2 mL.
(h) Courtesy of UCB Pharma, Inc. (i) Used with permisison of Abraxis BioScience, Inc.

Refer to Label H or I to answer questions 72–78.

72. The lot number for the drug on label I is _____.

73. Which label represents a combination drug? _____.

74. Which label represents a unit- or single-dose drug? _____.

75. The controlled substance schedule for the drug shown on label H is _____.

76. What is the route of administration for the drug shown on label H? _____.

77. Which label represents a drug that may be ordered by the number of tablets or capsules? _____.

78. What is the total volume of the vial as listed on label I? _____

NDC 10019-019-57

Lidocaine 2%
HCl Injection, USP

(20 mg/mL)   ℞ only
FOR INFILTRATION AND NERVE BLOCK
NOT FOR SPINAL OR EPIDURAL ANESTHESIA
50 mL Multiple Dose Vial

Baxter   **eSiLEDERLE™**
Mfd. for **Baxter Healthcare Corporation** affiliate
by: Elkins-Sinn, Cherry Hill, NJ 08003   400-747-01

Each mL contains lidocaine hydrochloride 20 mg, sodium chloride 6 mg
and methylparaben 1 mg in Water for
Injection. pH 5.0-7.0; sodium hydroxide and/or hydrochloric acid used,
if needed, for pH adjustment.
Usual Dosage: See package insert for
complete prescribing information.
Store at controlled room temperature
15°-30°C (59°-86°F).

Lot: Exp.:

Label J

Lidocaine 2 %.
Copyright Baxter Healthcare Corporation.

Refer to Label J to answer questions 79–80.

79. What is the supply dosage of the drug in label J, when expressed as a percentage? _____.

80. The supply dosage in label J is equivalent to _____ mg per mL.

Critical Thinking

A community pharmacy technician misread the handwriting on a prescription for 10 mg of Metadate ER and dispensed methadone 10 mg instead for a 7-year-old boy. Fortunately, the pharmacist read the information that accompanied the prescription and realized the error. It is the responsibility of the pharmacy technician to clarify any drug order that is doubtful in order to prevent medication errors.

1. If the handwriting on a prescription is not clear, what should a pharmacy technician do?

   _____

   _____

2. What are Metadate and methadone commonly prescribed for?

   _____

   _____

Percentage of Error Due to Equipment

OBJECTIVES

Upon completion of this chapter, you should be able to:

1. Calculate the smallest amount of medication to be measured by a specific device.
2. Determine the best instrument for measuring single-dose quantities and large amounts of medications.
3. Calculate and define percentage of error for weight and volume measurements.
4. Describe equipment used to measure weight and volume.

GLOSSARY

class A prescription balances – One- or two-pan balances that are commonly used by pharmacists; they may be electronic or torsion balances.

conical graduates – Cone-shaped containers with graduated markings for measuring liquids; their slanted sides may make estimations of quantity difficult.

cylindrical graduates – Cylinder-shaped containers with graduated markings for measuring liquids.

electronic balances – Scales that use electronic components and digital readouts to calibrate the weighing of different substances.

meniscus – The bottom portion of the concave surface of a liquid; used to measure the volume of a liquid in a container such as a graduate.

pipets – Graduated tubes used to transfer small volumes of liquids; also spelled *pipettes*.

OVERVIEW

The pharmacy technician must understand how to utilize the proper equipment to measure weight and volume for dosages. The ability to calculate percentage of error when weighing and conducting volumetric measurement is essential to the duties of the pharmacy technician. The demands of today's practice of pharmacy require skillful use of calculators when performing dosage calculations. State boards of pharmacy often require pharmacies to provide minimum lists of equipment for compounding prescriptions.

MEASUREMENT OF WEIGHT

Many types of equipment are available to measure weight in the pharmacy. Balances, scales, and metal weights are commonly utilized on a day-to-day basis. The correct equipment to use for each type of measurement is based on the task at hand. For example, prescription balances are commonly used in extemporaneous compounding, while electronic balances are used for assay tests. All weighing equipment must be calibrated and tested for accuracy and sensitivity.

Medicinal substances are usually weighed on Class A prescription balances. These balances are sensitive enough to weigh as little as 6 mg in each weighing pan and can weigh up to 120 grams in each weighing pan. They include torsion balances (see Figure 9-1) and electronic balances (see Figure 9-2).

Figure 9-1 Class A prescription balance.
© Cengage Learning 2013

Figure 9-2 Electronic balance.
© Cengage Learning 2013

A balance's *sensitivity requirement* is defined as the load that will cause a change of one division on its index plate. This is determined by first leveling the balance and then determining its rest point. Following this, the smallest weight that causes the rest point to shift one division on the index plate reveals the sensitivity requirement of the balance. High-precision electronic analytical balances are even more accurate for very small quantities. They are often able to weigh 0.1 mg of a substance, self-calibrate, and have easy-to-read digital displays. Metric weights used with balances are shown in **Figure 9-3**.

Figure 9-3 Metric weights used with balances.
© Cengage Learning 2013

MEASUREMENT OF VOLUME

In the pharmacy, the measurement of volume involves the use of a variety of equipment, including burettes, graduates, calibrated syringes, pipets, micropipets, and others. The level of precision needed determines the choice of the correct measuring instrument. Cylindrical and conical (cone-shaped) graduates are the most commonly used types of equipment for volumetric measurements.

Cylindrical graduates (see **Figure 9-4**) are calibrated in metric units. **Conical graduates** (see **Figure 9-5**) are usually calibrated in both metric and apothecary units. Graduates are made of glass or plastic and *usually* range in capacity from 5 to 1000 mL. To decrease errors, the smallest size graduate should be used to measure a specific quantity. In general, the thinner the graduate, the less error in reading the **meniscus** of the liquid contained (see **Figure 9-6**). To accurately read the amount of a substance inside a graduate, it should be placed on a flat, level surface.

Figure 9-4 Cylindrical graduates.
© Cengage Learning 2013

Figure 9-5 Conical graduates.
© Cengage Learning 2013

Figure 9-6 How to read the meniscus.
© Cengage Learning 2013

Both the *United States Pharmacopeia* and the *National Bureau of Standards Handbook* discuss how deviations affect errors in reading the meniscus when working with different sizes of graduates. It is essential that the pharmacy technician selects the proper type of graduate and also ascertains that its size is the most correct for the amount being measured. He or she must carefully observe the meniscus at eye level to achieve the desired measurement.

The household measurement system, while still used in homes throughout the United States, is highly inaccurate due to the discrepancies in sizes of manufactured equipment such as teaspoons and tablespoons. While teaspoons are (in general) equivalent to 5 mL, and tablespoons are considered to be 15 mL, calibrated droppers that can contain these quantities are preferred because they are more accurate and precise (see **Figure 9-7**). Calibrated dosage spoons, hypodermic syringes, and medicine cups are also preferred over household equipment (see **Figures 9-8** and **9-9**).

Figure 9-8 Calibrated spoon.
© Cengage Learning 2013

Figure 9-7 Calibrated dropper.
© Cengage Learning 2013

Figure 9-9 Oral syringe.
© Cengage Learning 2013

Remember

An oral syringe should never be confused with a syringe used for injections. Serious medication errors may occur as a result of such confusion.

Oral syringes are calibrated in both metric and household units. They are available in many different sizes to ensure accuracy for small dosages.

Medicine cups (see **Figure 9-10**) are preferred for larger dosages (usually from 2 teaspoons to 2 tablespoons).

Figure 9-10 Medicine cup with approximate equivalent measures.
© Cengage Learning 2013

Remember

It is important to make sure that, no matter what type of equipment is used for medication, the calibrations on the device match the calibrations listed in the dosage instructions.

Because drops are often used for medications, official medicine droppers are preferred because they better control the size of each drop. Droppers with round openings that have an external diameter of approximately 3 millimeters deliver accurate drop sizes when held vertically. These droppers are calibrated to deliver approximately 20 drops of water per mm.

PERCENTAGE OF ERROR

Pharmacy technicians as well as pharmacists must understand how inaccurate measurements may cause medication errors, and how these may vary in significance. Two quantities are important when measuring weight or volume:

1. The *apparent* weight or volume that is measured

2. The possible deficiency or excess of the actual quantity that is obtained

Percentage of error is the maximum potential error multiplied by 100 and then divided by the desired quantity:

$$\frac{\text{Error} \times 100\%}{\text{Desired quantity}} = \text{Percentage of error}$$

CALCULATING PERCENTAGE OF ERROR WHEN WEIGHING

The percentage of error when weighing is easily calculated using the preceding formula.

■ **EXAMPLE 1:**

If the maximum potential error is ± 5 mg in a total of 100 mg, what is the percentage of error?

$$\frac{5 \times 100\%}{100} = 5\%$$

Therefore, in this example, the percentage of error is 5%.

■ **EXAMPLE 2:**

A prescription calls for 600 mg of a substance. The amount is weighed, and the pharmacy technician double-checks it by using a more sensitive balance to weigh it again. This reveals the amount to be 575 mg. The difference is 25 mg, so what is the percentage of error?

$$\frac{25 \times 100\%}{600} = 4\%$$

Therefore, in this example, the percentage of error is 4%.

If a certain percentage of error is not to be exceeded, and the maximum potential error of a measuring instrument is known, you can calculate the smallest quantity that can be measured within the desired accuracy:

$$\frac{100 \times \text{Maximum potential error}}{\text{Permissible percentage of error}} = \text{Smallest quantity}$$

■ **EXAMPLE 3:**

On a balance that is sensitive to 6 mg, what is the smallest quantity that can be weighed with a potential error of no more than 5 percent?

$$\frac{100 \times 6\,\text{mg}}{5(\%)} = 120\,\text{mg}$$

Therefore, the smallest quantity that can be weighed with a potential error of no more than 5 percent is **120 mg**.

CALCULATING PERCENTAGE OF ERROR IN VOLUMETRIC MEASUREMENT

The percentage of error in volumetric measurement can be calculated easily, by relating the volume in error to the desired volume.

■ **EXAMPLE 1:**

A graduated cylinder is used to measure 30 mL of a medication. To double-check, the pharmacy technician uses a narrow-gauge burette and finds that 32 mL was actually measured. What is the percentage of error?

The volume of error is: 32 mL − 30 mL = 2 mL

Therefore,

$$\frac{2 \text{ mL} \times 100\%}{30 \text{ mL}} = 6.7\%$$

The percentage of error in this example is 6.7%.

Stop and Review
Answer the following questions.

1. What is the potential error (in terms of percentage) if 100 mg of a powdered medication is weighed on a balance with a sensitivity requirement of 6 mg?

   _____

   _____

2. If a 20-mL graduate weighs 85.49 grams, and 15 mL of distilled water is measured in it, the combined weight of the graduate and water is 100.28 grams. Because 15 mL of water should weigh 15 grams, calculate the weight of the measured water, and then express any deviation from 5 g as a percentage of error.

   _____

   _____

3. On a prescription balance with a sensitivity requirement of 0.06 g, what is the smallest amount that can be weighed with a maximum potential error of not more than 12%?

   _____

   _____

4. A pharmacy technician weighed 40 mg of menthol on a balance with a sensitivity requirement of 4 mg. Calculate the percentage of error that may have been incurred.

   _____

   _____

5. A pharmacy technician is directed to weigh 15 g of a substance in order to limit the percentage of error to 0.5%. What is the maximum potential error in milligrams the technician would not be allowed to exceed?

   _____

   _____

■ **EXAMPLE 1:**

CHAPTER 10

Dilutions and Solutions

OBJECTIVES

Upon completion of this chapter, you should be able to:

1. Describe how active ingredients and diluents are related if the amount of active ingredient remains constant yet the amount of diluent increases or decreases.
2. Define the term *stock solution*.
3. Explain the use of alligation methods in the pharmacy setting.
4. Determine the volume of a stock solution needed to prepare a given solution.
5. Understand how to use alligation for calculations and be able to proficiently perform calculations using this method.

GLOSSARY

alligation – A mathematical process that allows for calculation of amounts of substances based on their different percentage strengths.

diluents – Substances used to dilute another substance, solvents, used to prepare solutions; when added, they decrease concentrations.

dilutions – Parts of concentrate in total volume; they make a mixture weaker in concentration.

solvents – Materials (usually fluids) that can dissolve other substances; common solvents include water, alcohol, and acetone; often referred to as "diluents."

stock solutions – Concentrated solutions that are diluted to lower concentrations for actual use.

Test Your Knowledge

Answer the following questions.

1. A pharmacist weighed 0.075 g of a substance on a balance insensitive to quantities smaller than 0.005 g. What was the maximum potential error in terms of percentage?

_____

_____

2. A pharmacist weighed 500 mg of a substance on a balance of unknown accuracy. When checked on a more accurate balance, the weight was found to be 495 mg. Calculate the percentage of error in the first weighing.

_____

_____

3. A graduate weighs 42.85 g. When 10 mL of water is measured in it, the weight of the graduate and water is 45.95 g. Calculate the weight of the water and express any deviation from 10 g as the percentage of error.

_____

_____

4. A pharmacist prepared an ointment using 28.5 g of zinc oxide instead of the 30.5 grams required. Calculate the percentage of error on the basis of the desired quantity.

_____

_____

5. A pharmacist weighed 0.365 g of morphine sulfate on a balance of unknown accuracy. When checked on a better balance, the weight was found to be 0.385 g. Calculate the percentage of error in the first weighing.

_____

_____

6. A pharmacist measured 70 mL of a medication by difference, starting with 100 mL. He noted that the graduate used contained 35 mL of glycerin. Calculate the percentage of error incurred in the measurement.

_____

_____

7. A pharmacy technician did not calibrate a balance before weighing 225 mg of codeine sulfate. She later found that because of lack of calibration, a 10% error (over the desired amount) had occurred. If this error percentage is accurate, how much codeine sulfate was actually weighed?

_____

_____

8. A pharmacist measures 800 mL in a 1000-mL cylindrical graduate that is calibrated in 10 mL units. What is the percentage of error that might be incurred in the measurement?

_____

_____

9. How would you weigh .15 g of atropine sulfate and diluent of lactose with an error not greater than 5% if the prescription balance has a sensitivity requirement of 0.06 grams?

_____

_____

10. How would you weigh 0.006 g of a substance with an error not greater than 5% if the prescription balance has a sensitivity requirement of 0.004 grams?

_____

_____

Critical Thinking

A 4-year-old child has been on an oral antibiotic for 7 days. She still has all the same symptoms as when she started taking the antibiotic. Her mother called the pharmacy and spoke to a pharmacy technician. She tells him that though the antibiotic is supposed to continue for another 7 days, it is still almost $\frac{3}{4}$ full. The pharmacy technician asks the mother how she is administering the medication. She explains that she is administering one spoonful three times per day. The pharmacy technician asks what type of spoon she is using because the prescription was for "one teaspoonful three times per day". The mother says the child will only allow her to use a plastic spoon that was inside the packaging of her favorite doll.

1. What mistake has occurred in dosing?

_____

_____

2. Why is the child still exhibiting symptoms?

_____

_____

PART IV

LIQUID MEASURES, CONCENTRATIONS, AND DILUTIONS

OVERVIEW

Pharmacy technicians should be familiar with dilutions because many stock solutions must be diluted before they can be sold to patients. Diluted solutions have decreased concentrations and increased volumes. Pharmacy technicians often calculate mixtures of substances by using alligation. This is a mathematical process that allows for calculation of amounts of substances based on their different percentage strengths.

DILUTIONS

 Remember

The total volume = the parts of the concentrate + the parts of the diluent.

Solutions must often be diluted by adding water or a saline solution. Solvents are referred to as diluents. They decrease a solution's concentration and increase its volume. The formula $V_1 \times C_1 = V_2 \times C_2$ applies to dilutions with its V_2 and C_2 values, which usually represent the diluted solution. Often, powdered medications are diluted with normal saline or sterile water. Dilutions represent parts of concentrate in *total volume*.

STOCK SOLUTIONS FOR SOLIDS

Stock solutions are solutions of known concentration prepared by the pharmacist or pharmacy technician for convenience in dispensing. Weaker solutions are usually made from them. Stock solutions enable pharmacists to obtain the small quantities of medicinal substances that are to be dispensed in solution. They are usually prepared on a weight-in-volume basis. Their concentration is expressed as a ratio strength, or less frequently, as a percentage strength.

■ **EXAMPLE 1:**

How many milliliters of a 1:400 w/v stock solution are needed to make 4 L of a 1:2000 w/v solution? Remember that 4 L = 4000 mL. A 1:400 stock solution = 0.25%, while a 1:2000 solution = 0.05%. Using the standard formula to calculate this dilution,

$$X \text{ mL} \times 0.25\% = 4000 \text{ mL} \times 0.05\%$$

Therefore, by inverse proportion:

$$\frac{0.25\%}{0.05\%} = \frac{4000 \text{ mL}}{X \text{ mL}}$$

Or:

$$\frac{\frac{1}{400}}{\frac{1}{2000}} = \frac{4000 \text{ mL}}{X \text{ mL}}$$

The answer is 800 mL.

Stock Vials and Ampules

Vials and ampules commonly contain doses listed in milligrams per milliliter (mg/mL) or micrograms per milliliter (mcg/mL). Often, injectable products are mixed to concentrations for oral administration based on physician orders. The same method is usually used to calculate the amount of stock solution and diluent as is used to calculate the amount of active ingredient.

LIQUID DILUTIONS

A stock solution often contains a concentrate such as a medication and a diluent such as saline or sterile water. If 1 microliter of serum were mixed with 6 microliters of saline, the ratio would be 1:7. This means that there is 1 part concentrate out of a total of 7 parts (6 of which are the diluent). Remember that *dilution* is defined as parts concentrate in total volume.

■ **EXAMPLE 1:**

We need to make a 1 in 10 dilution of serum in saline. The total volume must be 150 microliters. What volume of serum and what volume of diluent are needed?

First, set up a proportion:

$$\frac{1 \text{ part serum}}{10 \text{ parts total volume}} = \frac{X \text{ parts serum}}{150 \text{ parts total volume}}$$

Cross-multiplying gives: $10X = 150$. Dividing both sides by 10 gives: $X = 15$.

Therefore, 15 parts serum are needed. Because the units are microliters, 15 microliters of serum are needed.

To determine how much diluent is needed, remember that parts concentrate plus parts diluent equal the total volume. Therefore,

$$15 \text{ (parts serum)} + X = 150$$

Solve by subtracting 15 from both sides, which gives: $X = 135$.

Therefore, we need 135 microliters of saline to make this solution. Notice that:

$$\frac{\text{Part serum}}{\text{Total volume}} = \frac{15 \text{ microliters}}{150 \text{ microliters}} = \frac{15}{150} = \frac{1}{10}$$

Therefore, a 1 in 10 dilution was achieved, which is what was required.

■ **EXAMPLE 2:**

Make a 1 in 8 dilution of insulin in water. The total volume must be 220 mL. What volume of insulin is needed?

Set up a proportion:

$$\frac{1 \text{ part insulin}}{8 \text{ parts total volume}} = \frac{X \text{ parts insulin}}{220 \text{ parts total volume}}$$

Cross-multiplying gives: 8X = 220. Dividing both sides by 8 gives: X = 27.5.

What volume of diluent is needed? We need 27.5 mL of insulin, and insulin plus diluent equals total volume, so 27.5 + X = 220. Subtracting 27.5 from both sides gives:

X = 192.5. Therefore, 192.5 mL of diluent is needed.

■ **EXAMPLE 3:**

Find the quantity of hydrogen peroxide in water in a 150-mL solution if the dilution is $\frac{1}{6}$.

$$\frac{1 \text{ hydrogen peroxide}}{6 \text{ total volume}} = \frac{X \text{ hydrogen peroxide}}{150 \text{ total volume}}$$

Cross-multiplying gives: 6X = 150. Dividing by 6 gives: X = 25. Therefore, for a 1:6 mixture, 25 mL of hydrogen peroxide are needed, mixed with 125 mL of water to reach the total volume of 150 mL.

■ **EXAMPLE 4:**

Find the quantity of liquid penicillin in a 50-mL solution if the dilution is $\frac{1}{5}$.

$$\frac{1 \text{ penicillin}}{5 \text{ total volume}} = \frac{X \text{ penicillin}}{50 \text{ total volume}}$$

Cross-multiplying gives: 5X = 50. Dividing by 5 results in X = 10. Therefore, for a 1:5 mixture, 10 mL penicillin are needed, mixed with 40 mL water to reach the total volume of 50 mL.

■ **EXAMPLE 5:**

For a 4 in 10 dilution, what is the ratio of serum to saline? Remember that serum plus diluent equals total volume. Therefore,

$$\frac{\text{Parts serum}}{\text{Total volume}} = \frac{4}{10}$$

So, 4 + X = 10, resulting in X = 6. This means that there are 6 parts of saline. The serum-to-saline ratio is $\frac{4}{6}$.

■ **EXAMPLE 6:**

For a 3 in 18 dilution, what is the ratio of ammonia to water? Remember that ammonia plus water equals total volume. Therefore,

$$\frac{\text{Parts ammonia}}{\text{Total volume}} = \frac{3}{18}$$

So, 3 + X = 18, resulting in X = 15. This means that there are 15 parts of water. The ammonia to water ratio is $\frac{3}{15}$.

Stop and Review

Fill in the blank and calculate the dilutions or stock solutions.

1. Solutions must often be diluted by adding _____ or a _____ solution.

2. Diluents are also known as _____.

3. Dilutions represent parts of concentrate in _____ volume.

4. Solutions of known concentration prepared for convenience in dispensing are known as _____ solutions.

5. If a microliter of serum were mixed with 6 microliters of saline, the ratio would be _____ : _____.

6. To make 4000 mL of a 1:2000 w/v solution using a 1:400 w/v stock solution, you need _____ mL of the stock solution.

7. To make 3000 mL of a 1:1000 w/v solution using a 1:500 w/v stock solution, you need _____ mL of the stock solution.

8. If a 1 in 5 dilution of insulin in water is required, and the total volume must be 200 mL, the volume of insulin needed is _____ mL.

9. For a 3 in 10 dilution, the ratio of serum to saline is _____ to _____.

10. 15 parts serum to 150 parts total volume signifies a dilution of _____ to _____.

ALLIGATION

Alligation is defined as a method of arithmetic that involves the mixing of solutions or mixtures of solids possessing different percentage strengths. Sometimes it is necessary to obtain the desired strength of a medication by compounding, mixing higher and lower concentrations of medications to be able to fill a specific prescription or medication order. This method is known as "alligation alternate" and offers a rapid method of calculation that is useful to pharmacists and pharmacy technicians.

All concentrations must be in a percentage form and the strength of the desired solution must lie between the stronger and weaker solutions available. In other words, the final mixture will be an average of the individual strengths. These will be calculated as proportional parts. If the concentration is not expressed in the percentage form, it must be converted to the percentage form. For example, a solution strength expressed as 1:200 must be converted to a percentage.

$$\frac{1}{200} \times 100 = 0.5\%$$

By using alligation, the number of parts of each component needed to prepare the final percentage concentration may be calculated. Lines are drawn during calculation to bind quantities together. The substance with a higher value than what is required is the one with the lower amount. The increase in the value or amount of one of the substances balances the decrease in value or amount of the other substances.

■ EXAMPLE 1:

The upper-right and lower-right corners of the X-shaped diagram are achieved by calculating the difference between the higher percentage (shown in the upper-left corner of the preceding example) and the desired percentage, as well as between the lower percentage (shown in the lower-left corner of the preceding example) and the desired percentage. The difference between these two figures is placed in the upper-right corner of the "X." Then, by adding the higher and lower parts, the total number of parts is calculated.

Alligation is useful in solving any type of dilution or concentration problem. Concentrations expressed in mg/mL, ratios, and even mixtures of liquids of known specific gravities, may be solved using alligation. The strengths of the preparations being mixed, as well as the final mixture, have to be expressed in a common denomination when the alligation formula is being set up. When diluting a preparation, the diluent's strength is considered as 0%. When the strength of a mixture is increased by adding more drug, the strength of this component is 100%. The final proportion allows a distinct correlation between the parts in the mixture and any specific denomination needed.

■ EXAMPLE 2:

The quantities of the higher and lower percentages of products may be achieved by using the following formula:

HIGHER quantity: $\dfrac{\text{Number of HIGHER Parts}}{\text{Total Number of Parts}} = \dfrac{X}{\text{Total Quantity for Compounding}}$

LOWER quantity: $\dfrac{\text{Number of LOWER Parts}}{\text{Total Number of Parts}} = \dfrac{X}{\text{Total Quantity for Compounding}}$

))) Remember

- Use alligation to determine the proper mixtures of solutions or solids with different percentage strengths.

- By using alligation, the final mixture will be an average of the individual strengths expressed as a percentage.

- The substance with a higher value (percentage) than what is required is the substance with the lower amount (strength).

- The increase in value of one of the substances balances the decrease in value of the other substances.

- Calculate the upper-right and lower-right corners by subtracting the desired amount from the higher concentration substance, and then subtracting the lower concentration substance from the desired amount.

- Add the higher and lower parts to determine the total number of parts.

■ **EXAMPLE 3:**

To find what proportion is required for a 1000 mL preparation containing 70% alcohol mixed with another that contains 20% alcohol, to produce a mixture of 35% strength, the following steps are taken:

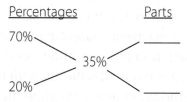

Percentages   Parts

70%

35%

20%

Remember:

Higher concentration parts $= 35 - 20 = 15$

Lower concentration parts $= 70 - 35 = 35$

Percentages   Parts

70%   15 parts HIGHER

35%

20%   35 parts LOWER

50 PARTS TOTAL

Therefore, the result will be as follows:

Amount of 70% solution:

$$\frac{15}{50} = \frac{X \text{ mL}}{1000 \text{ mL}} \quad X = 300 \text{ mL of 70% solution}$$

Amount of 20% solution:

$$\frac{35}{50} = \frac{X \text{ mL}}{1000 \text{ mL}} \quad X = 700 \text{ mL of 20% solution}$$

■ **EXAMPLE 4:**

To find what proportion is required for a preparation containing 10% of a drug mixed with another that contains 15% of a drug, to produce a mixture of 12% strength, the following steps are taken:

A. Understand that the 10% drug is 2% too weak. The 15% drug is 3% too strong. The excess strength of 3 parts of the stronger drug can be calculated to balance the deficient strength of 2 parts of the weaker drug, as follows:

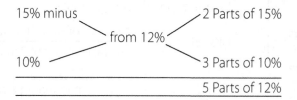

15% minus   2 Parts of 15%

from 12%

10%   3 Parts of 10%

5 Parts of 12%

The figure obtained from 12% − 10% is placed in the upper-right side of the equation. This is labeled as "2 parts of 15%."

The figure obtained from 15% − 12% is placed in the lower-right side of the equation. This is labeled as "3 parts of 10%."

This calculation produces a drug mixture of "5 parts of 12%," which is the desired strength.

Alligation calculations used to mix solutions may be checked by using the following formula:

$$\text{milliliters} \times \text{percent (as a decimal)} = \text{grams}$$

■ EXAMPLE 5:

Prepare 250 mL of dextrose 7.5%. To do this, you are required to use dextrose 5% (D_5W) and dextrose 50% ($D_{50}W$). Determine how many milliliters of each will be required.

As discussed previously, subtract the center number from the upper-left number and put it at the lower right. Then, subtract the lower-left number from the center number, and put it at the upper right.

The sum of the two numbers written at the right side of the equation, 2.5 + 42.5, equals 45, which is the total number of parts of the 7.5% final solution. Put in the terms of ratios, the ratio of the 5% solution to the 7.5% solution is 42.5: 45. The ratio of the 50% solution to the 7.5% solution is 2.5:45. Therefore, much less of the 50% solution is needed to make the 7.5% solution.

To calculate the volume needed of each dextrose solution, use the following equations:

50% Dextrose

$$\frac{x \text{ mL}}{2.5 \text{ parts}} = \frac{250 \text{ mL}}{45 \text{ parts}}$$

$$x \text{ mL} = \frac{(2.5 \text{ parts}) \times 250 \text{ mL}}{45 \text{ parts}}$$

$$x \text{ mL} = 13.89 \text{ mL } D_{50}W$$

5% Dextrose

$$\frac{x \text{ mL}}{42.5 \text{ parts}} = \frac{250 \text{ mL}}{45 \text{ parts}}$$

$$x \text{ mL} = \frac{(42.5) \times 250 \text{ mL}}{45 \text{ parts}}$$

$$x \text{ mL} = 236.11 \text{ mL } D_5W$$

Add the volumes of the two solutions; the sum should equal the required volume of 7.5% dextrose.

$$236.11 \text{ mL}$$
$$+ 13.89 \text{ mL}$$
$$\overline{250.00 \text{ mL}}$$

Check your answer using the following formula. The number of grams of solute should equal the sum of the grams of the solutes of the 50% solution and the 5% solution.

$$mL \times \% \; 5 \; g$$

$$250 \; mL \times 0.075 = 18.75 \; g \qquad 13.89 \; mL \times 0.5 = 6.945 \; g$$

$$236.11 \; mL \times 0.05 = 11.805 \; g$$

Now, add:

$$\begin{array}{r} 11.805 \; g \\ +6.945 \; g \\ \hline 18.75 \; g \end{array}$$

Stop and Review

Answer the following questions regarding alligation.

1. Ammoniated mercury ointment is available in 10% and 3%. A technician needs to prepare 450 g of a 5% ointment. How many grams of each of the 10% and 3% ointment will be needed?

   _____

2. How many mL of each of a 20% stock solution and a 30% stock solution will a technician need to make 500 mL of a 28% solution?

   _____

3. An order for 6 liters of 0.9% sodium chloride solution is to be prepared from 23.4% concentrated NaCl solution and sterile water for injection. How many milliliters of each will be used?

   _____

4. A technician is to prepare 250 mL of a 40% solution from a 60% stock solution and purified water. How many milliliters of each are needed?

   _____

5. A liter of $\dfrac{1}{3}$ NS is to be prepared from 0.9% concentrated sodium chloride solution and sterile water for injection. How many milliliters of each are to be used?

   _____

6. Stock solutions of 27% and 31% are available in the pharmacy. How many milliliters of each stock solution are needed to prepare 2 L of a 29% solution?

   _____

7. From two stock solutions, 18% and 42%, you are to prepare 1.5 L of a 34% solution. How many milliliters of each of the stock solutions do you need?

   _____

PART IV

LIQUID MEASURES, CONCENTRATIONS, AND DILUTIONS

CHAPTER 10
Dilutions and Solutions

OBJECTIVES

Upon completion of this chapter, you should be able to:

1. Describe how active ingredients and diluents are related if the amount of active ingredient remains constant yet the amount of diluent increases or decreases.

2. Define the term *stock solution*.

3. Explain the use of alligation methods in the pharmacy setting.

4. Determine the volume of a stock solution needed to prepare a given solution.

5. Understand how to use alligation for calculations and be able to proficiently perform calculations using this method.

GLOSSARY

alligation – A mathematical process that allows for calculation of amounts of substances based on their different percentage strengths.

diluents – Substances used to dilute another substance, solvents, used to prepare solutions; when added, they decrease concentrations.

dilutions – Parts of concentrate in total volume; they make a mixture weaker in concentration.

solvents – Materials (usually fluids) that can dissolve other substances; common solvents include water, alcohol, and acetone; often referred to as "diluents."

stock solutions – Concentrated solutions that are diluted to lower concentrations for actual use.

7. A pharmacy technician did not calibrate a balance before weighing 225 mg of codeine sulfate. She later found that because of lack of calibration, a 10% error (over the desired amount) had occurred. If this error percentage is accurate, how much codeine sulfate was actually weighed?

_____

_____

8. A pharmacist measures 800 mL in a 1000-mL cylindrical graduate that is calibrated in 10 mL units. What is the percentage of error that might be incurred in the measurement?

_____

_____

9. How would you weigh .15 g of atropine sulfate and diluent of lactose with an error not greater than 5% if the prescription balance has a sensitivity requirement of 0.06 grams?

_____

_____

10. How would you weigh 0.006 g of a substance with an error not greater than 5% if the prescription balance has a sensitivity requirement of 0.004 grams?

_____

_____

Critical Thinking

A 4-year-old child has been on an oral antibiotic for 7 days. She still has all the same symptoms as when she started taking the antibiotic. Her mother called the pharmacy and spoke to a pharmacy technician. She tells him that though the antibiotic is supposed to continue for another 7 days, it is still almost $\frac{3}{4}$ full. The pharmacy technician asks the mother how she is administering the medication. She explains that she is administering one spoonful three times per day. The pharmacy technician asks what type of spoon she is using because the prescription was for "one teaspoonful three times per day". The mother says the child will only allow her to use a plastic spoon that was inside the packaging of her favorite doll.

1. What mistake has occurred in dosing?

_____

_____

2. Why is the child still exhibiting symptoms?

_____

_____

Test Your Knowledge

Answer the following questions.

1. A pharmacist weighed 0.075 g of a substance on a balance insensitive to quantities smaller than 0.005 g. What was the maximum potential error in terms of percentage?

    _____

    _____

2. A pharmacist weighed 500 mg of a substance on a balance of unknown accuracy. When checked on a more accurate balance, the weight was found to be 495 mg. Calculate the percentage of error in the first weighing.

    _____

    _____

3. A graduate weighs 42.85 g. When 10 mL of water is measured in it, the weight of the graduate and water is 45.95 g. Calculate the weight of the water and express any deviation from 10 g as the percentage of error.

    _____

    _____

4. A pharmacist prepared an ointment using 28.5 g of zinc oxide instead of the 30.5 grams required. Calculate the percentage of error on the basis of the desired quantity.

    _____

    _____

5. A pharmacist weighed 0.365 g of morphine sulfate on a balance of unknown accuracy. When checked on a better balance, the weight was found to be 0.385 g. Calculate the percentage of error in the first weighing.

    _____

    _____

6. A pharmacist measured 70 mL of a medication by difference, starting with 100 mL. He noted that the graduate used contained 35 mL of glycerin. Calculate the percentage of error incurred in the measurement.

    _____

    _____

Test Your Knowledge

Answer the following questions.

1. To create a desired concentration, we must have a 2 mg substance for each 6-mL solution. How much substance is needed to make a 10-mL solution?

   _____

   _____

2. To create a desired concentration, we must have a 3 mg substance for each 10-mL solution. How much substance is needed to make a 50-mL solution?

   _____

   _____

3. To create a desired concentration, we must have 4 mg substance for every 60-mL solution. How much substance is needed to make a 100-mL solution?

   _____

   _____

4. To create a desired concentration, we must have 8 mg substance for every 20-mL solution. How much substance is needed to make 250-mL solution?

   _____

   _____

5. For a 2 in 7 dilution, what is the ratio of serum to saline? What is the ratio of serum to total volume?

   _____

   _____

6. For a 3 in 10 dilution, what is the ratio of urine to water? What is the ratio of water to total volume?

   _____

   _____

7. For a 4 in 15 dilution, what is the ratio of urine to water? What is the ratio of water to total volume?

   _____

   _____

8. For a 5 in 12 dilution, what is the ratio of serum to saline? What is the ratio of saline to total volume?

   _____

   _____

9. One microliter serum is added to 6 microliters diluent. Give the dilution of the solution. What is the serum-to-total volume ratio?

   _____

   _____

10. Three milliliters urine are added to 11-mL diluent. Give the dilution of the solution. What is the urine-to-total volume ratio?

    _____

    _____

11. Two milliliters urine are added to 15-mL diluent. Give the dilution of the solution. What is the urine-to-total volume ratio?

    _____

    _____

12. Five milliliters serum are added to 18-mL diluent. Give the dilution of the solution. What is the serum-to-total volume ratio?

    _____

    _____

13. The serum-to-water ratio is 2:3. Find the solution dilution.

    _____

    _____

14. The alcohol-to-water ratio is 5:8. Find the solution dilution.

    _____

    _____

15. The alcohol-to-water ratio is 1:10. Find the solution dilution.

    _____

    _____

16. The serum-to-water ratio is 3:10. Find the solution dilution.

    _____

    _____

17. Explain how a healthcare professional would make a 270-mL urine in water solution if the dilution is to be $\dfrac{9}{15}$.

    _____

    _____

18. Explain how a healthcare professional would make a 100-mL urine in water solution if the dilution is to be $\dfrac{2}{5}$.

    _____

    _____

19. Explain how a healthcare professional would make an 80-mL urine in water solution if the dilution is to be $\frac{5}{8}$.

    _____

    _____

20. Three parts serum are added to nine parts water. Find the solution dilution.

    _____

    _____

21. Two parts urine are added to 12 parts water. Find the solution dilution.

    _____

    _____

22. Two parts serum are added to 5 parts water. Find the solution dilution.

    _____

    _____

23. A technician needs to make a 1 in 8 dilution of serum. The total volume must be 120 microliters. What volume of serum is needed? What volume of diluent is needed?

    _____

    _____

24. Four milliliters urine are to be used to make a 2 in 9 dilution. What will be the total volume of the solution? What volume of diluent is needed?

    _____

    _____

25. A technician needs to make a 1 in 15 dilution of serum. The total volume is to be 150 microliters. What volume of serum is needed? What volume of diluent is needed?

    _____

    _____

26. Three milliliters urine are to be used to make a 2 in 8 dilution. What will be the total volume of the solution? What volume of diluent is needed?

    _____

    _____

27. How would a scientist make 500 mL of a $\frac{3}{5}$ dilution of concentrate?

    _____

    _____

28. How would a scientist make 400 microliters of a $\frac{2}{5}$ dilution of concentrate?

_____

_____

29. We have 50 microliters of a $\frac{1}{4}$ dilution of serum. How much serum would be present?

_____

_____

30. How would a scientist make 250 microliters of a $\frac{1}{2}$ dilution of concentrate?

_____

_____

31. We have 20 microliters of a $\frac{1}{10}$ dilution of serum. How much serum would be present?

_____

_____

32. Five milliliters concentrate will make how much of a $\frac{2}{5}$ dilution?

_____

_____

33. How many grams of 20% and 15% stock ichthammol ointments are needed to prepare 60 g of a 17.5% ichthammol ointment?

_____

_____

34. Rx: zinc oxide 10% ointment 60 g
How many grams of zinc oxide 20% ointment and zinc oxide 5% ointment should you mix to prepare the order?

_____

_____

35. Rx: coal tar 5% ointment 160 g
You have coal tar 10% ointment and coal tar 2% ointment. How many grams of each will you use to prepare the final product?

_____

_____

36. Rx: benzocaine 5% ointment 4 oz
How many grams of benzocaine 2% ointment should you mix with 25 g of benzocaine 10% ointment to prepare the order?

_____

_____

37. How much 10% hydrocortisone cream and 0.5% hydrocortisone cream will you need to prepare 90 g of 2.5% hydrocortisone cream?

_____

_____

38. Prepare 2 L of a 20% alcohol solution using a 90% alcohol and a 10% alcohol.

_____

_____

39. You are asked to prepare 4 L of a 30% strength solution. Your pharmacy stocks the active ingredient in 8 oz bottles of 60%. How many bottles of the active ingredient will you need to open to complete the order?

_____

_____

40. Prepare 1 L of a 7.5% dextrose solution using sterilized water or injection (SWFI) and dextrose 10% in water (D10W).

_____

_____

41. How many grams of petrolatum should you add to 60 g of hydrocortisone 2.5% ointment to reduce its strength to 2%? The percent strength of petrolatum is zero.

_____

_____

42. Prepare 480 mL of a 1:20 solution using a 1:10 solution and a 1:50 solution.

_____

_____

Critical Thinking

You must prepare 400 mL of a solution that requires a 1:8 dilution. The diluent to be used is sterile water.

1. How would you calculate this dilution?

_____

2. How many milliliters of water must be added to the solution to achieve the desired dilution?

_____

CHAPTER 11

Concentrations

OBJECTIVES

Upon completion of this chapter, you should be able to:

1. Determine final concentrations.
2. Determine what dilution was performed.
3. Use the formula $V_1 \times C_1 = V_2 \times C_2$ to solve dilution problems.
4. Determine the ratio strength of a given product when the active ingredient remains constant and the amount of diluent is increased or decreased.

GLOSSARY

concentrate – A highly condensed drug product that is diluted prior to administration.

concentration – The amount of a particular substance in a given volume.

normal saline – A general term referring to a sterile solution of sodium chloride in water.

ratio strength – A numerator expressing an active ingredient and a denominator expressing the number of parts of a whole preparation.

solute – The substance being dissolved in a solvent to form a solution.

OVERVIEW

When a solution is diluted, it will have a decreased concentration as well as an increased volume. Two volumes and two concentrations may be related by using the formula:

$$V_1 \times C_1 = V_2 \times C_2$$

In this formula, V_1 and C_1 represent the original volume and concentration. Likewise, V_2 and C_2 represent the volume and concentration of the diluted solution.

CONCENTRATION

The term **concentration** refers to the amount of a particular substance in a given volume. The greater the substance in a given volume, the more concentrated the solution becomes. Therefore, the less the amount of a substance in a given volume, the less concentrated the solution becomes. For example, in a 15% solution, the entire solution consists of 15% of a certain substance. To dilute this into a one-third solution, the dilution would be referred to as $\frac{"1"}{3}$. It is easy to see that $\frac{1}{3}$ of 15% is 5%. This can also be represented as the following formula:

$$15\% \times \frac{1}{3} =$$

$$\frac{15\%}{1} \times \frac{1}{3} = \frac{15\%}{3} = 5\%$$

Therefore, the original concentration × the dilution = the final concentration.

■ EXAMPLE 1:

Remember

Original concentration ×
dilution = final concentration

Find the final concentration if a solution consisting of 20% solution is diluted using a $\frac{1}{5}$ dilution.

$$20\% \text{ solution} \times \frac{1}{5} = \frac{20\%}{5} = 4\% \text{ solution}$$

■ EXAMPLE 2:

Find the final concentration if a solution consisting of 25% is diluted using a $\frac{1}{10}$ dilution.

$$25\% \text{ solution} \times \frac{1}{10} = \frac{25\%}{10} = 2.5\% \text{ solution}$$

■ EXAMPLE 3:

If a 15% solution is diluted $\frac{1}{30}$, what is the final concentration?

$$15\% \text{ solution} \times \frac{1}{30} = \frac{15\%}{30} = 0.5\% \text{ solution}$$

EXAMPLE 4:

If a solution has an original concentration of 40% and is diluted so that the final concentration is 10%, what amount of dilution was performed?

Original concentration		Dilution		Final concentration
(40%)	$\times$	(X)	$=$	(10%)

When this equation is rewritten, we have $40x = 10$. After dividing by 40, we find:

$$X = \frac{10}{40} = \frac{1}{4}$$

Therefore, a dilution of $\frac{1}{4}$ was performed.

Concentrations and Volumes of Solutions

The mathematical formula used to determine concentrations and volumes of two solutions is the following:

$$\frac{V_1}{V_2} = \frac{C_2}{C_1}$$

When this formula is cross-multiplied, it becomes

$$V_1 \times C_1 = V_2 \times C_2$$

This formula can be used to find the volumes and concentrations of original and resulting solutions when they change as a result of adding a diluent.

EXAMPLE 5:

If $V_1 = 10$ mL, $V_2 = 15$ mL, and $C_1 = 30\%$, find C_2 in the following equation:

$$V_1 \times C_1 = V_2 \times C_2$$

After substituting the given values, we have:

$$10 \text{ mL} \times 30\% = 15 \text{ mL} \times C_2$$

When the left side of the equation is simplified, we have:

$$3 = 15 \times C_2$$

Dividing both sides by 15 results in:

$$\frac{3}{15} = C_2$$

Simplifying, we find that:

$$C_2 = 0.20 \text{ or } 20\%$$

Therefore, the concentration of the diluted solution is 20%.

EXAMPLE 6:

There are 12 mL of a 3% solution. This solution is added to water, totaling 60 mL. What is the concentration of the 60-mL solution? Use the equation $V_1 \times C_1 = V_2 \times C_2$. $V_1 = 12$ mL, $C_1 = 3\%$, and $V_2 = 60$ mL.

Therefore, we begin with:

$$12 \times 0.03 = 60 \times C_2$$

Simplifying the left side results in:

$$0.36 = 60 \times C_2$$

Dividing both sides by 60 results in:

$$C_2 = 0.006$$

Therefore, the concentration of the diluted solution is 0.006

■ EXAMPLE 7:

There are 10 mL of a 5% solution. This solution is added to water to make a total of 50 mL. What is the concentration of the 50-mL solution? Use the same equation as in the preceding examples. $V_1 = 10$ mL, $C_1 = 5\%$, and $V_2 = 50$ mL.

Therefore, we begin with:

$$10 \times 0.05 = 50 \times C_2$$

Simplifying the left side results in:

$$0.5 = 50 \times C_2$$

Dividing both sides by 50 results in:

$$C_2 = 0.01 = 1\%$$

Therefore, the concentration of the diluted solution is 1%.

■ EXAMPLE 8:

The ordered solution is 200 mL of a 2% solution via dilution of an 8% solution. How many milliliters of the 8% solution are needed? $V_1 = 200$, $C_1 = 2\%$, and $C_2 = 8\%$. In this example, remember that we are solving for V_2.

Therefore, we begin with:

$$200 \times 0.02 = V_2 \times 0.08$$

Simplifying the left side results in:

$$4 = V_2 \times 0.08$$

Dividing both sides by 0.08 results in:

$$V_2 = 50 \text{ mL}$$

Therefore, take 50 mL of the 8% solution and dilute it to a total of 200 mL by adding 150 mL of the desired diluent.

■ EXAMPLE 9:

A pharmacy technician poured a 5% solution into a container that already held a solution of an unknown volume. If the total volume of the mixed solution in the container is 100 mL, and its concentration is 2%, how many milliliters of the 5% solution were poured into the container? In this example, $C_1 = 5\%$, $C_2 = 2\%$, and $V_2 = 100$ mL. We are trying to solve for V_1.

Therefore, we begin with:

$$V_1 \times 0.05 = 100 \times 0.02$$

Simplifying the right side results in:

$$V_1 \times 0.05 = 2$$

Dividing both sides by 0.05 results in:

$$V_1 = 40 \text{ mL.}$$

Therefore, 40 mL of the 5% solution were poured into the container.

 Stop and Review

Write your answers to each question on the line following the question.

1. A physician prescribed an antibiotic to be mixed in white petrolatum to produce a 25% antibiotic preparation. The physician later changed the protocol to be only 12.5%. How much white petrolatum must be mixed with each 6-oz ointment container of 25% preparation to make the new 12.5% preparation? Calculate your answer in grams

   _____

2. How much silver nitrate (in grams) must be used in preparing 600 mL of a solution such that 20 mL diluted to 1 L will yield a 1:5000 solution?

   _____

3. A pharmacy technician prepares 3 L of 15% neomycin solution. A 25% solution is available. How much stock solution and how much water does he need?

   _____

WEIGHT/WEIGHT

The term *percent* means "per 100". A *percent weight per unit weight* is abbreviated as *% w/w*. A percent weight per unit weight is defined as:

$$\frac{\text{Unit weights of solute}}{100 \text{ unit weights of solution}} = \frac{\text{Grams of solute}}{100 \text{ grams of solution}}$$

A **solute**, as described in the preceding equation, is the substance being dissolved in the solution. A solute is often a medication. Therefore, the phrase *5% w/w* means that 5% of the total mass of an entire solution is the mass of the solute or medication itself.

■ **EXAMPLE 1:**

150 grams of a medication in a 20% w/w solution are required. How would this be made?

Use the *% w/w* formula.

Therefore, we begin with:

$$0.20 = \frac{X \text{ g solute}}{100 \text{ g solution}}$$

If we multiply both sides by 100, we have:

$$X = 20 \text{ g}$$

To make a solution containing 100 g of medication, you need to have 20 g of solute. To find out how to make a solution containing 150 g of medication, use the following proportions:

$$\frac{20 \text{ g solute}}{100 \text{ g solution}} = \frac{X \text{ g solute}}{150 \text{ g solution}}$$

After cross-multiplying, we have:

$$100X = 3000$$

After dividing by 100, we have:

$$X = 30$$

Therefore, to make the solution containing 150 g of medication (such as an ointment or cream), you would mix 30 g of solute (active ingredient) with 120 g of diluent (base) to get a total of 150 g.

 ## Stop and Review

Find the missing value in the following question.

1. A pharmacist added 15 g of 20% w/w calamine cream to 300 g of Aquaphor®. What is the percent strength w/w of the final calamine product?

_____

VOLUME/VOLUME

A *percent volume per unit volume* is abbreviated % *v/v* and defined as:

$$\frac{\text{mL concentrate}}{100\text{-mL solution}} = \frac{\text{mL concentrate}}{100\text{-mL solution}}$$

The term concentrate refers to a concentrated solution. A 25% v/v solution means that 25% of the entire solution is the solute itself.

■ EXAMPLE 1:

If a solution of 50 mL of 60% v/v solution of hydrogen peroxide in water is required, how would it be made?

Use the % *v/v* formula.

Therefore, we begin with:

$$0.60 = \frac{X \text{ mL hydrogen peroxide}}{100\text{-mL solution}}$$

Multiplying both sides by 100 results in X = 60. Therefore, 60 mL of hydrogen peroxide should be added to 40 mL water to get a 100-mL solution that has a 60% v/v. If 50 mL were desired, use proportions to solve this:

$$\frac{60 \text{ mL}}{100 \text{ mL}} = \frac{X \text{ mL}}{50 \text{ mL}}$$

By cross-multiplying, we find that X = 30. Therefore, 30 mL of hydrogen peroxide should be added to 20 mL water to get a 50-mL solution with a 60% v/v.

Remember

The *amount* of solution is less important than the *percentage* strength of the solution.

■ EXAMPLE 2:

How many milliliters of alcohol are in 40 mL of a 60% v/v solution? The concentration remains the same, so you can solve this with proportions:

$$\frac{60 \text{ mL alcohol}}{100\text{-mL solution}} = \frac{X \text{ mL alcohol}}{40\text{-mL solution}}$$

Cross-multiplying results in 100X = 2400. Dividing by 100, we have X = 24.

Therefore, 24 mL alcohol are in 40 mL of a 60% v/v solution.

Stop and Review

Calculate the volume needed for each of the following % v/v questions.

1. 1000 mL of a 7% solution are needed, but only a 10% solution is in stock. How many mL of the 10% solution are required to make 1000 mL of the 7% solution?

_____

2. A 5% solution has been poured into a container already containing some solution. The total volume is now 300 mL and its concentration is 4.5%. How many mL of the 5% solution were poured in?

_____

3. A 10% solution has been poured into a container already containing some solution. The total volume is now 400 mL and its concentration is 6%. How many mL of the 10% solution were poured in?

_____

4. A 9% solution was poured into a test tube already containing some solution. The total volume is now 300 mL and its concentration is 5%. How many mL of the 9% solution were poured in?

_____

5. A 7% solution was poured into a flask already containing some solution. The total volume is now 200 mL and its concentration is 5.5%. How many mL of the 7% solution were poured in?

_____

WEIGHT/VOLUME

A *percent weight per unit volume* is abbreviated % *w/v* and defined as:

$$\frac{\text{Grams of solute}}{100\text{-mL solution}} = \frac{\text{Grams of solute}}{100\text{-mL solution}}$$

Therefore, 5% w/v means that a 100-mL solution would contain 5 g solute. This type of calculation is probably the most common type used in the

> **Remember**
>
> Weight/volume is also expressed as a function of grams per 100 mL.

pharmacy setting. Many medications are solutions prepared as a ratio of the amount of medicine (as weight) to the volume of solution

■ **EXAMPLE 1:**

If 350 mL of a 12% w/v Duramorph solution are required, how would it be made? Use the *% w/v* formula.

Therefore, we begin with:

$$0.12 = \frac{X \text{ grams}}{100 \text{ mL}}$$

Multiply by 100, which gives us: X = 12. Therefore, 12 g of Duramorph would be dissolved in 100 mL of diluent (usually water) to get 100 mL. However, 350 mL are desired. Use proportions to solve this:

$$\frac{12 \text{ g}}{100 \text{ mL}} = \frac{X \text{ g}}{350 \text{ mL}}$$

By cross-multiplying, we have: 100X = 4,200. Dividing by 100 results in X = 42. Therefore, for this example, dissolve 42 g of Duramorph in 350 mL diluent. This is a 12% solution.

■ **EXAMPLE 2:**

If 200 mL of a 70% w/v lidocaine solution are desired, how would it be made? Use the same formula as that used in Example 1.

Therefore, we begin with:

$$0.70 = \frac{X \text{ g}}{100 \text{ mL}}$$

We then have: X = 70. Therefore, 12 g lidocaine would be dissolved in 100 mL water to get 100 mL. However, 200 mL are needed. Use proportions to solve this:

$$\frac{70 \text{ g}}{100 \text{ mL}} = \frac{X \text{ g}}{200 \text{ mL}}$$

Cross-multiplying gives us: 100X = 14,000. Dividing by 100 gives us X = 140. Therefore, for this example, dissolve 140 g of lidocaine in 200 mL water. This is a 70% solution.

■ **EXAMPLE 3:**

If 1000 mL of a 5% dextrose w/v solution are desired, how would it be made? Use the same formula as that used in Example 1.

Therefore, we begin with:

$$0.05 = \frac{X \text{ g}}{100 \text{ mL}}$$

We then have: X = 5. Therefore, for this example, dissolve 5 g dextrose in 100 mL water to get 100 mL. However, 1000 mL are desired. Use proportions to solve this:

$$\frac{5 \text{ g}}{100 \text{ mL}} = \frac{X \text{ g}}{1000 \text{ mL}}$$

Cross-multiplying gives: 100X = 5000. Dividing by 100 gives: X = 50. Therefore, dissolve 50 g dextrose in 1000 mL water. This is a 5% solution.

■ EXAMPLE 4:

How many grams of sodium chloride (NaCl) are in 25 mL of a 0.9% w/v solution (known as a **normal saline** solution). This solution contains 0.9 grams of sodium chloride in every 100 mL. Use proportions to solve this:

$$\frac{0.9 \text{ g NaCl}}{100\text{-mL solution}} = \frac{X \text{ g NaCl}}{25\text{-ml solution}}$$

Cross-multiplying gives: 100X = 22.5 and dividing by 100 gives: X = 0.225.

Therefore, there is 0.225 g NaCl in 25 mL of a 0.9% w/v NaCl solution. Note that this is less than a 1% solution.

■ EXAMPLE 5:

A 500-mL solution contains 50 g ibuprofen. What is the percentage of ibuprofen in this solution?

$$\text{The radio is } \frac{50 \text{ g ibuprofen}}{500\text{-mL solution}}$$

Because the percent formula is % w/v =

$$\frac{\text{Grams of solute}}{100\text{-mL solution}}$$

Set up the following proportion:

$$\frac{X \text{ grams of ibuprofen}}{100\text{-mL solution}} = \frac{50 \text{ grams of ibuprofen}}{500\text{-mL solution}}$$

Cross-multiplying gives: 500X = 5000.

Dividing by 500 gives: x = 10 (the percentage of drug in the solution). Observe that $\frac{50}{500} = 0.1 = 10\%$.

■ EXAMPLE 6:

How many mL of a 5% dextrose w/v solution can be made by using 20 grams of dextrose? A 5% dextrose w/v solution is made up of:

$$\frac{5 \text{ g dextrose}}{100 \text{ mL}}$$

Use proportions to find the amount of mL that can be made by using 20 g dextrose:

$$\frac{5 \text{ g dextrose}}{100 \text{ mL}} = \frac{20 \text{ g dextrose}}{X \text{ mL}}$$

Cross-multiplying gives: 5X = 2000.

Dividing by 5 gives: x = 400. So, 400 mL of a 5% dextrose w/v solution can be made from 20 g dextrose. Observe that $\frac{20}{400} = 0.05 = 5\%$.

Stop and Review

Use % w/v to calculate the following.

1. Prepare one dose of 0.6 mg kanamycin in 2 mL diluted from a stock solution of 20 mg/mL. How much kanamycin and how much diluent are used?

   _____

2. Furosemide is packaged as 10 mg/mL. A pharmacy technician must make a preparation totaling 25 mL of 2 mg/mL concentration. How much drug and how much diluent are used?

   _____

3. Bactocill comes packaged as a powder for reconstitution at 250 mg/mL. You must prepare 20 mL of a 25 mg/mL dilution. How many milligrams of the drug are needed, and what volume of diluent is needed?

   _____

4. You are asked to prepare 20 mL of a 50 mg/mL drug dilution from a stock of 2 g/5 mL. How many milliliters of diluent will be needed?

   _____

5. You must prepare 10 mL of a 4 mcg/mL-solution of magnesium sulfate. You have 10 mcg/mL on hand. How much concentrate will you need?

   _____

6. You need 5 mL of heparin 100 units/mL. In stock are 10,000 units/mL in a 20 mL vial. How much concentrate will you need?

   _____

7. Tobramycin 2 mL of 80 mg/mL is ordered. The pharmacy has 160 mg/mL tobramycin in stock. How much concentrate will you need?

   _____

8. A patient needs 50 mL of 5% dextrose. You have 70% dextrose 1000 mL on hand. How much concentrate will you need?

   _____

RATIO STRENGTH

The term **ratio strength** is defined as the concentration of weak solutions. All percentages are a ratio of parts per hundred. In a ratio, the numerator expresses the strength of an active ingredient and the denominator expresses the strength of a whole preparation. A ratio strength is commonly used to express the concentration of weak solutions or liquid preparations.

It is another way of expressing the percentage strength of solutions or liquid preparations, and sometimes mixtures of solids. For example, 10% means that 10 parts per 100 can be expressed as 10:100, which can be reduced to 1:10.

To calculate ratio strength of a solution by diluting or concentrating it, the following steps may be followed:

■ EXAMPLE 1:

If 500 mL of a 15% v/v solution are diluted to 1500 mL, what is the percentage strength?

Begin with:

$$500 \text{ mL} \times 15\% = 1500 \text{ mL} \times X\%$$

Calculate the left side first:

$$75 = 1500 \times X\%$$

Divide both sides by 1500:

$$0.05 = X\%$$

Therefore, X = 5%. This can also be solved by *inverse proportion:*

$$\frac{1500 \text{ mL}}{500 \text{ mL}} = \frac{15\%}{X\%}$$

This can also be solved by *calculating the active ingredient:*

$$\frac{1500 \text{ mL}}{75 \text{ mL}} = \frac{100\%}{X\%}$$

By any method of calculation, the preceding answer is still 5%.

■ EXAMPLE 2:

A 50 mL of 1:20 w/v solution is diluted to 1000 mL. What is the ratio strength w/v?

Begin with:

$$1:20 = 5\%$$

Therefore,

$$50 \text{ (mL)} \times 5 \text{ (\%)} = 1000 \text{ (mL)} \times X \text{ (\%)}$$

This gives:

$$2.5 = 1000 \times X\%$$

Dividing by 1000 produces the following answer:

$$X = 0.25\% \text{ or } 1:400$$

Again, this example may also be solved by inverse proportion or by calculating the active ingredient.

Test Your Knowledge

Calculate the following concentrations.

1. What is the final concentration of a 15% solution diluted $\frac{1}{10}$?

   _____

2. What is the final concentration of an 8% solution diluted $\frac{1}{10}$?

   _____

3. What is the final concentration of a 25% solution diluted $\frac{1}{5}$?

   _____

4. What is the final concentration of a 50% solution diluted $\frac{1}{2}$?

   _____

5. What is the final concentration of a 12% solution diluted $\frac{1}{8}$?

   _____

6. A 10% solution was diluted to a 2% solution. Determine the dilution performed.

   _____

7. A 20% solution was diluted to a 10% solution. Determine the dilution performed.

   _____

8. An 8% solution was diluted to a 2% solution. Determine the dilution performed.

   _____

9. A 12% solution was diluted to a 4% solution. Determine the dilution performed.

   _____

10. A 20% solution is diluted by $\frac{1}{10}$. It is diluted again by $\frac{1}{10}$. What is the final concentration?

   _____

11. An 8% solution is diluted by $\frac{1}{2}$. It is diluted again by $\frac{1}{4}$. What is the final concentration?

_____

12. A 40% solution is diluted by $\frac{1}{2}$. It is diluted again by $\frac{1}{2}$. What is the final concentration?

_____

Calculate the following concentrations and volumes of solutions.

13. If $V_1 = 16$ mL, $V_2 = 20$ mL, and $C_1 = 6\%$, find C_2.

_____

14. If $V_1 = 10$ mL, $V_2 = 20$ mL, and $C_1 = 15\%$, find C_2.

_____

15. If $V_1 = 30$ mL, $C_1 = 60\%$, and $C_2 = 20\%$, find V_2.

_____

16. If $V_1 = 150$ mL, $C_1 = 7\%$, and $C_2 = 12\%$, find V_2.

_____

17. If $V_2 = 200$ mL, $C_1 = 80\%$, and $C_2 = 50\%$, find V_1.

_____

18. If $V_2 = 80$ mL, $C_1 = 25\%$, and $C_2 = 30\%$, find V_1.

_____

19. If 60 mL of a 2.5% solution are diluted to 120 mL, what is its concentration?

_____

20. If 50 mL of a 3% solution are diluted to 300 mL, what is its concentration?

_____

21. If 80 mL of a 3.5% solution has another 80 mL added to make a total of 160 mL, what is this concentration?

_____

22. A 40 mL medication has a 4.5% concentration. It is diluted to 240 mL. What is its concentration?

_____

23. On hand are 100 mL of a 2% solution. It is diluted to 500 mL. What is its concentration?

_____

24. You need 500 mL of a 4% solution, and a 5% solution must be added to do this. How many mL of the 5% solution are required?

_____

25. You need 200 mL of a 6% solution. Because only 7% solution is in stock, how many mL of the stock solution are needed to make 200 mL of the 6% solution?

_____

26. You need 300 mL of a 7% solution. A 9% solution must be used to dilute it. How many mL of the 9% solution are required?

_____

27. You need 1200 mL of a 7% solution. Only a 12% solution is in stock. How many mL of the 12% solution are needed to make 1200 mL of the 7% solution?

_____

Calculate the w/w, v/v, or w/v equations.

28. Calculate how to make 125 g of an 18% w/w NaOH solution.

_____

29. Calculate how to make 250 g of a 15% w/w NaOH solution.

_____

30. Calculate how to make 75 g of a 9% w/w NaCl solution.

_____

31. Calculate how to make 300 g of a 30% w/w NaCl solution.

_____

32. Calculate how to make 250 mL of an 18% v/v solution of isopropyl alcohol in water.

_____

33. Calculate how to make 200 mL of a 20% v/v solution of isopropyl alcohol in water.

_____

34. Calculate how to make 225 mL of a 10% v/v solution of isopropyl alcohol in water.

_____

35. Calculate how to make 70 mL of a 70% v/v solution of isopropyl alcohol in water.

_____

36. Calculate how to make 150 mL of a 25% w/v NaCl solution.

_____

37. Calculate how to make 200 mL of a 6% w/v ampicillin solution.

_____

38. Calculate how to make 50 mL of a 2% w/v NaCl solution.

_____

39. Calculate how to make 125 mL of a 12% w/v cephapirin solution.

_____

40. Calculate how to make 150 mL of a 14% w/v cephapirin solution.

_____

41. How many grams of dextrose are contained in 10 dL of a 15% w/v NaCl solution?

_____

42. How many grams of dextrose are contained in 45 dL of a 30% w/v NaCl solution?

_____

43. How many grams of NaCl are in 20 mL of a 10% w/v solution?

_____

44. How many grams of NaCl are in 250 mL of an 8% w/v solution?

_____

45. How many mL of a 5% dextrose w/v solution can be produced by using 30 g of dextrose?

_____

46. How many mL of a 5% dextrose w/v solution can be produced by using 50 g of dextrose?

_____

47. How many mL of a 6% dextrose w/v solution can be produced by using 35 g of dextrose?

_____

48. How many mL of a 6% dextrose w/v solution can be produced by using 15 g of dextrose?

_____

49. If a 1000-mL solution contains 30 g of a drug, what is the percentage of the drug in this solution?

_____

50. If a 1000-mL solution contains 80 g of kanamycin, what is the percentage of kanamycin in this solution?

_____

51. If a 200-mL solution contains 12 g of a drug, what is the percentage of the drug in this solution?

_____

52. If a 300-mL solution contains 25 g of a drug, what is the percentage of the drug in this solution?

_____

53. If a 500-mL solution contains 100 g of acetaminophen, what is the percentage of acetaminophen in this solution?

_____

54. If an 800-mL solution contains 150 g of ibuprofen, what is the percentage of ibuprofen in this solution?

_____

Oral Medication Labels and Dosage Calculation

OBJECTIVES

Upon completion of this chapter, you should be able to:

1. List the common information found on drug labels.
2. Explain the United States Pharmacopoeia and the National Formulary.
3. Demonstrate how to calculate dosages for tablets and capsules.
4. Explain the measurement of oral solutions.

GLOSSARY

capsules – Solid oral dosage forms in which a medication is enclosed in a hard or soft soluble container, usually made of gelatin.

National Formulary – A part of the United States Pharmacopeia that contains public pharmacopeia standards.

scored – Manufactured with a groove or indentation so that it may be easily broken; scored tablets are designed to be broken into one or more pieces so that lower dosages can be administered.

tablets – Solid oral dosage forms containing a medication with or without a diluent.

United States Pharmacopeia (USP) – An organization that sets official public standards for all prescription and OTC medications, dietary supplements, and other health care products.

OVERVIEW

It is vital to understand the information on drug labels. This information includes the drug's name, dosage strength, form, total amount contained, route of administration, storage requirements, warnings, manufacturing information, and references. The **United States Pharmacopeia (USP)** sets official public standards for all prescription and OTC medications, dietary supplements, and other health care products. The **National Formulary** is part of the USP. The *United States Pharmacopeia – National Formulary (USP-NF)* is a book containing public pharmacopeia standards.

Tablet and capsule labels contain information about the dosage contained. To calculate tablet and capsule dosages, you must know the desired dose, dose on hand, and dosage unit. Oral solutions are often ordered for children, the elderly, and for patients who have trouble swallowing. Pharmacy technicians must calculate the volume of these solutions so that the prescribed dosage of the drug is administered.

TABLET AND CAPSULE LABELS AND CALCULATIONS

When a prescriber orders medications in tablet or capsule form, the pharmacy technician must determine if the strength or dosage on hand is the same strength as the dosage ordered or in multiples of the dosage ordered. Sometimes patients should divide the tablet in half or, less commonly, into quarters. **Figure 12-1** shows Biaxin tablets in two different strengths (scored and non-scored).

(a)

(b)

Figure 12-1 (a) Biaxin 250 mg (b) Biaxin 500 mg.
(a) *Courtesy of Abbott Laboratories* (b) *Courtesy of Abbott Laboratories*

■ EXAMPLE 1:

The doctor's order reads: *Biaxin 500 mg p.o. q12h.*

Biaxin comes in tablet strengths of 250 milligrams per tablet (or filmtab), and 500 milligrams per tablet. When both strengths are available, the pharmacy technician should select the 500 milligram strength, and give one whole tablet for each dose.

■ EXAMPLE 2:

The order reads: *Clonazepam 1.5 mg p.o. t.i.d.*

Clonazepam comes in strengths of 0.5 mg, 1 mg, and 2 mg tablets (**Figure 12-2**). When the three strengths are available, the pharmacy technician should select one 1 mg tablet and one 0.5 mg tablet (1 mg + 0.5 mg = 1.5 mg). This provides the ordered dosage of 1.5 mg and is the least number of tablets (2 tablets total) for the patient to swallow. However, another option would be to give three 0.5 mg tablets, which also equal 1.5 mg.

(a)

(b)

(c)

Figure 12-2 (a) Clonazepam .5 mg (b) Clonazepam 1 mg (c) Clonazepam 2 mg.
(a) © *Cengage Learning 2013* (b) © *Cengage Learning 2013* (c) © *Cengage Learning 2013*

Another option for the pharmacy technician is to halve the 2 mg tablets to obtain two 1 mg parts, and pair one-half with a 0.5 mg tablet. This would also equal 1.5 mg, and would amount to $1\frac{1}{2}$ tablets. However, cutting any tablet in half may produce slightly unequal halves. It is preferable to give whole, undivided tablets when they are available. In practice, only scored tablets should be cut in half.

In some instances it may be necessary to convert between systems of measurement to accurately calculate the dosage. Previously, you learned a formula for dosage calculations, as follows:

$$\frac{D}{H} \times Q = X$$

$$\frac{D \text{ (desired)}}{H \text{ (have)}} \times Q \text{ (quantity)} = X \text{ (amount)}$$

To convert dosages, ensure that all measurements are in the same system of measurement and the same size unit of measurement. If not, convert before proceeding.

■ EXAMPLE 3:

The drug order reads: *Ampicillin 0.5 g p.o. q6h.*

Available on hand: *Ampicillin 500 mg per capsule*

This medication order is written and supplied in the same system (metric) but in different size units (g and mg). A drug order written in grams but supplied in milligrams will have to be converted to the same size unit. You must convert 0.5 gram to milligrams, as follows:

$$1 \text{ g} = 1000 \text{ mg}$$

Remember, you are converting from a larger to a smaller unit. Therefore, you will multiply by the conversion factor of 1000 or move the decimal point three places to the right.

$$0.5 \text{ g} = 0.5 \times 1000 = 500 \text{ mg, or } 0.5 \text{ g} =$$

$$0.500 = 500 \text{ mg}$$

Order: *Ampicillin 500 mg p.o. q6h*

On hand: *Ampicillin 500 mg per capsule*

You would give the patient one ampicillin 500 mg capsule by mouth every 6 hours.

■ EXAMPLE 4:

The drug order reads: *Lopressor 100 mg p.o. b.i.d.*

The medication container is labeled "Lopressor 50 mg per tablet."

Calculate one dose.

Lopressor 50 mg.
Courtesy of Norvatis

$$\frac{D}{H} \times Q = \frac{100 \text{ mg}}{50 \text{ mg}} \times 1 \text{ tablet}$$

$$\frac{100 \text{ mg}}{50 \text{ mg}} = \frac{2 \text{ mg}}{1 \text{ mg}} \times 1 \text{ tablet} = 2 \times 1 \text{ tablet}$$

$$= 2 \text{ tablets, given orally, twice daily}$$

■ EXAMPLE 5:

The drug order reads: *V-Cillin K 0.5 g p.o. q.i.d.*

Available on hand: *V-Cillin K 250 mg per tablet*

How many tablets should you give to the patient per dose?

V-Cillin K 250 mg.
© *Copyright Eli Lilly and Company. Used with permission.*

As you know, 1 g = 1000 mg

$$0.5 \text{ g} = 0.5 \times 1000 = 0.500 = 500 \text{ mg}$$

Now you have the ordered drug and the on-hand drug measured in the same size units.

Ordered: *V-Cillin K 0.5 g = 500 mg*

On hand: *V-Cillin K 250 mg tablets*

$$\frac{500 \text{ mg}}{250 \text{ mg}} \times 1 \text{ tablet} = 2 \times 1 \text{ tablet} = 2 \text{ tablets, given orally 4 times daily}$$

EXAMPLE 6:

The drug order reads: *Codeine sulfate gr $\frac{3}{4}$ p.o. q4h p.r.n., pain.*

The drug on hand is: *Codeine sulfate 30 mg per tablet*

Calculate one dose.

Codeine 30 mg.
Used with permission of Roxane Laboratories, Inc.

$$gr\ I\ =\ 60\ mg$$

$$gr = \frac{3}{4} = \frac{3}{4} \times 60 = \frac{3 \times 60}{4} = 45 \text{ mg}$$

Therefore, order: Codeine gr $\frac{3}{4}$ = 45 mg

Then calculate:

$$\frac{D}{H} \times Q = \frac{45}{30} \times 1 \text{ tablet} = \frac{3}{2} \text{ tablets}$$

$$= 1\frac{1}{2} \text{ tablets}$$

Therefore, $1\frac{1}{2}$ tablets are to be given every 4 hours as needed for pain.

EXAMPLE 7:

The order is: *Synthroid 0.05 mg p.o. q.d.*

The tablets available are 25 mcg. How many tablets will you give?

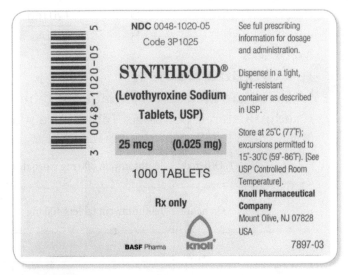

Synthroid 25 mcg.
Courtesy of Abbott Laboratories, 2002

1 mg = 1000 mcg. Conversion factor is 1000.

$$0.05 \text{ mg} = 0.05 \times 1000 = 0.050 = 50 \text{ mcg}$$

Order: *Synthroid 0.05 mg = 50 mcg*

On hand: *Synthroid 25 mcg tablets*

$$\frac{D}{H} \times Q = \frac{50 \text{ mcg}}{25 \text{ mcg}} \times 1 \text{ tablet} = 2 \text{ tablets, given orally once a day}$$

■ **EXAMPLE 8:**

A patient uses codeine gr ii orally. The label on the available codeine bottle tells you that each tablet provides 30 mg. How much will you give the patient?

Codeine 30 mg.
Used with permission of Roxane Laboratories, Inc.

Approximate equivalent gr 1 = 60 mg. The conversion factor is 60.

$$gr \frac{1}{60} \times 60 = \frac{60}{60} = 1 \text{ mg}$$

Ordered: Codeine gr ii orally p.r.n., pain

On hand: Codeine 30 mg tablet

Calculate how much you will give as needed for pain:

$$\frac{D}{H} \times Q = \frac{120 \text{ mg}}{30 \text{ mg}} = 4 \text{ tablets}$$

Stop and Review

Calculate the correct number of tablets or capsules to be administered per dose. Tablets are scored.

1. Ordered:	Telithromycin 800 mg p.o. q.d.
On hand:	Telithromycin tablets 400 mg
Give:	_____

2. Ordered:	Pravachol 20 mg p.o. q.h.s.
On hand:	Pravachol 10 mg tablets
Give:	_____
3. Ordered:	ferrous sulfate (FeS_{o4}) 300 mg p.o. q.d.
On hand:	ferrous sulfate tablets 5 gr (324 mg)
Give:	_____
4. Ordered:	Codeine 60 mg p.o.; q3h p.r.n.
On hand:	Codeine tablets 15 mg ($\frac{1}{4}$ gr)
Give:	_____
5. Ordered:	Nitroglycerin $\frac{1}{150}$ gr S.L. p.r.n.
On hand:	Nitrostat tablets 0.4 mg ($\frac{1}{150}$ gr)
Give:	_____
6. Ordered:	Quinidine 0.6 g p.o. q4h
On hand:	Quinidine 200 mg tablets
Give:	_____
7. Ordered:	Prednisone 7.5 mg p.o. q.d.
On hand:	Prednisone 5 mg scored tablets
Give:	_____

8. Ordered:	Aldomet 250 mg p.o. b.i.d.
On hand:	Aldomet 125 mg tablets
Give:	_____
9. Ordered:	Duricef 0.5 g p.o. b.i.d.
On hand:	Duricef 500 mg tablets
Give:	_____
10. Ordered:	Coumadin 5 mg p.o. q.d.
On hand:	Coumadin 2 mg scored tablets
Give:	_____

Calculate one dose for each of the medication orders in questions 11 through 19. The labels lettered A through I are the drugs you have available. Indicate the letter corresponding to the label you select.

11. Order:	*verapamil sustained release 240 mg p.o. q.d.*
Select:	_____
Give:	_____
12. Order:	*carbamazepine 0.2 g p.o. t.i.d.*
Select:	_____
Give:	_____
13. Order:	*Lopressor 50 mg p.o. b.i.d.*
Select:	_____
Give:	_____

14. Order:	potassium chloride 16 mEq p.o. q.d.
Select:	_____
Give:	_____
15. Order:	procainamide hydrochloride 1 g p.o. q6h
Select:	_____
Give:	_____
16. Order:	cephalexin 0.5 g p.o. q.i.d.
Select:	_____
Give:	_____
17. Order:	levothyroxine sodium 0.2 mg p.o. q.d.
Select:	_____
Give:	_____
18. Order:	digoxin 0.5 mg p.o. q.d.
Select:	_____
Give:	_____
19. Order:	allopurinol 0.1 g p.o. t.i.d.
Select:	_____
Give:	_____

Label A

Allopurinol 100 mg.
Courtesy of Mylan Pharmaceuticals Inc.

Label B

Calan SR 240 mg.
Courtesy of Pharmacia Corporation, Peapack, NJ

Label C

Procainamide hydrochloride 1000 mg.
© Cengage Learning 2013

Label D

Synthroid 100 mcg.
Courtesy of Abbott Laboratories

Label E

Keflex 250 mg.
Copyright Eli Lilly and Company. Used with permission.

Label F

Lopressor 50 mg.
Courtesy of Norvatis

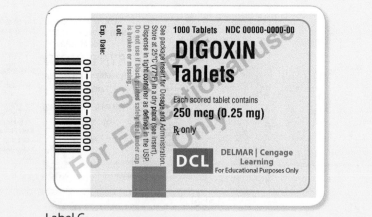

Label G

Digoxin 250 mcg.
© Cengage Learning 2013

Label H

Potassium Chloride extended release tablets
USP, 100 tablets.
© Cengage Learning 2013

Label I

Carbamazepine USP 100 mg, chewable tablets.
© Cengage Learning 2013

ORAL SOLUTION LABELS

Oral solutions are liquids usually ordered for children, elderly people, or patients who are not able to swallow tablets or capsules. Each oral solution contains a specific amount of medication in a given volume as written on the label (**Figures 12-3a** through **c**, listed next).

(a)

(b)

(c)

Figure 12-3 (a) Cefaclor 125 mg (b) Cefaclor 250 mg (c) Cefaclor 375 mg.
(a) © *Cengage Learning 2013* (b) © *Cengage Learning 2013* (c) © *Cengage Learning 2013*

MEASUREMENT OF ORAL SOLUTIONS

In solid form, the drugs can be calculated by the number of tablets or capsules that contain the prescribed dosage. In liquid form, pharmacy technicians must calculate the volume of the liquid that contains the prescribed dosage of the drug. The supply dosage is written on the label, indicating the amount of drug per 1 mL of solution; example amounts are as follows: 125 mg per 5 mL, 250 mg per 5 mL, or 375 mg per 5 mL.

■ **EXAMPLE 1:**

The prescriber orders *Cefaclor 100 mg p.o. q.i.d.*

To calculate this prescription, look at the label of Ceclor available in Figure 12–3a. See Figure 12–3a.

$$\frac{D}{H} \times Q = X$$

$$\frac{100 \text{ mg}}{125 \text{ mg}} \times 5 \text{ mL} = \frac{4}{5} \times 5 \text{ mL} = \frac{20}{5} = 4 \text{ mL}$$

given orally 4 times a day

■ **EXAMPLE 2:**

If you select the same drug order as in Example 1, Cefaclor 100 mg p.o. q.i.d., as a stronger solution (Cefaclor 250 mg per 5 mL), you must calculate as follows:

$$\frac{D}{H} \times Q = \frac{100 \text{ mg}}{250 \text{ mg}} \times 5 \text{ mL}$$

$$\frac{2}{5} \times 5 \text{ mL} = 2 \text{ mL}$$

given orally 4 times a day

You realize that in both Example 1 and Example 2, the supply quantity is the same (5 mL), but the dosage strength (weight) of the drug is different (125 mg per 5 mL vs. 250 mg per 5 mL) because of each liquid's concentration. The more concentrated solution must be given to the patient, offering less volume per dose for the same dosage.

Stop and Review

Calculate the following drugs ordered for one dose.

1. Ordered:	Zovirax susp 400 mg p.o. b.i.d.
On hand:	Zovirax 200 mg/5 mL suspension 10 mL
Give:	_____ mL

2. Ordered:	Artane 3 mg p.o. t.i.d. a.c.
On hand:	Artane Elixir 2 mg/5 mL
Give:	_____ mL
3. Ordered:	Depakene syrup 125 mg p.o. q12h
On hand:	Depakene syrup 250 mg/5 mL
Give:	_____ mL
4. Ordered:	Amoxil 100 mg p.o. q.i.d.
On hand:	80 mL bottle suspension (125 mg per 5 mL)
Give:	_____ mL
5. Ordered:	Zofran 8 mg p.o. b.i.d.
On hand:	Zofran liquid 4 mg/5 mL
Give:	_____ mL
6. Ordered:	Compazine syr 10 mg p.o. t.i.d.
On hand:	Compazine syrup 5 mg/5 mL
Give:	_____ mL
7. Ordered:	erythromycin suspension 600 mg p.o. q6h
On hand:	erythromycin 400 mg/5 mL
Give:	_____ mL

8. Ordered:	Ceclor suspension 225 mg p.o. b.i.d.	
On hand:	Ceclor suspension 375 mg per 5 mL	
Give:	_____ mL	
9. Ordered:	Dilantin-125 p.o. b.i.d.	
On hand:	Dilantin-125 suspension 125 mg/5 mL	
Give:	_____ mL	
10. Ordered:	digoxin elixir 0.25 mg p.o. q.d.	
On hand:	digoxin elixir 50 mcg/mL	
Give:	_____ mL	
11. Ordered:	Pepcid 20 mg p.o. q.i.d.	
On hand:	Pepcid 80 mg/10 mL	
Give:	_____ mL	
12. Ordered:	Grifulvin V 500 mg p.o. b.i.d.	
On hand:	Grifulvin V suspension 125 mg/5 mL	
Give:	_____ mL	
13. Ordered:	Mycostatin 250,000 units p.o. q.i.d.	
On hand:	Mycostatin 100,000 units per mL	
Give:	_____ mL	
14. Ordered:	Dicloxacillin: 100 mg q.i.d.	
On hand:	Dicloxacillin 62.5 mg per 5 mL	
Give:	_____ mL	

15. Ordered:	Augmentin 0.5 g, p.o. t.i.d.
On hand:	Augmentin 250 mg/5 mL
Give:	_____ mL
16. Ordered:	Vistaril 10 mg p.o. q.i.d.
Give:	_____ mL

Vistaril 25 mg/5mL.
Label reproduced with permission of Pfizer Inc.

17. Ordered:	Cephalexin 50 mg p.o. q.i.d.
Give:	_____ mL

Cephalexin 125 mg.
© Cengage Learning 2013

18. Ordered:	Digoxin elixir 0.25 mg p.o. q.d.
Give:	_____ mL

Digoxin 50 mcg.
© *Cengage Learning 2013*

19. Ordered:	OxyFast (oral solution concentrate) 15 mg p.o. q.i.d. p.r.n.
Give:	_____ mL

OxyFast 20 mg 1 mL.
Courtesy of Purdue Pharma L.P.

20. Ordered: Valproic acid 0.5 g p.o. t.i.d.

Give: _____ mL

Valproic acid syrup, USP 250 mg per 5 mL.
© *Cengage Learning 2013*

21. Ordered: Biaxin 75 mg p.o. b.i.d.

Give: _____

Biaxin granules 125 mg.
Courtesy of Abbott Laboratories

Test Your Knowledge

Calculate the oral medication dosages.

1.   Ordered: calcium carbonate 1.5 grams P.O. t.i.d.

On hand: calcium carbonate labeled "750 mg capsules"

Give: _____

2. Ordered: allopurinol 0.6 gram P.O. every day

   On hand: allopurinol 300 mg tablets

   Give: _____

3. Ordered: anastrozole 1000 mcg P.O. once daily

   On hand: anastrozole 1 mg tablets

   Give: _____

4. Ordered: levothyroxine sodium 0.15 mg by mouth each morning

   On hand: levothyroxine sodium 150 mcg tablets

   Give: _____

5. Ordered: acetaminophen 160 mg P.O. b.i.d.

   On hand: acetaminophen 325 mg tablets

   Give: _____

6. Ordered: cefaclor 0.5 gram P.O. t.i.d.

   On hand: cefaclor 250 mg capsules

   Give: _____

7. Ordered: oxcarbazepine 600 mg b.i.d.

   On hand: oxcarbazepine 150 mg tablets

   Give: _____

8. Ordered: busulfan 8000 mcg per day as a single oral dose

   On hand: busulfan 2 mg tablets

   Give: _____

9. Ordered: zidovudine 0.1 gram every 4 hours

   On hand: zidovudine 100 mg capsules

   Give: _____

10. Ordered: OxyContin $\frac{1}{3}$ grain P.O., b.i.d. for 7 days

    On hand: OxyContin 20 mg tablets

    Give: _____

11. Ordered: zafirlukast 0.020 gram P.O. b.i.d.

    On hand: zafirlukast 10 mg tablets

    Give: _____

12. Ordered: codeine sulfate 1 grain P.O. q.i.d., p.r.n.

    On hand: codeine sulfate 30 mg tablets

    Give: _____

13. Ordered: clonidine hydrochloride 200 mcg

    On hand: clonidine hydrochloride 0.2 mg extended release tablets

    Give: _____

14. Ordered: clonazepam 0.25 mg P.O. every morning

    On hand: clonazepam 125 mcg tablets

    Give: _____

15. Ordered: triamcinolone hexacetonide 0.004 gram P.O. t.i.d.

    On hand: triamcinolone hexacetonide 2 mg tablets

    Give: _____ per dose

16. Ordered: clorazepate dipotassium 7.5 mg P.O. b.i.d.

    On hand: clorazepate dipotassium 3.75 mg tablets

    Give: _____

17. Ordered: pyridoxine 0.2 gram P.O. every day

    On hand: pyridoxine 50 mg tablets

    Give: _____ per dose

18. Ordered: naproxen sodium 0.75 gram P.O. every day

    On hand: naproxen sodium 375 mg tablets

    Give: _____

19. Ordered: propylthiouracil 200 mg P.O. q.i.d.

    On hand: propylthiouracil 50 mg tablets

    Give: _____

20. Ordered: nitroglycerin sublingual 300 mcg at first sign of chest pain

    On hand: sublingual nitroglycerin 0.3 mg tablets

    Give: _____

21. Ordered: gatifloxacin 400 mg P.O. daily for 5 days

    On hand: gatifloxacin oral suspension with a concentration of
               200 mg/5 mL

    Give: _____

22. Ordered: haloperidol 3 mg P.O. at bedtime

    On hand: haloperidol oral concentrate 2 mg/mL

    Give: _____ at bedtime

23. Ordered: oxycodone elixir 5 mg every 4 hours for pain

    On hand: oxycodone elixir concentration of 5 mg/5 mL

    Give: _____

24. Ordered: furosemide 100 mg P.O.

    On hand: furosemide oral solution 40 mg/5 mL

    Give: _____

25. Ordered: guaifenesin oral liquid 300 mg every 4 hours

    On hand: guaifenesin oral liquid concentration 200 mg/5 mL

    Give: _____

26. Ordered: ibuprofen oral suspension 75 mg P.O., q.i.d. for fever

    On hand: ibuprofen oral suspension concentration 50 mg/1.25 mL

    Give: _____

27. Ordered: haloperidol 0.5 mg P.O. b.i.d.

    On hand: haloperidol oral solution 2 mg/2 mL

    Give: _____

28. Ordered: isoniazid 300 mg P.O. once daily

    On hand: isoniazid syrup 50 mg/5 mL

    Give: _____ per dose

29. Ordered: lansoprazole 15 mg P.O. solution daily

    On hand: lansoprazole 2.5 mg/mL oral solution

    Give: _____

30. Ordered: memantine 5 mg P.O. per day

    On hand: memantine 2 mg/2 mL oral solution

    Give: _____

31. Ordered: vancomycin 0.125 gram P.O. q.i.d.

    On hand: vancomycin 250 mg/5 mL of oral solution

    Give: _____

32. Ordered: methadone 2.5 mg P.O. every 3–4 hours p.r.n.

    On hand: methadone 5 mg/5 mL

    Give: _____

33. Ordered: mycophenolate mofetil 1 gram P.O., b.i.d.

    On hand: mycophenolate mofetil oral suspension concentration
              200 mg/mL

    Give: _____

34. Ordered: tetracycline 500 mg P.O., q.i.d.

    On hand: tetracycline syrup 125 mg/5 mL

    Give: _____

35. Ordered: amoxicillin 275 mg P.O.

    On hand: amoxicillin suspension 250 mg/5 mL

    Give: _____

36. Ordered: azithromycin 300 mg P.O. for 5 days

    On hand: azithromycin 450 mg in 5 mL

    Give: _____

37. Ordered: amprenavir 1350 mg P.O., b.i.d.

    On hand: amprenavir oral liquid 15 mg/mL

    Give: _____ per dose

38. Ordered: amoxicillin / clavulanate potassium 100 mg P.O. b.i.d.

    On hand: amoxicillin / clavulanate potassium 150 mg in a 5 mL
    suspension

    Give: _____

39. Ordered: cetirizine 2.5 mg daily

    On hand: cetirizine syrup containing 1 mg/mL

    Give: _____

40. Ordered: clindamycin 300 mg P.O., q.i.d.

    On hand: clindamycin 75 mg/5 mL oral solution

    Give: _____

Critical Thinking

The physician ordered Inderal 120 mg P.O. q.d. The pharmacy technician supplied 20 mg tablets. The nurse did not think about the reasonable amount that should be taken in a 1-day period and mistook "q.d." for "q.i.d.", and then calculated the dosage as follows:

$$\frac{\text{Desired}}{\text{Have}} \times \text{Quantity} = \text{Amount}$$

So,

$$\frac{120 \text{ mg}}{20 \text{ mg}} \times 4 = 24 \text{ tablets (incorrect)}$$

1. If the nurse gave the patient 24 tablets of 20 mg per tablet Inderal, how many milligrams will the patient receive over a 24-hour period? Is it the correct dosage?

_____

_____

Reconstitution of Powdered Drugs

OBJECTIVES

Upon completion of this chapter, you should be able to:

1. Calculate the volume of reconstituted medication that is required when the medication is supplied in powdered form.

2. Determine whether an in-stock vial contains enough medication to fill an order.

3. Demonstrate reconstitution of single- and multiple-strength solutions.

4. Calculate amounts of solutes and solvents needed to prepare various desired strengths and quantities.

5. Demonstrate reconstitution from package insert directions.

6. Define the terms *diluent, solute,* and *solution.*

7. Reconstitute and label medications supplied in powdered or dry form.

GLOSSARY

reconstitution – The return of a substance to its original liquid state.

solution – A liquid preparation of several soluble chemical substances, often dissolved in water.

OVERVIEW

Many medications come in powdered form, including parenteral medications. Normal saline, sterile water, or some other diluent is mixed with the powder to convert these medications into liquid form. Powdered drugs that must be reconstituted are used because, in this form, they retain their potency longer than after they have been reconstituted.

Usually, the **reconstitution** of powdered drugs is done by clinical pharmacies, but it is important to understand procedures for reconstitution and how to correctly label drugs with a correct expiration date and time. Drug labels and instructional package inserts provide this specific information. You must understand the properties of various types of solutions.

RECONSTITUTION OF A SINGLE-STRENGTH SOLUTION

Using the label shown in **Figure 13-1**, notice that the directions for reconstitution of this single-strength solution are on the left side of the label. A solute is the substance dissolved in a solvent to form a solution.

Figure 13-1 Solu-Medrol 500 mg.
Used with permission from Pharmacia Corporation, Peapack, NJ.

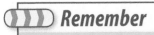

Remember

After *reconstitution*, it is important to understand how long the reconstituted solution may be stored and the correct storage methods.

An order is given to "Reconstitute with 8 mL Bacteriostatic Water for injection with Benzyl Alcohol." In this example, the *diluent* is the bacteriostatic water. In **Figure 13-1**, notice that the reconstituted medication can be stored at room temperature, but it must be used within 48 hours after reconstitution.

Once you have reconstituted a medication, print your initials on the label to identify yourself as the person who reconstituted the drug. Add the expiration date and time to the label.

The total dosage strength is 500 mg. The individual dosage strength is four 125 mg doses. Because 8 mL of diluent has been injected, this is

> **)))) Remember**
>
> Most reconstituted volumes are not exactly equal to the amount of diluent added. The medication itself has a certain volume, so, combined, the total volume is larger than the amount of diluent injected.

approximately 2 mL for each 125 mg dose. However, as you should in every instance, check the small print on the label. It says that the individual dosage is 62.5 mg per mL. Therefore, if 62.5 mg is ordered, you need 1 mL. If 125 mg is ordered, you must have 2 mL. If 250 mg is ordered, you must have 4 mL. If 500 mg is ordered, you must have 8 mL.

■ EXAMPLE 1:

A physician orders 400 mg of Zithromax IV. The vial that is in stock lists the following instructions: "Constitute to 100 mg/mL with 4.8 mL of Sterile Water for Injection." The single-dose vial contains 500 mg. What volume must be given?

Apply the dosage formula, based on the following:

Desired dose (D) is 400 mg.

On-hand amount (H) is 100 mg.

Vehicle (V) is 1 mL.

Therefore,

$$\frac{D}{H} \times V = A$$

So

$$\frac{400 \text{ mg}}{100 \text{ mg}} \times 1 \text{ mL} = 4 \times 1 \text{ mL} = 4 \text{ mL}$$

Apply proportions by substituting given values into the formula D/A = H/V:

$$\frac{400 \text{ mg}}{A} = \frac{100 \text{ mg}}{1 \text{ mL}}$$

Cross-multiply, which gives:

$$A \times 100 \text{ mg} = (400 \text{ mg})(1 \text{ mL})$$

Divide by 100, which gives:

$$A = \frac{(400)(1 \text{ mL})}{100} = \frac{400 \text{ mL}}{100} = 4 \text{ mL}$$

Apply dimensional analysis to determine the quantity in milliliters:

$$\frac{100 \text{ mg}}{\text{mL}} \text{ as } \frac{1 \text{ mL}}{100 \text{ mg}}$$

Therefore,

$$400 \,(1 \text{ mL}/100) = \frac{400 \text{ mL}}{100} = 4 \text{ mL}$$

Therefore, add 4.8 mL sterile water to the vial contents and mix. Draw 4 mL of the reconstituted solution into a syringe for IV administration. The vial contains 500 mg and the order is for 400 mg, so there is enough for a full dose. Notice, however, that there is not enough for a second dose.

■ EXAMPLE 2:

An order is placed for 125,000 units penicillin for IM injection. If a vial on hand contains 50,000 units/mL penicillin, how many mL should be administered? Again, you can apply the dosage formula, apply proportions, or apply dimensional analysis to solve this example. Regardless of the method used, we find that:

$$\frac{125,000 \text{ units} \times 1 \text{ mL}}{50,000 \text{ units}} = \frac{125,000 \text{ mL}}{50,000} = 2.5 \text{ mL}$$

Therefore, from 3 single vials, you must draw 2.5 mL into a syringe for IM administration. Because one vial contains 50,000 units and the order is for 125,000 units, a total of 3 vials are needed. Notice that only ½ of the third vial will be used.

■ EXAMPLE 3:

An order is placed for 250 mg of a medication for IM injection. On hand is a vial that contains 1 g of the powdered medication. The directions on the vial note that 2.5 mL diluent should be added, resulting in a concentration of 300 mg/mL. What volume should be administered? (Because the order is in mg, you must first convert 1 g to milligrams.) Regardless of the method of calculation, we find that:

$$\frac{250 \text{ mg}}{300 \text{ mg}} \times 1 \text{ mL} = 0.83 \times 1 \text{ mL} = 0.8 \text{ mL}$$

Therefore, you must add 2.5 mL diluent to the vial contents and mix. Draw 0.8 mL of the reconstituted solution into a 1 mL syringe for IM administration.

■ EXAMPLE 4:

An order is placed for 2,000,000 units penicillin for IM injection. On hand is a vial containing 5,000,000 units penicillin. The vial instructions list the following:

- The concentration will be 250,000 units/mL if 18.2 mL diluent is added.

- The concentration will be 500,000 units/mL if 8.2 mL diluent is added.

- The concentration will be 1,000,000 units/mL if 3.2 mL diluent is added.

Because 3 mL is the maximum volume an adult should receive as an IM injection in a large muscle, which of the three sets of directions should be used for this order? Use the D/H x V formula.

- We will need 8 mL if 18.2 mL is added.

- We will need 4 mL if 8.2 mL is added.

- We will need 2 mL if 3.2 mL is added.

Because a 2 mL syringe is less than a 3 mL syringe, 2 mL is the syringe size that should be chosen. Measure 2 mL of penicillin reconstituted to 1,000,000 units per milliliter for IM administration.

Stop and Review

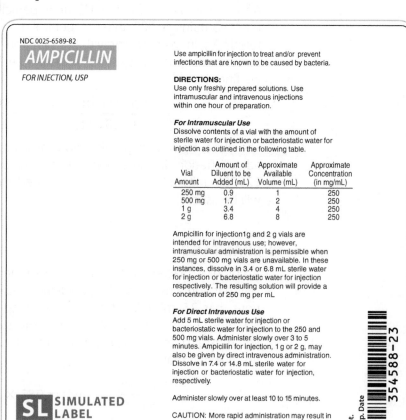

Ampicillin.
© Cengage Learning 2013

Using the Ampicillin label, answer the following questions:

1. What types of diluent may be used for reconstitution? _____

2. What volume of diluent is specified for a 250 mg vial? _____

3. How much diluent is needed for a 500 mg vial? _____

4. How much diluent is needed for a 1 g vial? _____

5. How much diluent is needed for a 2 g vial? _____

6. What is the mL dosage strength of all four reconstituted solutions?
   _____

7. How much diluent must be added to the 250 mg vial and to the 500 mg vial? _____

8. List the stipulation for direct IV administration of the 250 and 500 mg reconstituted solution. _____

9. Locate the caution pertaining to rapid IV administration. _____

SEE ACCOMPANYING PRESCRIBING INFORMATION.	NDC 0049-0530-28	USUAL DOSAGE 6 to 40 million units daily by intravenous infusion only.

RECOMMENDED STORAGE IN DRY FORM.

Store below 86°F (30°C).

Buffered with sodium citrate and citric acid to optimum pH.

AFTER RECONSTITUTION, SOLUTION SHOULD BE REFRIGERATED. DISCARD UNUSED SOLUTION AFTER 7 DAYS.

Rx only

MADE IN USA
7488

Buffered

Pfizerpen®
(penicillin G potassium)

For Injection

TWENTY MILLION UNITS **20**

FOR INTRAVENOUS INFUSION ONLY

Pfizer **Roerig**
Division of Pfizer Inc, NY, NY 10017

mL diluent added	Approx. units per mL of solution
75 mL	250,000 u/mL
33 mL	500,000 u/mL
11.5 mL	1,000,000 u/mL

PATIENT_____

ROOM_____

DATE/_____
TIME
BY_____

05-4211-00-8

Pfizerpen 20 mil units.
Used with permission from Pfizer, Inc.

Using the Pfizerpen label, answer the following questions:

10. If 75 mL of diluent is added, what dosage strength should be printed on the label? _____

11. Does this prepared solution need to be refrigerated? _____

12. If reconstituted at 2 p.m. on June 1, what expiration date and time must be printed on the label? _____

13. What is the vial's total dosage strength? _____

14. Besides the dosage strength, what else must be printed on the label? _____

15. Where can you find information on the diluent that should be used? _____

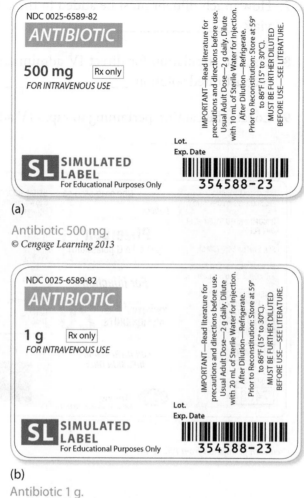

(a)

Antibiotic 500 mg.
© *Cengage Learning 2013*

(b)

Antibiotic 1 g.
© *Cengage Learning 2013*

PREPARATION AND STABILITY
At the time of use, reconstitute by adding either 10 mL of Sterile Water for Injection to the 500-mg vial or 20 mL of Sterile Water for Injection to the 1-g vial of dry, sterile powder. Vials reconstituted in this manner will give a solution of 50 mg/mL. FURTHER DILUTION IS REQUIRED.
After reconsition, the vials may be stored in a refrigerator for 14 days without significant loss of potency. Reconstituted solutions containing 500 mg must be diluted with at least 100 mL of diluent. Reconstituted solutions containing 1g must be diluted with at least 200 mL of diluent, The desired dose, diluted in this manner, should be administered by intermittent intravenous infusion over a period of at least 60 minutes.

(c)

Preparation and Stability.
© *Cengage Learning 2013*

Using the three antibiotic labels, answer the following questions:

16. To reconstitute a 500 mg vial, how much diluent is needed?

_____

17. For a 1 g vial, how much diluent is needed? _____

18. What kind of diluent is specified? _____

19. For both solutions, what is the reconstituted dosage per mL?
    _____

20. If refrigerated, how long can the solution be used? _____

21. If reconstituted at 1350 hours on May 4, what expiration date and time should be printed on the label? _____

22. What else must be printed on the label? _____

Ceftriaxone sodium 1 g.
© *Cengage Learning 2013*

Using the Ceftriaxone sodium label, answer the following questions:

23. What is the vial's total dosage? _____

24. For reconstitution, what volume of diluent is needed? _____

25. What is the dosage strength of 1 mL of reconstituted solution?
    _____

Levothyroxine 200 mcg.
Used with permission from Bedford Laboratories, A Division of Ben Venue Laboratories. A Boehringer-Ingelheim Company.

Using the Levothyroxine label, answer the following questions:

26. What is this vial's total strength in mcg and mg? _____

27. To prepare the solution for use, what volume of diluent must be added? _____

28. What kind of diluent is required? _____

29. How long will this reconstituted solution be potent? _____

30. What is this reconstituted solution's per mL strength? _____

31. Where can you find average dosage instructions? _____

CYTARABINE FOR INJECTION USP

FOR INTRAVENOUS, SUBCUTANEOUS, OR INTRATHECAL USE

1 gram

Rx ONLY

NDC 55390-133-01   LYOPHILIZED

See package insert for complete prescribing information.

Each vial contains cytarabine 1 g and, if necessary, hydrochloric acid and/or sodium hydroxide for pH adjustment.

When reconstituted with 10 mL Bacteriostatic Water for Injection USP with benzyl alcohol, each mL contains 100 mg cytarabine. **Do not use a diluent containing benzyl alcohol for intrathecal and high dose investigational use.**

Store both powder and reconstituted solution at 25°C (77°F); excursions permitted to 15° to 30°C (59° to 86°F) [see USP Controlled Room Temperature].

Use reconstituted solution within 48 hours. Discard solution if a slight haze develops.

Manufactured for:
Bedford Laboratories™
Bedford, OH 44146

Manufactured by:
Ben Venue Laboratories, Inc.
Bedford, OH 44146   CYB-VC05

Cytarabine 1 g.

Used with permission from Bedford Laboratories, A Division of Ben Venue Laboratories. A Boehringer-Ingelheim Company.

Using the Cytarabine label, answer the following questions:

32. How much diluent is needed for reconstitution? _____

33. What type of diluent should be used? _____

34. What is the total dosage of this vial? _____

35. What temperature should be used to store this medication? _____

36. What dosage will be contained in each mL? _____

37. What is this reconstituted solution's expiration time? _____

38. If reconstituted at 0840 hours on Feb. 14, what is the expiration date to be printed on the label? _____

Vfend® I.V. 200 mg.
Used with permission from Pfizer, Inc.

Using the Vfend IV label, answer the following questions:

39. How much diluent is required for reconstitution? _____

40. What diluent must be used? _____

41. What is the strength of each mL of the reconstituted solution?

_____

42. What is this vial's total dosage? _____

Vantin 100 mg.
Used with permission from Pharmacia Corporation, Peapack, NJ.

Using the Vantin label, answer the following questions:

43. To reconstitute this medication, how much diluent is required?

_____

44. What type of diluent must be used? _____

45. How must the diluent be added? _____

46. What is the reconstituted dosage strength? _____

47. How long will the reconstituted medication be potent? _____

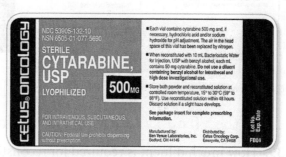

Cytarabine 500 mg.
Used with permission from Bedford Laboratories, A Division of Ben Venue Laboratories. A Boehringer-Ingelheim Company.

Using the Cytarabine label, answer the following questions:

48. What is this medication's total strength? _____

49. What diluent is needed for reconstitution? _____

50. How much diluent is needed? _____

51. What is the dosage per mL after reconstitution? _____

52. How long does this reconstituted medication remain potent at room temperature? _____

Drug package inserts contain much more information than do labels, including specific uses for diagnosed conditions, dosage recommendations if the vial label does not contain them, and information about untoward or adverse reactions. While no standard way is used to feature all of this information, it is included somewhere in the package insert and must be located and studied carefully.

RECONSTITUTION OF MULTIPLE-STRENGTH SOLUTIONS

Because some powdered drugs offer different dosage strengths, you must understand how to choose the most appropriate strength for the dosage ordered. In **Figure 13-2**, the penicillin label shows dosage strengths on the right side. Three different dosage strengths are listed: 250,000 units, 500,000 units, and 1,000,000 units per mL.

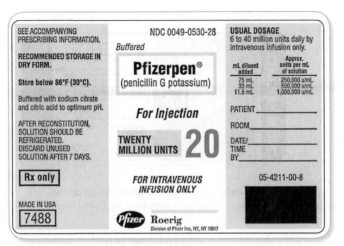

Figure 13-2 Pfizerpen 20 mil units.
Used with permission from Pfizer, Inc.

Remember

After reconstituting a multiple-strength solution, you must add the dosage strength you have just mixed to the label.

If 500,000 units were ordered, it would be most appropriate to mix 500,000 units per mL. The information on the label indicates that to achieve this, you should add 33 mL of diluent.

Test Your Knowledge

Acyclovir 500 mg.
Used with permission from Bedford Laboratories, A Division of Ben Venue Laboratories. A Boehringer-Ingelheim Company.

Using the Acyclovir label, answer the following questions:

1. For reconstitution, what type of diluent is needed? _____

2. How much diluent is needed? _____

3. What is this vial's total dosage strength? _____

4. How soon must this medication be used? _____

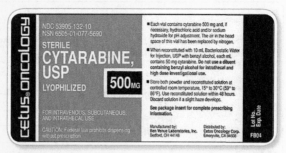

Cytarabine 500 mg.

Used with permission from Bedford Laboratories, A Division of Ben Venue Laboratories. A Boehringer-Ingelheim Company.

Using the Cytarabine label, answer the following questions:

5. What is this vial's total dosage strength? _____

6. What volume of diluent is needed? _____

7. What kind of diluent is needed? _____

8. What is the reconstituted dosage strength per mL?

   _____

9. How long will this medication be potent? _____

Pfizerpen 1 mill units.

Used with permission from Pfizer, Inc.

Using the Pfizerpen label, answer the following questions:

10. What is this vial's total dosage strength? _____

11. To prepare a 100,000 units/mL strength, how much diluent is needed?

    _____

12. To prepare a 500,000 units/mL strength, how much diluent is needed?

    _____

13. To prepare a 50,000 units/mL strength, how much diluent is needed? _____

14. Where can the information on the type of diluent for this medication be found? _____

15. How must this medication be stored? _____

16. If this medication is reconstituted at 1:10 a.m. on Dec. 18, what must be printed on the label? _____

17. What else must be printed on the label? _____

18. Why should the label be printed and not handwritten? _____

Store at or below 86°F (30°C).

DOSAGE AND USE
See accompanying prescribing information.
Constitute to 100 mg/mL* with
4.8 mL of Sterile Water For Injection.

Must be further diluted before use.
For appropriate diluents and storage
recommendations, refer to prescribing information.

*Each mL contains azithromycin dihydrate
equivalent to 100 mg of azithromycin,
76.9 mg of citric acid, and sodium hydroxide
for pH adjustment.   05-5191-32-0

CAUTION: Federal law prohibits
dispensing without prescription.

NDC 0069-3150-83

Zithromax®
(azithromycin for injection)

For IV infusion only
STERILE
equivalent to
500 mg
of azithromycin
Distributed by

Pfizer **Pfizer Labs**
Division of Pfizer Inc., NY, NY 10917

Zithromax 500 mg.
Used with permission from Pfizer, Inc.

Using the Zithromax label, answer the following questions:

19. What is the generic name for Zithromax? _____

20. What is this vial's dosage strength? _____

21. For reconstitution, what diluent is specified? _____

22. How much diluent is needed? _____

23. After reconstitution, what is the dosage strength? _____

Parenteral Medication Labels and Dosage Calculation

OBJECTIVES

Upon completion of this chapter, you should be able to:

1. Read and understand metric solution labels.
2. Read and understand percent and ratio solution labels.
3. Calculate solutions in international units and milliequivalents.
4. Calculate parenteral drug dosages.
5. Perform accurate insulin injection dosage calculations.

GLOSSARY

parenteral – Injectable; this term indicates medications that are administered other than by the oral (enteral) route.

percentage solutions – Liquid mixtures that may be calculated with percentages pertaining to mass/mass, mass/volume, or volume/volume.

OVERVIEW

Parenteral forms of medication are selected when a rapid response time to medication is desired or if the patient is not able to take the medication orally. Injectable drug forms may be available as a solution or a powder. Some vitamins, a few antibiotics, and biologics such as vaccines are expressed in terms of units. The U.S. Food & Drug Administration (FDA) approved the measures of potency for these substances, as set forth in the *United States Pharmacopeia (USP)*. They also conform to international standards (*international units*).

READING METRIC SOLUTION LABELS

It is important for the pharmacy technician to be able to read and interpret metric solution labels. The most common units of measurement seen on medication labels are metric units, including milligrams, grams, milliliters, and so forth.

■ EXAMPLE 1:

See the label for Vistaril in **Figure 14-1**. Note that the generic name of the drug is hydroxyzine hydrochloride and its trade name is Vistaril. Its dosage strength is 50 mg per mL and the total contents of the vial are 10 mL. Most intramuscular and subcutaneous dosages consist of one-half to double the average dosage strength. For this IM Vistaril, this is 50 mg per mL. Therefore, the following applies:

• For 25 mg, 0.5 mL would be administered.

• For 50 mg, 1 mL would be administered.

• For 75 mg, 1.5 mL would be administered.

• For 100 mg, 2 mL would be administered.

These dosages are within the common 0.5 to 3 mL IM volume.

Figure 14-1 Vistaril 50 mg/mL.
Labels reproduced with permission of Pfizer, Inc.

■ EXAMPLE 2:

Figure 14-2 shows a Robinul (glycopyrrolate) label, with a dosage strength of 0.2 mg/mL. Therefore, the following applies:

• If the dosage was 0.1 mg, 0.5 mL would be administered.

• If the dosage was 100 mcg, 0.5 mL would be administered.

- If the dosage was 0.2 mg, 1 mL would be administered.
- If the dosage was 200 mcg, 1 mL would be administered.
- If the dosage was 0.4 mg, 2 mL would be administered.
- If the dosage was 400 mcg, 2 mL would be administered.

Figure 14-2 Robinul 0.2 mg/mL.
Courtesy of ESI Lederle, Philadelphia, PA

PERCENT AND RATIO SOLUTION LABELS

Percent and ratio solution labels are used for drugs labeled as percentage solutions. These solutions often express the dosage strength in metric measures as well as in percentage strength. **Figure 14-3** shows a lidocaine label available as a 2% solution. Notice that below this information is listed 20 mg/mL. Lidocaine hydrochloride is usually ordered in milligrams, but when used as a local anesthetic, it may be used as a percentage strength solution.

Figure 14-3 Lidocaine 2%.
Copyright Baxter Healthcare Corporation.

SOLUTIONS MEASURED IN INTERNATIONAL UNITS

Many medications are measured in international units, including insulin, penicillin, heparin, and others. These medications are usually expressed in units per milliliter.

Insulin Injections

Insulin is a hormone released from the pancreas. It is essential for glucose, proteins, and fat metabolism. Patients who suffer from insulin-dependent diabetes are required to receive insulin injections each day. Insulin is measured in units and the most frequent supply dosage is 100 units per mL. U-100 is the abbreviation of 100 units per mL.

Pharmacy technicians must remember that accuracy in insulin preparation and administration is critical. Potentially life-threatening situations may result from inaccuracy of the measurement. The information on the insulin label must be correctly interpreted and the correct size syringe must be selected for administration of insulin. These are the two most important factors for the pharmacy technician to understand regarding insulin injections.

Types of Insulin

There are several sources of insulin, which include the following:

1. Human insulin (the most common type)

   a. Biosynthetic—bacteria genetically altered to create human insulin

   b. Semisynthetic—pork insulin chemically altered to produce human insulin

2. Beef insulin—from the pancreas of a cow (no longer commonly used)

3. Pork insulin—from the pancreas of a pig (no longer commonly used)

4. Beef-pork mixture—a combination of beef and pork insulin (no longer commonly used)

Timing of Action

Insulins are classified by the timing of their action. **Figures 14-4a** through **e** illustrate various insulin labels arranged by the three action times:

- Rapid-acting (Regular, Lispro)

- Intermediate-acting (NPH, or Neutral Protamine Hagedorn)

- Long-acting (Lantus, Levemir)

The two most common types of insulin used are Regular and NPH insulin. You can see the uppercase, bold letters on each insulin label as follows: R for Regular insulin; and N for NPH insulin. These letters are important visual identifiers when selecting the insulin type.

Insulin Labels

Insulin labels are identified by the manufacturer, the brand and generic names, storage information, the supply dosage or concentration, and the expiration date (**Figure 14-5**).

Figure 14-4 (a) Humulin® R 10 mL (b) Humalog 10 mL (c) Novolin® R (d) Humulin® N 10 mL (e) Novolin® N 10 mL.

(a) © Copyright Eli Lilly and Company. Used with permission. (b) © Copyright Eli Lilly and Company. Used with permission. (c) Courtesy of Novo Nordisk Pharmaceuticals, Inc. (d) © Copyright Eli Lilly and Company. Used with permission. (e) Courtesy of Novo Nordisk Pharmaceuticals, Inc.

Figure 14-5 Humulin® R.
© Copyright Eli Lilly and Company. Used with permission.

Mixing Insulins

Premixed insulin combinations, including Humalog mixtures, that are commercially available are $\frac{70}{30}$ U-100 insulin and $\frac{50}{50}$ U-100 insulin (**Figure 14-6**). The $\frac{70}{30}$ insulin concentration means there are 70% NPH insulin and 30% Regular insulin in each unit. Therefore, if the prescriber

(a)   (b)

Figure 14-6 (a) Novolin $\frac{70}{30}$ (b) Humulin $\frac{50}{50}$.

(a) *Courtesy of Novo Nordisk Pharmaceuticals, Inc.* (b) © *Copyright Eli Lilly and Company. Used with permission.*

orders 10 units of $\frac{70}{30}$ insulin, the patient would receive 7 units of NPH insulin (70% or 0.7×10 units = 7 units) and 3 units of Regular insulin (30% or 0.3×10 units = 3 units) in the $\frac{70}{30}$ concentration.

The $\frac{50}{50}$ insulin concentration means each unit has 50% NPH insulin and 50% Regular insulin. Therefore, if the physician orders 16 units of $\frac{50}{50}$ insulin, the patient would receive 8 units of NPH insulin (50% or 0.5×12 units = 8 units) and 8 units of Regular insulin (50% or 0.5×16 units = 8 units).

Measuring Insulin in an Insulin Syringe

Measuring insulin with the insulin syringe is quite simple. The insulin syringe obtains a correct dosage without mathematical calculation. The syringes are the *standard* (100-unit) capacity and the *lo-dose* (50-unit and 30-unit) capacities.

Standard U-100 Insulin Syringe

The Standard U-100 insulin syringe is a dual-scale syringe with 100 units/mL capacity. It is calibrated on one side in even-numbered, 2-unit increments (2, 4, 6 . . .) with every 10 units labeled (10, 20, 30 . . .). It is calibrated on the reverse side in odd-numbered, 2-unit increments (1, 3, 5 . . .) with every 10 units labeled (5, 15, 25 . . .). The measurement of 73 units of U-100 insulin is shown in **Figure 14-7**.

Figure 14-7 Standard U-100 insulin syringe measuring 73 units.
© *Cengage Learning 2013*

Lo-Dose U-100 Insulin Syringes

The Lo-Dose U-100 insulin syringe is a single-scale syringe with 50 units/0.5 mL capacity. It is calibrated in 1-unit increments with every 5 units (5, 10, 15 . . .) labeled up to 50 units. The enlarged 50-unit calibration of this

Figure 14-8 50 U Lo-Dose U-100 insulin syringe measuring 32 units.
© *Cengage Learning 2013*

syringe makes it easy to read 32 units. To measure 32 units, withdraw 100 units of insulin to the 32-unit mark (**Figure 14-8**).

The Lo-Dose U-100 insulin syringe is another single-scale syringe with 30 units/0.3 mL capacity. It is calibrated in 1-unit increments with every 5 units (5, 10, 15 . . .) labeled up to 30 units. The enlarged 30-unit calibration accurately measures very small amounts of insulin, such as for children. To measure 12 units, withdraw 100 units of insulin to the 12-unit mark (**Figure 14-9**).

Figure 14-9 30 U-Lo Dose U-100 insulin syrginge measuring 12 units.
© *Cengage Learning 2013*

Combination Insulin Dosage

Some patients may use two types of insulin that have been ordered to be administered at the same time. To avoid injecting the patient twice, it is common practice to draw up both insulins in the same syringe.

■ EXAMPLE 1:

Ordered: *Novolin R Regular U-100 insulin 12 units with Novolin N NPH U-100 insulin 40 units SC with breakfast*

To accurately draw up both insulins into the same syringe, the pharmacy technician must know the total units of both insulins: 12 + 40 = 52 units. Withdraw 12 units of the Regular U-100 insulin (clear) and then withdraw 40 more units of the NPH U-100 insulin (cloudy) up to the 52-unit mark (**Figure 14-10**). In this case, the smallest capacity syringe that can be used is the Standard U-100 insulin syringe.

The second example gives step-by-step directions for this procedure. Look closely at **Figure 14-11** and **14-12** to demonstrate the procedure as you study Example 2. Notice that to withdraw Regular insulin (clear) first and then NPH insulin (cloudy), you must inject the dose amount of air into the NPH insulin before you inject the dose amount of air into the Regular insulin.

Figure 14-10 (a) Combination insulin dosage (b) Novolin ® R (c) Novolin ® N 10 mL.
(a) © Cengage Learning 2013 (b) *Courtesy of Novo Nordisk Pharmaceuticals, Inc.* (c) *Courtesy of Novo Nordisk Pharmaceuticals, Inc.*

Figure 14-11 Procedure for drawing up combination insulin dosage: 10 U Regular
U-100 insulin with 30 U NPH U-100 insulin.
© Cengage Learning 2013

Figure 14-12 Combination insulin dosage.
© Cengage Learning 2013

■ EXAMPLE 2:

A prescriber orders Novolin R Regular U-100 insulin 10 units with Novolin N NPH

U-100 insulin 30 USC $\frac{1}{2}$ hour before dinner.

1. Draw back and inject 30 units of air into the NPH insulin vial (cloudy liquid). Remove the needle.

2. Draw back and inject 10 units of air into the Regular insulin (clear liquid) and leave the needle in the vial.

3. Turn the vial of Regular insulin upside down, and draw out the insulin to the 10-unit mark on the syringe. Make sure all air bubbles are removed.

4. Roll the vial of the NPH insulin in your hands to mix; do not shake it. Insert the needle into the NPH insulin vial, turn the vial upside down and slowly draw back to the 40-unit mark, being careful not to exceed the 40-unit calibration. 10 units of Regular + 30 units of NPH = 40 units of insulin total.

Stop and Review

Read the following labels. Identify the insulin brand name and its action time (rapid-acting, intermediate-acting, or long-acting).

1. Insulin brand name	_____	
Action time	_____	

Humulin® R.

2. Insulin brand name _____

Action time _____

Novolin® N 10 mL.
Courtesy of Novo Nordisk

3. Insulin brand name _____

Action time _____

Humulin® U.
© *Copyright Eli Lilly and Company. Used with permission.*

4. Insulin brand name _____

Action time _____

Humalog 10 mL.
© *Copyright Eli Lilly and Company. Used with permission.*

5. Insulin brand name	_____
Action time	_____

Humulin® L 10 mL.
© Copyright Eli Lilly and Company. Used with permission.

6. Describe the three syringes available to measure U-100 insulin.

_____

7. What would be your preferred syringe choice to measure 24 units of U-100 insulin?

_____

8. What would be your preferred syringe choice to measure 35 units of U-100 insulin?

_____

9. There are 60 units of U-100 insulin per _____ mL.

10. There are 25 units of U-100 insulin per _____ mL.

11. 65 units of U-100 insulin should be measured in a(n) _____ syringe.

12. The 50-unit Lo-Dose U-100 insulin syringe is intended to measure U-50 insulin only.

_____ (True or False)

Identify the U-100 insulin dosage indicated by the colored area of the syringe.

13. _____ units

14. _____ units

15. _____ units

16. _____ units

Draw an arrow on the syringe to identify the given dosages.

17. 80 units U-100 insulin

18. 15 units U-100 insulin

19. 66 units U-100 insulin

© Cengage Learning 2013

20. 16 units U-100 insulin

© Cengage Learning 2013

21. 32 units of U-100 insulin

© Cengage Learning 2013

Draw arrows and label the dosage for each of the combination insulin orders to be measured in the same syringe. Label and measure the insulins in the correct order, indicating which insulin will be drawn up first.

22. Novolin R Regular U-100 insulin 21 units with Novolin N NPH U-100 insulin 15 units SC stat

© Cengage Learning 2013

23. Humulin R Regular U-100 insulin 16 units with Humulin N NPH U-100 insulin 42 units SC stat

© Cengage Learning 2013

24. Humulin R Regular U-100 insulin 32 units with Humulin N NPH U-100 insulin 40 units SC with dinner

© Cengage Learning 2013

25. Humulin R Regular U-100 insulin 8 units with Humulin N NPH U-100 insulin 12 units SC stat

© Cengage Learning 2013

SOLUTIONS MEASURED AS MILLIEQUIVALENTS

Other medications are measured as milliequivalents (mEq). An example of a medication measured in mEq is calcium gluconate (see **Figure 14-13**). This medication has a 10% strength, and the vial contains a dosage of 0.465 mEq/mL.

Figure 14-13 Calcium Gluconate 10 mL.
© Cengage Learning 2013

Stop and Review

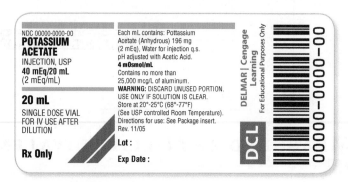

© Cengage Learning 2013

Use the above label to answer the following questions.

1. For this vial, what are the total dosage and volume?

_____

2. List the dosage in mEq per mL. _____

3. What volume would be drawn up if you were asked to prepare 15 mEq for addition to an IV? _____

Potassium Acetate.
© Cengage Learning 2013

Use the above label to answer the following questions.

4. In mEq per mL, what is the strength of this solution?

_____

5. What volume would you draw up in the syringe if you were asked to prepare 40 mEq for addition to an IV solution? _____

6. For a dosage of 20 mEq, what volume would you need?

_____

Sodium Bibarbonate.
© Cengage Learning 2013

Use the above label to answer the following questions.

7. In mEq/mL, what is the dosage strength?

   _____

8. What is this vial's total volume, and how many mEq does it contain?

   _____

9. What is the strength per mL in grams? _____

10. What volume would you draw up in a syringe if you were asked to prepare 10 mL of an 8.4% sodium bicarbonate solution?

    _____

CALCULATING PARENTERAL DRUG DOSAGES

Parenteral medications are measured in proper syringes. The amount of solution delivered is called the desired dose of drug. The dosage strength on an injectable drug's label represents the amount of medication contained within a volume of solution. For example, xylocaine 1% (label drug) can be interpreted as 100 mL contains 1g of xylocaine. Another example is Compazine 5 mg/mL, which means 1 mL contains 5 mg of Compazine.

When the dosage ordered and the dose on hand have different units, the dosage ordered must be converted to the desired dose. Use this formula to calculate the amount of an injectable drug by the formula method:

$$\frac{D \text{ (desired)}}{H \text{ (have)}} \times Q \text{ (quantity)} = X \text{ (amount)}$$

■ EXAMPLE 1:

Measure 0.33 mL in a 1 mL syringe.

0.33 mL

© Cengage Learning 2013

■ EXAMPLE 2:

Round 1.33 mL to 1.3 mL, and measure in a 3 mL syringe.

© *Cengage Learning 2013*

■ EXAMPLE 3:

Measure 0.6 mL in either a 1 mL or 3 mL syringe.

(Notice that the amount is measured in tenths, but the 1 mL syringe would be preferable.)

(a)

© *Cengage Learning 2013*

(b)

© *Cengage Learning 2013*

■ EXAMPLE 4:

Measure 0.65 mL in a 1 mL syringe. (Notice that the amount is measured in hundredths and is less than 1 mL.)

© *Cengage Learning 2013*

An amber color has been added to selected syringe drawings throughout the text to represent a specific amount of medication, as indicated in the example or problem. Because the color used may not correspond to the actual color of the medication named, it must not be used as a reference for identifying medications.

The following are some examples of parenteral dosage calculations.

■ **EXAMPLE 5:**

Ordered: *Vistaril 100 mg IM stat*

On hand: Vistaril IM solution 50 mg/mL in a 10 mL multiple-dose vial

The amount that should be administered to the patient follows:

$$\frac{D}{H} \times Q = \frac{100 \text{ mg}}{50 \text{ mg}} \times 1 \text{ mL} = 2 \text{ mL}$$

Give intramuscularly immediately.

Vistaril 50 mg/mL.
Label reproduced with permission of Pfizer, Inc.

Select a 3 mL syringe and measure 2 mL of Vistaril 50 mg/mL. Look carefully at the illustration to clearly identify the part of the black rubber stopper that measures the exact dosage.

© Cengage Learning 2013

■ **EXAMPLE 6:**

Ordered: *heparin 8,000 units SC b.i.d.*

On hand: A vial of heparin sodium injection 10,000 units/1 mL

$$\frac{D}{H} \times Q = \frac{8,000 \text{ U}}{10,000 \text{ U}} \times 1 \text{ mL} = \frac{8}{10} \text{ mL} = 0.8 \text{ mL}$$

given subcutaneously twice daily.

Heparin 1 mL.
Courtesy of ESI Lederle, a Business Unit of Wyeth Pharmaceuticals, Philadelphia, PA

Select a 1 mL or a 3 mL syringe and measure 0.8 mL of heparin 10,000 units/mL. Heparin is a very potent anticoagulant drug. It is safest to measure it in a 1 mL syringe.

© Cengage Learning 2013

■ EXAMPLE 7:

Ordered: *Cleocin Phosphate 150 mg IM q12h*

On hand: Cleocin Phosphate (clindamycin injection) 300 mg/2 mL

Cleocin Phospahte 300 mg.
Label reproduced with permission of Pfizer, Inc.

$$\frac{D}{H} \times Q = \frac{150 \text{ mg}}{300 \text{ mg}} \times 2 \text{ mL} = \frac{2}{2} = 1 \text{ mL}$$

given intramuscularly every 12 hours.

Select a 3 mL syringe, and measure 1 mL of Cleocin 300 mg/2 mL.

© Cengage Learning 2013

■ EXAMPLE 8:

Ordered: *Robinul 150 mcg IM stat*

On hand: Robinul 0.2 mg/mL

$$0.2 \times 1000 = 200 \text{ mcg}$$

Equivalent : 1 mg = 1000 mcg

Robinul 0.2 mg/mL.
Courtesy of ESI Lederle, Philadelphia, PA

$$\frac{D}{H} \times Q = \frac{150 \text{ mcg}}{200 \text{ mcg}} \times 1 \text{ mL} = \frac{3}{4} = 0.75 \text{ mL}$$

given intramuscularly immediately.

Select a 1 mL syringe, and measure 0.75 mL of Robinul 0.2 mg/mL.

0.75 mL

© Cengage Learning 2013

■ EXAMPLE 9:

Ordered: *morphine sulfate gr* $\frac{1}{6}$ *IM q3–4h p.r.n.*

The label on the dosette vial states morphine sulfate 10 mg/mL.

On hand: morphine sulfate 10 mg/mL

Equivalent: gr i = 60 mg

Morphine 10 mg/mL.
Courtesy of Baxter Healthcare Corporation

$$gr \frac{1}{6} \times \frac{60}{1} = 10 \text{ mg}$$

$$\frac{D}{H} \times Q = \frac{10 \text{ mg}}{10 \text{ mg}} \times 1 \text{ mL} = 1 \text{ mL}$$

given intramuscularly every 3 to 4 hours as needed for pain.

1 mL

© Cengage Learning 2013

Test Your Knowledge

Calculate one dose of each of the drug orders numbered 1 through 12. Draw an arrow on the syringe, indicating the calibration line that corresponds to the dose to be administered. The labels provided following these questions are the drugs that are on hand. Indicate dosages that must be administered.

1. Haldol 1.5 mg IM q8h

Give: _____ mL

Haldol 1 mL.
Courtesy of Ortho-McNeil Pharmaceuticals

2. Thorazine 40 mg IM q6h

Give: _____ mL

Thorazine 25 mg/mL.
Reprinted with permission from GlaxoSmithKline

3. Inapsine 1 mg IV stat.

Give: _____ mL

Inapsine 5 mg/mL.
Courtesy of Akorn Inc

4. Nebcin 100 mg IM q8h.

Give: _____ mL

Nebcin® 1.2 g.
© Copyright Eli Lilly and Company. Used with permission.

5. Epoetin alpha 12,000 units SC q.d. × 10 days

Give: _____ mL

Epoetin alfa recombinant M10.
© Cengage Learning 2013

6. Humulin Regular U-100 insulin 22 units SC stat

Give: _____ units

Humulin® R.
© Copyright Eli Lilly and Company. Used with permission.

7. Meperidine 60 mg IM q3–4h p.r.n., pain

Give: _____ mL

Meperidine 75 mg/mL.
Courtesy of Baxter Healthcare Corporation

8. Phenergan 15 mg IM q3–4h p.r.n., nausea and vomiting

Give: _____ mL

Phenergan 25 mg/mL.
Courtesy of Wyeth Pharmaceuticals, Phildadelphia, PA

9. Reglan 7 mg IM stat

   Give: _____ mL

Reglan Injectable.
Courtesy of ESI Lederle, Philadelphia, PA

10. Filgrastim 225 mcg SC q.d. × 2 weeks

    Give: _____ mL

Filgrastim 480 mcg.
© Cengage Learning 2013

11. Novolin R Regular U-100 insulin 32 units with Novolin N NPH U-100 insulin 54 units SC with breakfast.

Give: _____ units

Novolin® N 10 mL/Novolin® R.
Courtesy Novo Nordisk

12. Novolin $\frac{70}{30}$ U-100 insulin 46 units SC with dinner.

Give: _____ units

Novolin $\frac{70}{30}$.
Courtesy Novo Nordisk

Calculate the amount you will prepare for one dose. Indicate the syringe you will select to measure the medication.

13. Ordered: *Demerol 35 mg IM q4h p.r.n., pain*

On hand: Demerol 50 mg/1 mL

Give: _____ mL   Select: _____ syringe

14. Ordered: *Atarax 40 mg IM q4–6h p.r.n., agitation*

    On hand: Atarax 50 mg/mL

    Give: _____ mL   Select: _____ syringe

15. Ordered: *Garamycin 40 mg IM q8h*

    On hand: Garamycin 80 mg/2 mL

    Give: _____ mL   Select: _____ syringe

16. Ordered: *heparin 3500 units SC q12*

    On hand: heparin 5000 units/mL

    Give: _____ mL   Select: _____ syringe

17. Ordered: *Lasix 60 mg IV stat*

    On hand: Lasix 20 mg per 2 mL ampule

    Give: _____ mL   Select: _____ syringe

18. Ordered: *Phenergan 35 mg IM q4h p.r.n., nausea and vomiting*

    On hand: Phenergan 50 mg/1 mL

    Give: _____ mL   Select: _____ syringe

19. Ordered: *vitamin B12 0.75 mg IM q.d.*

    On hand: vitamin B12 1000 mcg/mL

    Give: _____ mL   Select: _____ syringe

20. Ordered: *lidocaine 50 mg IV stat*

    On hand: lidocaine 2%

    Give: _____ mL   Select: _____ syringe

21. Ordered: *morphine sulfate gr $\frac{1}{4}$ IM stat*

    On hand: morphine sulfate 10 mg/mL

    Give: _____ mL   Select: _____ syringe

22. Ordered: *Cleocin 300 mg IM q.i.d.*

    On hand: Cleocin 0.6 g/4 mL

    Give: _____ mL   Select: _____ syringe

23. Ordered: *Dilantin 25 mg IV q8 h*

    On hand: Dilantin 100 mg/2 mL ampule

    Give: _____ mL   Select: _____ syringe

24. Ordered: *heparin 6000 units SC q12h*

    On hand: heparin 10,000 units/mL vial

    Give: _____ mL   Select: _____ syringe

25. Ordered: *atropine gr $\frac{1}{150}$ IM on call to O.R.*

    On hand: atropine 0.4 mg/mL

    Give: _____ mL   Select: _____ syringe

26. Ordered: *Thorazine 10 mg deep IM q.i.d.*

    On hand: Thorazine 25 mg/mL

    Give: _____ mL   Select: _____ syringe

27. Ordered: *Epogen 1400 units SC tiw*

    On hand: Epogen 2000 units/mL

    Give: _____ mL   Select: _____ syringe

28. Ordered: *Adrenalin 0.2 mg SC stat*

    On hand: Adrenalin 1:2000 solution

    Give: _____ mL   Select: _____ syringe

29. Ordered: *Brethine 0.25 mg SC stat*

    On hand: Brethine 1 mg/mL

    Give: _____ mL   Select: _____ syringe

30. Ordered: *magnesium sulfate 250 mg IM q.d.*

    On hand: magnesium sulfate 10% solution

    Give: _____ mL   Select: _____ syringe

31. Ordered: *Calciferol 24,000 IU IM q.d.*

    On hand: Calciferol 500,000 IU/5 mL

    Give: _____ mL   Select: _____ syringe

32. Ordered: *Robinul 0.15 mg IM stat*

    On hand: Robinul 0.2 mg/mL

    Give: _____ mL   Select: _____ syringe

Critical Thinking

Describe how to prevent a medication error in the following example.

A patient presents with nausea, and a physician orders oral Compazine liquid. Due to the patient's difficulty in taking the medication normally, the physician has instructed that a needleless syringe be supplied along with the medication, which the patient can use to self-administer the medication. The pharmacy technician processing the order accidentally packages it with needles so that the medication may be self-injected, along with appropriate self-injection instructions.

1. If the patient followed these instructions and did self-inject the medication, how would the medication be absorbed?

   _____

2. What could possibly develop at the site of the injection as a result of the self-injection?

   _____

CHAPTER 15

Intravenous Flow Rate Calculations

OBJECTIVES

Upon completion of this chapter, you should be able to:

1. Distinguish components of intravenous solutions.
2. Understand common IV components and solutions.
3. Calculate the adjustment of IV flow rates.
4. Calculate flow rates in drops per minute and milliliters per hour by using the formula method.
5. Calculate infusion times and completion times.
6. Calculate IV flow rates for electronic regulation.
7. Calculate IV flow rates from units per hour ordered.
8. Calculate units per hour infusing from IV flow rate.

GLOSSARY

continuous IV infusion – Replaces or maintains fluids and electrolytes and serves as a vehicle for medication administration.

controllers – Devices that are often referred to as electronic flow clamps because they control infusion rate by either drop counting or volumetric delivery, using gravity to maintain desired flow rates.

D$_5$W (Dextrose 5% in water) – In this mixture, the solute is dextrose, and the solvent is water.

heparin lock – A device attached to the hub of the IV catheter that allows access to the vein for IV push medications; also known as a saline lock or an intermittent peripheral infusion device.

infusion pump – A device that maintains flow by displacing fluid at an ordered rate, rather than relying on gravity.

intermittent intravenous infusion – Medication administration as a single dose into a vein that has been maintained open with an IV catheter.

intermittent peripheral infusion device – A device attached to the hub of the IV catheter that allows access to the vein for IV push medications; also known as a heparin lock or a saline lock.

IV bolus – A quantity of IV fluid that can be run over a specified period of time through an IV setup attached to the lock.

IV push – Drugs that are administered by the direct IV injection route.

saline lock – A device attached to the hub of the IV catheter that allows access to the vein for IV push medications; also known as a heparin lock or an intermittent peripheral infusion device.

syringe pump – A kind of electronic infusion pump used to infuse fluids or medications directly from a syringe.

OVERVIEW

Intravenous (IV) fluids and drugs may be administered for many different reasons. Intravenous therapy is prescribed to persons requiring electrolyte replacement, fluid, calories, vitamins, or other nutritional substances. It may also be prescribed for administration of medications, chemotherapy, or for transfusion of blood products. There are about 200 different manufactured IV fluids. Approximately 90 percent of all hospitalized clients, some outpatients, and some health-care clients receive IV therapy. Regulation of IV fluids is normally not a responsibility of pharmacy technicians. Pharmacists and technicians are involved with compounding IV fluids. This chapter explains the basic concepts of IV therapy.

Calculation errors can have serious, even fatal, consequences. Drug information inserts must be read carefully, and attention must be paid to the amount of drug that can be given per minute. If the drug is administered into the blood circulation at a rate faster than that specified in the drug literature, adverse reactions to the medication are likely to occur.

Heparin is an anticoagulant that inhibits new blood clot formation or the extension of already-existing clots. It is often mixed in IV solutions for postoperative administration to prevent clot formation from venous stasis. Heparin dosages are based on body weight (in kilograms) or on a patient's clotting time, which is checked frequently during administration. Pharmacy technicians may be involved with heparin intravenous calculations in compounding.

IV PUSH

Drugs that are administered by the IV injection route are often referred to as IV push. This route has a rapid onset of action, and calculation errors can have serious or even fatal consequences. Calculating the amount of drug needed to infuse by direct IV infusion can be determined by using the ratio and proportion method.

■ **EXAMPLE 1:**

Ordered: Dilantin 200 mg IV stat

On hand: Dilantin 250 mg/5 mL; IV infusion not to exceed 50 mg/min

Give: $\dfrac{D}{H} \times V = \dfrac{200}{250} \times 5 = 4\,mL$

or

$$H : V :: D : X$$

$$250\,mg : 5\,mL :: 200\,mg : X\,mL$$

$$250X = 5 \times 200 = 1000$$

$$X = \frac{1000}{250}$$

$$X = 4\,mL$$

$$Minutes :: desired\ drug : desired\ minutes$$

$$50\,mg : 1\,minute :: 200\,mg : x\,minutes$$

$$50X = 200$$

$$X = 4\,minutes$$

■ **EXAMPLE 2:**

Ordered: furosemide 120 mg IV stat

On hand: furosemide 10 mg/mL; IV infusion not to exceed 40 mg/min

a. $H : V :: D : X$

$$10\,mg : 1\,mL :: 120\,mg : X$$

$$10X = 120$$

$$X = 12\,mL\ of\ Lasix$$

or

$$\frac{D}{H} \times V = \frac{1\,mL \times 120\,mg}{10\,mg \times 1} = 12\,mL\ of\ Lasix$$

b.   On hand: minutes :: desired drug : desired minutes

$$40\,mg : 1\,min :: 120\,mg : X$$

$$40X = 120$$

$$X = 3\,min$$

■ **EXAMPLE 3:**

Ordered: Ativan 3 mg IV push 20 min preoperatively

On hand: Ativan 4 mg/mL with drug literature guidelines of "IV infusion not to exceed 2 mg/min"

How much Ativan should you prepare? Use the formula:

$$\frac{D}{H} \times Q = \frac{3\,mg}{4\,mg} \times 1\,mL = 0.75\,mL$$

What is a safe infusion time?

$$\frac{D}{H} \times Q = \frac{3\,mg}{2\,mg} \times 1\,min = \frac{3}{2} = 1\frac{1}{2}\,min$$

Administer 0.75 mL over 1.5 min

■ EXAMPLE 4:

Ordered: Cefizox 1500 mg IV push q8h

On hand: Cefizox 2 g powder with directions: "For direct IV administration, reconstitute each 1 g in 10 mL sterile water and give slowly over 3–5 minutes"

How much Cefizox should you prepare?

$$2\,g = 2 \times 1000 = 2000\,mg$$

$$\frac{D}{H} \times Q = \frac{1500\,mg}{2000\,mg} \times 20\,mL = 15\,mL$$

What is a safe infusion time?

$$\frac{D}{H} \times Q = \frac{1500\,mg}{1000} \times 5\,min = \frac{15}{2} = 7.5\,min$$

Administer 15 mL over 7.5 min.

Stop and Review
Calculate the following IV Push Rates.

1. Ordered:	morphine sulfate 6 mg IV push q3h p.r.n., pain
On hand:	morphine sulfate 10 mg/mL with a written drug reference recommendation: "IV infusion not to exceed 2.5 mg/min"
Give:	_____ mL/_____ min/_____ sec
2. Ordered:	Oxacillin Sodium 900 mg in 125 mL D$_5$W IV PB to be infused over 45 min
Instructions:	Use an infusion pump.
Flow rate:	_____ mL/hr

3. Ordered:	Versed 1.5 mg IV push stat
On hand:	Versed 1 mg/1 mL
Instructions:	Slowly titrate to the desired effect using no more than 1.5 mg initially given over 2-min period.
Prepare:	_____ mL Versed
Give:	_____ mL/15 sec
4. Ordered:	Merrem 1 g in 100 mL D$_5$W IV PB to be infused over 50 min
Instructions:	Use an infusion pump.
Flow rate:	_____ mL/hr
5. Ordered:	Unasyn 1.5 g in 50 mL D$_5$W IV PB to be infused over 15 min
Drop factor:	15 gtt/min
Flow rate:	_____ gtt/min
6. Ordered:	Keflin 500 mg in 50 mL NS IV PB to be infused over 20 min
Drop factor:	10 gtt/mL
Flow rate:	_____ gtt/min
7. Ordered:	Ancef 1 g in 100 mL D$_5$W IV PB to be infused over 45 min
Drop factor:	60 gtt/mL
Flow rate:	_____ gtt/min
8. Ordered:	Zosyn 1.3 g in 100 mL D5W IV PB to be infused over 30 min
Drop factor:	60 gtt/mL
Flow rate:	_____ gtt/min

9. Ordered:	Dilantin 150 mg IV push stat
On hand:	Dilantin 250 mg/5 mL with drug insert, which states "IV infusion not to exceed 50 mg/min"
Given:	_____ mL/_____ min
10. Ordered:	Cimetidine 300 mg IV push stat
On hand:	Tagamet (cimetidine) 300 mg/2 mL
Instructions:	For direct IV injection, dilute 300 mg in 0.9% NaCl to a total volume of 20 mL. Inject over at least 2 minutes.
Prepare:	_____ mL Tagamet
Dilute with:	_____ mL 0.9% NaCl for a total of 20 mL of solution
Administer:	_____ mL/15 sec

CONTINUOUS INTRAVENOUS INJECTIONS

Continuous IV infusions replace or maintain fluids and electrolytes and serve as a vehicle for medication administration. IV fluids can be supplied in plastic solution bags or glass bottles with the volume of the IV fluid container typically varying from 50 mL to 1000 mL (**Figure 15-1**). Some IV bags may

Figure 15-1 IV solutions come in various sizes.
© *Cengage Learning 2013*

even contain more than 1000 mL. Solutions used for total parenteral nutrition usually contain 2000 mL or more in a single bag. The IV solution bag or bottle will be labeled with the exact components and amount of the IV solution. Pharmacy technicians often use abbreviations when communicating about the IV solution. Therefore, it is important for the technicians to know the common IV solution components and the solution concentration strengths represented by such abbreviations (**Table 15-1**).

TABLE 15–1 Common IV Components and Solutions

Abbreviation	Solution	Component
D5W	Dextrose 5% in water	5% dextrose
D5NS	Dextrose 5% in normal saline	5% dextrose in 0.9% sodium chloride
D5 ½ NS	Dextrose 5% in 0.45% normal saline	5% dextrose in 0.45% sodium chloride
NS	Normal Saline 0.9%	0.9% sodium chloride
½ NS	Normal Saline 0.45%	0.45% sodium chloride
LR, RL, RLS	Lactated Ringer's solution, Ringer's lactated solution	Electrolytes

■ EXAMPLE 1:

Suppose an order includes D_5W, which means "Dextrose 5% in Water" and it is supplied as 5% dextrose injection (**Figure 15-2**). This means that the solution strength of the solute (dextrose) is 5%. The solvent is water. Read the IV bag label and notice that "each 100 mL contains 5 g dextrose…." For every 100 mL of solution, there are 5 g of dextrose.

Figure 15-2 Dextrose Injection 5% USP.
© Cengage Learning 2013

◼ EXAMPLE 2:

Suppose a physician writes D$_5$LR on the prescription. This abbreviation means "Dextrose 5% in Lactated Ringer's" and is supplied as lactated Ringer's and 5% dextrose injection, as shown in **Figure 15-3**.

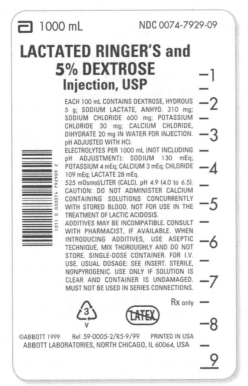

Figure 15-3 D5LR.
Photography courtesy of Abbott Laboratories

◼ EXAMPLE 3:

A physician orders D$_5$NS 1000 mL IV q8h. This order is translated as "administer 1000 mL of 5% dextrose in normal saline intravenously every 8 hours." It is supplied as 5% dextrose and 0.9% sodium chloride. The common term for 0.9% sodium chloride is *normal saline* (also known as *physiologic saline*). In normal saline, the concentration of sodium chloride is 0.9 g (which is equal to 900 mg) per 100 mL of solution.

Solution Additives

In some cases, electrolytes, nutrients, and medications can be added and mixed with IV solutions. Antibiotics, potassium chloride, and water-soluble vitamins such as B and C are common additives. If additives are not prepackaged in the solution, the pharmacy technician needs to mix the additive and IV solution. The prescriber's order will explain how much additive is to be given, the amount and type of basic IV solution to use, or how long it should be infused.

◼ EXAMPLE 4:

The physician orders *D$_5$NS 20 mEq KCl/L*. This means to add 20 milliequivalents of potassium chloride per liter of 5% dextrose and 0.9% sodium chloride IV solution.

Stop and Review

For each of the following IV solutions labeled A through H, specify the letter of the illustration corresponding to the fluid abbreviation, list the solute(s) of each solution, identify the strength (g/mL) of each solute, and identify the osmolarity (mOsm/L) of each solution.

	Letter of Matching Illustration	Components and Strength	Osmolarity (mOsm/L)
1. NS	_____	_____	_____
2. D_5W	_____	_____	_____
3. D_5NS	_____	_____	_____
4. $D_5\frac{1}{2}NS$	_____	_____	_____
5. $D_5\frac{1}{4}NS$	_____	_____	_____
6. D_5LR	_____	_____	_____
7. $D_5\frac{1}{2}NSc$ 20 mEq KCl/L	_____	_____	_____
8. $\frac{1}{2}NS$	_____	_____	_____

Label A

5% Dextrose and sodium chloride.
Photography courtesy of Abbott Laboratories

Label B

20 mEq Potassium Chloride.
Photography courtesy of Abbott Laboratories

Label C

.9% Sodium Chloride.
Photography courtesy of Abbott Laboratories

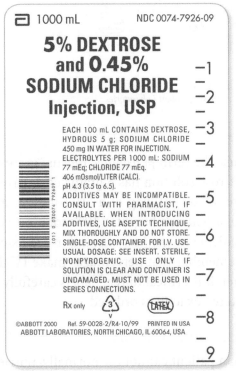

Label D

5% Dextrose and .45% Sodium Chloride.
Photography courtesy of Abbott Laboratories

Label E

Dextrose Injection 5% USP.
© Cengage Learning 2013

Label F

.45% Sodium Chloride Injection.
© Cengage Learning 2013

Label G

5% Dextrose and .9% sodium chloride.
Photography courtesy of Abbott Laboratories

Label H

Lactated Ringer's and 5% Dextrose.
Photography courtesy of Abbott Laboratories

Percentage in IV Fluids

Because the term *percentage* means "grams of drug per 100 mL of fluid," a 5% dextrose solution has 5 grams of dextrose in each 100 mL of solution. Therefore, a 500 mL bag of a 5% solution contains 25 grams of dextrose. Likewise, a 500 mL bag of a 10% solution contains 50 grams of dextrose. All ingredients in any bag of solution are listed on the IV label. It is important to remember that percentages make IV fluids extremely different from each other. It is critical to read labels carefully and make sure that each IV is administered exactly as ordered.

Parenteral Nutrition

When a patient cannot eat normally, nutrients can be administered via a central vein. This is called *parenteral nutrition*. In general, parenteral nutrition solutions contain high calories and various amounts of amino acids, glucose, and (sometimes) fat emulsions. Common types of parenteral nutrition include the following:

- Total parenteral nutrition (TPN)

- Partial parenteral nutrition (PPN)

- Hyperalimentation (nutrition that is in excess of maintenance needs)

Solutions that contain lipids appear opaque white and are usually infused slowly over a period of less than 24 hours. This is because they can spoil and support bacterial growth if infused over 24 hours or longer. General intravenous administration precautions apply to parenteral nutrition, but greater care must be taken to prevent infection. These solutions are infused similarly to other IV solutions, with similar flow rates and infusion times.

CALCULATING IV COMPONENTS AS PERCENTAGES

The concept of calculating components of an IV solution by expressing them as a percentage is important because it helps in understanding that IV solutions provide much more than fluid. They also provide other components.

■ EXAMPLE 1:

Ordered: *D₅W 1000 mL*

Calculate the amount of dextrose in 1000 mL D₅W. This can be calculated using ratio and proportion. Recall that % indicates g per 100 mL; therefore, 5% dextrose is 5 g dextrose per 100 mL of solution.

$$\frac{5\,g}{100\,mL} = \frac{X\,g}{1000\,mL}$$

$$100X = 5000$$

$$X = \frac{5000}{100} = 50\,g$$

■ EXAMPLE 2:

Ordered: $D_5\frac{1}{4}NS\ 500\,mL$

Calculate the amount of dextrose and sodium chloride in 500 mL.

$$\frac{5\,g}{100\,mL} = \frac{X\,g}{500\,mL}$$

$$100X = 2500$$

$$X = \frac{2500}{100} = 25\,g\,dextrose$$

$$\frac{1}{4}\,NS = 0.225\%\ NaCl = 0.225\ g\ NaCl\ per\ 100\ mL$$

Recall that NS, or Normal Saline, is 0.9% NaCl; therefore, $\frac{1}{2}$ NS is 0.45% NaCl and $\frac{1}{4}$ NS is 0.225% NaCl.

$$\frac{0.225\,g}{100\,mL} = \frac{Xg}{500\,mL}$$

$$100X = 112.5$$

$$X = 1.125\,g\ NaCl$$

500 mL D$_5$¼ NS contains 25 g dextrose and 1.125 g sodium chloride.

Stop and Review

Calculate the amount of dextrose and/or sodium chloride in each of the following IV solutions.

1. 250 mL NS

    sodium chloride _____ g

2. 3 L of D$_5$NS

    dextrose _____ g

    sodium chloride _____ g

3. 500 mL of D$_5$ 0.33% NaCl

    dextrose _____ g

    sodium chloride _____ g

4. 250 mL of D10W

    dextrose _____ g

5. 1000 mL of D$_5$NS

    dextrose _____ g

    sodium chloride _____ g

6. 750 mL of NS

    sodium chloride _____ g

7. 0.75 L of 0.45% NaCl

    sodium chloride _____ g

8. 300 mL of D12 0.9% NaCl

    dextrose _____ g

    sodium chloride _____ g

9. 500 mL of $D_5\frac{1}{2}NS$

    dextrose _____ g

    sodium chloride _____ g

10. 0.5 L of $D10\frac{1}{4}NS$

    dextrose _____ g

    sodium chloride _____ g

Calculating IV Flow Rates

Intravenous fluids are administered via an intravenous infusion set. This primary line usually includes the sealed bottle or bag containing the fluids, a drip chamber connected to the bag or bottle by a small tube or spike, a roller clamp, and tubing that leads from the roller clamp down to and connecting with the needle or catheter at the site of insertion into the patient (**Figure 15-4**).

Injection Port

Drip Chamber

Roller Clamp

IV Solution Bag

Figure 15-4 Standard IV set-up.
© Cengage Learning 2013

Figure 15-5 Piggyback IV set-up.
© Cengage Learning 2013

The nurse can regulate the rate either by using the roller clamp or by placing the tubing in an electronic infusion pump. Another type of IV tubing (the secondary intravenous tubing) is used when medications are administered by "piggybacking" into the primary line (**Figure 15-5**).

IV fluids are usually ordered for a certain volume to run for a stated period of time, such as *125 mL/h* or *1000 mL/8h*. The nurse may use electronic or manual regulating equipment to monitor the flow rate. The calculations performed to set the flow rate will depend on the equipment used to administer the IV solutions. It is important to note that in most settings, nurses will use IV pumps and not gravity-fed tubing.

The infusion of intravenous fluids is monitored in many different ways. Most times, for manual regulation, the bag containing the intravenous solution is hung 36 inches above the patient's heart so that gravity will draw the fluid into the patient. When the infusion is regulated, the roller clamp is used to adjust the rate of delivery. Therefore, the nurse manually regulates the IV rate. To calculate the ordered IV rate based on a certain number of drops per minute (gtt/min), understand that this actually represents the ordered milliliters per hour. For calculating flow rate manually, you must count the number of drops falling into the drip chamber while holding a watch next to the drip chamber, to see how many drops fall in one minute (gtt/min). The number of drops dripping per minute into the IV drip chamber are controlled and counted by opening and closing the roller clamp. The drop factor is the number of drops per milliliter (gtt/mL) that a particular IV tubing set will deliver. It is written on the IV tubing package (**Figure 15-6**) and varies according to the manufacturer of the IV equipment. Standard or macrodrop IV tubing sets have a drop factor of 10, 15, or 20 gtt/mL. All microdrip IV tubing has a drop factor of 60 gtt/mL.

Figure 15-6 Primany Intravenous infusion set.
Photography courtesy of Abbott Laboratories

Figure 15-7 compares macrodrops and microdrops. Figure 15-8 illustrates the size and number of drops in 1 mL for each drop factor. Notice that the fewer the number of drops per milliliter, the larger the actual drop size.

(a)   (b)

Figure 15-7 Intravenous drip chambers: (a) macrodrops; (b) microdrops.
© Cengage Learning 2013

| 1 mL | 1 mL | 1 mL | 1 mL |
| 10 gtt/mL | 15 gtt/mL | 20 gtt/mL | 60 gtt/mL |

Standard or Macrodrop Calibration   Microdrop Calibration

Figure 15-8 Comparison of calibrated drop factors.
© Cengage Learning 2013

Stop and Review

Identify the drop factor calibration of the IV tubing pictured.

LATEX-FREE

No. 4967

PRIMARY I.V. SET,
Convertible Pin, 80 Inch
with Backcheck Valve
and 2 Injection Sites
Piggyback

15 DROPS/mL

Courtesy of Abbott Laboratories

1. Primary IV Set

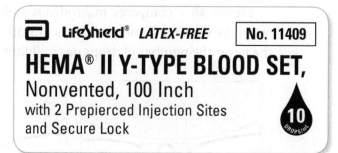

Courtesy of Abbott Laboratories

2. Hema II Y-type Blood Set

_____

Courtesy of Abbott Laboratories

3. Continu-Flo

_____

Courtesy of Abbott Laboratories

4. Primary IV Set

_____

Courtesy of Baxter Healthcare Corporation

5. Continu-Flo Solution Set

Calculating Flow Rates Using Ratio and Proportion

In this procedure, the flow rate is calculated in drops per minute (gtt/min) from the gtt/mL calibration of the required IV set. This is either 10, 15, 20, or 60 gtt/mL, with a specified order of milliliters per hour (mL/hr).

■ EXAMPLE 3:

An IV is ordered to infuse at a rate of 125 mL/hr. The IV set is calibrated at 10 gtt/mL. What is the gtt/min flow rate?

First, convert the 125 mL/hr ordered to mL/min. This is done by dividing 125 mL by 60 minutes, which gives you approximately 2 mL/min.

Then calculate the gtt/min rate for 2 mL/min. Enter the 10 gtt/mL set calibration as the first ratio in this proportion. The X gtt in 2 mL is then entered:

$$\frac{10\,gtt}{1\,mL} = \frac{X\,gtt}{2\,mL} = 20\,gtt$$

This is the same as the following:

$$10\,gtt : 1\,mL = X\,gtt : 2\,mL$$

This also gives you the answer of X = 20 gtt

Therefore, to infuse an IV at 125 mL/hr using a 10 gtt/mL calibrated set, you should set the drip rate at 20 gtt/min.

■ EXAMPLE 4:

If an IV of 150 mL must be infused over 1 hour using an IV set calibrated at 15 gtt/mL, calculate the gtt/min flow rate.

First, convert the 150 mL/hr to mL/min. To do this, divide 150 mL by 60 minutes, which gives you 2.5 mL/min.

Then calculate the gtt/min rate for 2.5 mL/min as follows:

$$\frac{15\,gtt}{1\,mL} = \frac{X\,gtt}{2.5\,mL} = 37.5 = 38\,gtt$$

This is the same as the following:

$$15\,gtt : 1\,mL = X\,gtt : 2.5\,mL$$

The same answer is achieved:

$$X = 37.5 \text{ or } 38 \text{ gtt}$$

So to infuse 150 mL/hr using a set calibrated at 15 gtt/mL, set the drip rate at 38 gtt/min.

▇ EXAMPLE 5:

An IV of 2500 mL must be infused over 24 hours using a 20 gtt/mL calibrated set. What is the gtt/min flow rate?

First, convert 2500 mL/24 hr to mL/hr:

$$2500 \text{ mL} \div 24 \text{ hr} = 104.1 = 104 \text{ mL/hr}$$

Convert 104 mL/hr to mL/min:

$$104 \text{ mL} \div 60 \text{ min} = 1.73 = 1.7 \text{ mL/min}$$

Calculate the gtt/min rate for 1.7 mL/min:

$$\frac{20 \text{ gtt}}{1 \text{ mL}} = \frac{X \text{ gtt}}{1.7 \text{ mL}} = 34 \text{ gtt}$$

Or:

$$20 \text{ gtt} : 1 \text{ mL} = X \text{ gtt} : 1.7 \text{ mL}$$

$$X = 34 \text{ gtt}$$

Therefore, to infuse an IV of 2500 mL in 24 hr using an IV set calibrated at 20 gtt/mL, set the flow rate at 34 gtt/min.

▇ EXAMPLE 6:

1000 mL must be infused IV over 5 hr using an IV set calibrated at 15 gtt/mL.

Convert 1000 mL/5 hr to mL/hr:

$$1000 \text{ mL} \div 5 \text{ hr} = 200 \text{ mL/hr}$$

Convert 200 mL/hr to mL/min:

$$200 \text{ mL} \div 60 \text{ min} = 3.3 \text{ mL/min}$$

Calculate the gtt/min rate for 3.3 mL/min:

$$\frac{15 \text{ gtt}}{1 \text{ mL}} = \frac{X \text{ gtt}}{3.3 \text{ mL}} = 49.5 \text{ (or 50) gtt}$$

Or:

$$15 \text{ gtt} : 1 \text{ mL} = X \text{ gtt} : 3.3 \text{ mL}$$

$$X = 49.5 = 50 \text{ gtt}$$

Therefore, to infuse 1000 mL in 5 hr using a set calibrated at 15 gtt/mL, set the rate at 50 gtt/min.

Stop and Review

Calculate the gtt/min flow rates in the following scenarios.

1. A nurse starts to infuse an IV of 2000 mL in 12 hr using a 10 gtt/mL set.

   How many gtt/min should be given? _____

2. A physician orders an infusion of 500 mL in 3 hr using a 15 gtt/mL set.

   How many gtt/min should be given? _____

3. If an IV of 750 mL is ordered to infuse in 8 hr on a 10 gtt/mL set, how many gtt/min should be given? _____

4. A practitioner ordered 3000 mL volume to be infused in 24 hr on a set calibrated at 20 gtt/mL.

   How many gtt/min should be given? _____

5. A physician ordered 3500 mL to be infused in 24 hr using a set calibrated at 20 gtt/mL.

   How many gtt/min should be given? _____

6. 1500 mL must be infused in 5 hr using a 15 gtt/mL set.

   How many gtt/min should be given? _____

Calculating Flow Rates Using Dimensional Analysis

In dimensional analysis, calculations include two values: drops (gtt) and minutes (min), as follows.

■ EXAMPLE 7:

Calculate a gtt/min flow rate for the infusion of 125 mL/hr using an IV set calibrated at 10 gtt/mL.

First, enter the gtt/min to be calculated as a common fraction:

$$\frac{gtt}{min}$$

Begin ratio entries as in calculating only the gtt numerator. Find the ratio containing gtt (the 10 gtt/mL set calibration). Enter 10 gtt as the numerator to match the gtt numerator being calculated. Therefore, 1 mL becomes the denominator:

$$\frac{gtt}{min} = \frac{10\ gtt}{1\ mL}$$

Match the mL denominator with the 125 mL (of the 125 mL/hr ordered). Therefore, 1 hr becomes the denominator:

$$\frac{gtt}{min} = \frac{10\ gtt}{1\ mL} \times \frac{125\ mL}{1\ hr}$$

A conversion ratio can then be entered, showing that 1 hr equals 60 minutes. The numerator will be 1 hr and the denominator will be 60 min. Notice that the minutes being calculated is easily placed as the final denominator of this equation:

$$\frac{gtt}{min} = \frac{10 \, gtt}{1 \, mL} \times \frac{125 \, mL}{1 \, hr} \times \frac{1 \, hr}{60 \, min}$$

Cross-multiply to cancel out the mL and hr in the equation. Do the math.

This results in 1250 divided by 60 = 20.8 or 21 gtt/min.

Therefore, to infuse 125 mL/hr using a 10 gtt/mL infusion set, the flow rate is 21 gtt/min.

■ **EXAMPLE 8:**

To infuse 90 mL/hr, a 20 gtt/mL set is to be used. What is the gtt/min flow rate?

$$\frac{gtt}{min} = \frac{20 \, gtt}{1 \, mL}$$

$$\frac{gtt}{min} = \frac{20 \, gtt}{1 \, mL} \times \frac{90 \, mL}{1 \, hr}$$

$$\frac{gtt}{min} = \frac{20 \, gtt}{1 \, mL} \times \frac{90 \, mL}{1 \, hr} \times \frac{1 \, hr}{60 \, min}$$

After cancelling out the mL and hr, you find that:

1800 divided by 60 = 30 gtt/min.

Therefore, to infuse 90 mL/hr using a 20 gtt/mL set, the rate is 30 gtt/min.

Stop and Review

Calculate the gtt/min flow rates in the following scenarios using dimensional analysis.

1. An order of 1250 mL must be infused in 12 hr using a 15 gtt/mL set.

   How many gtt/min should be given? _____

2. A physician ordered an IV of 2500 mL to be infused in 18 hr on a set calibrated at 10 gtt/mL.

   How many gtt/min should be given? _____

3. An order of 1000 mL must be infused in 6 hr using a 5 gtt/mL set.

   How many gtt/min should be given? _____

4. An order of 2750 mL must be infused in 22 hr on a 15 gtt/mL set.

   How many gtt/min should be given? _____

5. A physician ordered 500 mL in 3 hr using a 15 gtt/mL set.

   How many gtt/min should be given? _____

6. An IV of 1000 mL must be infused in 6 hr using a 10 gtt/mL set.

   How many gtt/min should be given? _____

Calculating Flow Rates Using the Formula Method

The formula method is used to determine the flow rate in drops per minute (gtt/min).

$$\frac{V}{T} \times C = R$$

$$\frac{Volume\,(mL)}{Time\,(\min)} \times Calibration\,or\,drop\,factor\,(gtt/mL)$$

$$= Rate\,(gtt/min)$$

In this formula:
V = volume per hour to be infused in mL ordered by the prescriber
T = time converted to minutes ordered by the prescriber
C = calibration of tubing (drop factor) in gtt/mL
R = rate of the flow in gtt/min

▓ EXAMPLE 9:

The prescriber orders 1000 mL to be infused over 8 hours, with a drip factor of 30 gtt/mL. First determine the mL/hour. 1000 mL/8 hours = 125 mL per hour. Then use this formula:

$$\frac{mL/hour \times gtt/mL}{60\ minutes}$$

Therefore,

$$\frac{125\,mL/h \times 30\,gtt/mL}{60\ minutes} = \frac{3750}{60}$$

$$= 62.5\ gtt/min$$

▓ EXAMPLE 10:

The physician orders 500 mL to be infused over 24 hours, with a drip factor of 60 gtt/mL.

$$\frac{500\,mL}{24\,hours} = 20.8\ mL\ per\ hour$$

$$\frac{20.8\,mL/hr \times 60\,gtt/mL}{60\,minutes} = \frac{1248}{60}$$

$$= 20.8\ gtt/min$$

(may be rounded to 21 drops per minute)

■ **EXAMPLE 11:**

The physician orders 250 mL to be infused over 3 hours, with a drip factor of 15 gtt/mL. 250 mL/3 hours = 83.3 mL per hour

$$\frac{83.3\,mL/hr \times 15\,gtt/mL}{60\,minutes} = \frac{1249.5}{60}$$

$$= 20.8\ gtt/min$$

■ **EXAMPLE 12:**

The prescriber orders 350 mL to be infused over 4 hours, with a drip factor of 8 gtt/mL. 350 mL/4 hours = 87.5 mL per hour

$$\frac{87.5\,mL/hr \times 8\,gtt/mL}{60\,minutes} = \frac{700}{60}$$

$$= 11.7\ gtt/min\ (rounded\ to\ 12\ gtt/min)$$

 ## Stop and Review

Calculate the flow rate or watch count in gtt/min in the following scenarios using the formula method.

1. Ordered:	D_5 NS IV at 150 mL/hr
Drop factor:	20 gtt/mL
Flow rate:	_____ gtt/min
2. Ordered:	3500 mL D_5 LR IV to run at 160 mL/h
Drop factor:	15 gtt/mL
Flow rate:	_____ gtt/min
3. Ordered:	80 mL D_5W antibiotic solution IV to infuse in 60 min
Drop factor:	60 gtt/mL
Flow rate:	_____ gtt/min

4. Ordered:	250 mL LR IV at 50 mL/hr
Drop factor:	60 gtt/mL
Flow rate:	_____ gtt/min
5. Ordered:	480 mL packed red blood cells IV to infuse in 4 hours
Drop factor:	10 gtt/mL
Flow rate:	_____ gtt/min
6. Ordered:	2500 mL LR IV at 165 mL/hr
Drop factor:	20 gtt/mL
Flow rate:	_____ gtt/min
7. Ordered:	100 mL NS bolus IV to infuse in 60 min
Drop factor:	20 gtt/mL
Flow rate:	_____ gtt/min
8. Ordered:	Two 500 mL units of whole blood IV to be infused in 4 hours. Infusion set is calibrated to 20 drops per milliliter.
Flow rate:	_____ gtt/min

Calculating Flow Rates Using the Shortcut Method

This method is used when converting the volume and time in the formula method to mL/hr (or mL/60 min) to use as a shortcut for calculating flow rate.

■ **EXAMPLE 13:**

Dr. Smith has ordered 125 mL/hr IV with a 20 gtt/mL infusion set. You can calculate this example using the following formula:

$$\frac{125\,mL}{60\,min} \times 20\,gtt/mL = \frac{125\,gtt}{3\,min}$$

$$= 41.7\,gtt/min = 42\,gtt/min$$

■ **EXAMPLE 14:**

Ordered: Normal Saline 1000 mL IV at 125 mL/hr with a microdrop infusion set calibrated for 60 gtt/mL.

Use the formula:

$$\frac{V}{T} \times C = R$$

$$\frac{125\,mL}{60\,min} \times 60\,gtt/mL = \frac{125\,gtt}{1\,min}$$

$$= 125\,gtt/min$$

Stop and Review

Calculate the IV flow rate in gtt/min in the following scenarios using the shortcut method.

1. Ordered:	650 mL D$_5$ 0.33% NaCl IV to infuse in 10 hr
Drop factor:	10 gtt/mL
Flow rate:	_____ gtt/min
2. Ordered:	500 mL D$_5$W 0.45% Saline IV to infuse at 165 mL/hr
Drop factor:	10 gtt/mL
Flow rate:	_____ gtt/min
3. Ordered:	3L NS IV to infuse at 125 mL/hr
Drop factor:	15 gtt/mL
Flow rate:	_____ gtt/min

4. Ordered:	400 mL D₅W IV to infuse at 50 mL/hr
Drop factor:	10 gtt/mL
Flow rate:	_____ gtt/min
5. Ordered:	0.5 L 0.45% NaCl IV to infuse in 20 hr
Drop factor:	60 gtt/mL
Flow rate:	_____ gtt/min
6. Ordered:	1000 mL D₅W IV to infuse at 200 mL/hr
Drop factor:	15 gtt/mL
Flow rate:	_____ gtt/min
7. Ordered:	2L NS IV to infuse at 60 mL/hr with microdrop infusion set of 60 gtt/mL
Flow rate:	_____ gtt/min
8. Ordered:	500 mL D₅ LR to infuse in 6 hr
Drop factor:	20 gtt/mL
Flow rate:	_____ gtt/min

Adjusting Intravenous Flow Rates

When IV fluids are added with medicines, the rate of flow must be carefully calculated and close observation at regular intervals must be conducted. Various situations such as gravity, condition, and movement of the patient can alter the set flow rate of an IV, causing the IV to run ahead of or behind schedule. Therefore, the flow rate per minute may be adjusted by up to 25% more or less than the original rate, depending on the condition of the patient. In such cases, assess the patient. If the patient is stable, recalculate the flow rate to administer the total milliliters remaining over the number of hours remaining of the original order. If the patient is not stable, the physician must assess the rate of flow of IV fluids.

Use the following formula to recalculate the mL/hr and gtt/min for the time remaining and the percentage of variation.

First:

$$\text{Recalculated mL/hr} = \frac{\text{Remaining volume}}{\text{Remaining hours}}$$

Then:

$$\frac{V}{T} \times C = \text{gtt/min}$$

Last:

$$\frac{\text{Adjusted gtt/min} - \text{ordered gtt/min}}{\text{Ordered gtt/min}} = \%\text{ variation}$$

■ EXAMPLE 15:

The prescriber has ordered 500 mL LR to run over 10 hr at 50 mL/hr. The drop factor is 60 gtt/mL and the IV is correctly infusing at 50 gtt/min. After $2\frac{1}{2}$ hours, you find 300 mL remaining. Almost half of the total volume has already infused in about one-quarter the time. This IV infusion is ahead of schedule. You would compute a new flow rate of 300 mL to complete the IV fluid order in the remaining $7\frac{1}{2}$ hours. The patient would require close assessment for fluid overload.

Step 1.

$$\frac{\text{Remaining volume}}{\text{Remaining hours}} = \text{Recalculate mL/hr}$$

$$\frac{300\,\text{mL}}{7.5} = 40\,\text{mL/hr}$$

Step 2.

$$\frac{V}{T} \times C = \frac{40\,\text{mL}}{60\,\text{min}} \times 60\,\text{gtt/mL} = 40\,\text{gtt/min}$$

(adjusted flow rate)

Step 3.

$$\frac{\text{Adjusted gtt/min} - \text{Ordered gtt/min}}{\text{Ordered gtt/min}}$$

$$= \%\text{ of variation}$$

$$\frac{40 - 50}{50} = \frac{-10}{50} = -0.2 = -20\%$$

within the acceptable 25% of variation

Stop and Review

Compute the flow rate in drops per minute. Hospital policy permits recalculation of IVs when off schedule, with a maximum variation in rate of 25% for stable patients. Compute the % of variation.

1. Ordered:	2000 mL NS IV for 16 hr at 125 mL/hr
Drop factor:	15 gtt/mL
Original flow rate:	_____ gtt/min

After 6 hours, 650 mL of fluid have infused; explain your next action.

Solution remaining:	_____ mL
Time remaining:	_____ hr
Recalculated flow rate:	_____ mL/hr
Recalculated flow rate:	_____ gtt/min
Variation:	_____ %
Action:	_____
2. Ordered:	1000 mL D$_5$W IV for 10 hr at 100 mL/hr
Drop factor:	60 gtt/mL
Original flow rate:	_____ gtt/min

After 5 hours, 500 mL are remaining; explain your next action.

Time remaining:	_____ hr
Recalculated flow rate:	_____ mL/hr
Recalculated flow rate:	_____ gtt/min
Variation:	_____ %
Action:	_____
3. Ordered:	1000 mL NS IV for 8 hr at 125 mL/hr
Drop factor:	10 gtt/mL
Original flow rate:	_____ gtt/min

After 4 hours, 750 mL are remaining; describe your next action.

Time remaining:	_____ hr
Recalculated flow rate:	_____ mL/hr
Recalculated flow rate:	_____ gtt/min
Variation:	_____ %
Action:	_____
4. Ordered:	500 mL D_5 NS IV for 5 hr at 100 mL/hr
Drop factor:	20 gtt/mL
Original flow rate:	_____ gtt/min

After 2 hours, 250 mL are remaining; describe your next action.

Time remaining:	_____ hr
Recalculated flow rate:	_____ mL/hr
Recalculated flow rate:	_____ gtt/min
Variation:	_____ %
Action:	_____
5. Ordered:	1500 mL lactated Ringer's IV for 12 hr at 125 mL/hr
Drop factor:	20 gtt/mL
Original flow rate:	_____ gtt/min

After 6 hours, 850 mL are remaining; explain your next action.

Time remaining:	_____ hr
Recalculated flow rate:	_____ mL/hr
Recalculated flow rate:	_____ gtt/min
Variation:	_____ %
Action:	_____
6. Ordered:	1000 mL D$_5$W IV for 8 hr at 125 mL/hr
Drop factor:	20 gtt/mL
Original flow rate:	_____ gtt/min

After 4 hours, 800 mL are remaining; explain your next action.	
Time remaining:	_____ hr
Recalculated flow rate:	_____ mL/hr
Recalculated flow rate:	_____ gtt/min
Variation:	_____ %
Action:	_____
7. Ordered:	1 L NS IV for 20 hr at 50 mL/hr
Drop factor:	15 gtt/mL
Original flow rate:	_____ gtt/min
After 10 hours, 600 mL are remaining; explain your next action.	
Time remaining:	_____ hr
Recalculated flow rate:	_____ mL/hr
Recalculated flow rate:	_____ gtt/min
Variation:	_____ %
Action:	_____
8. Ordered:	1000 mL lactated Ringer's IV for 6 hr at 167 mL/hr
Drop factor:	15 gtt/mL

Original flow rate:	_____ gtt/min
After 4 hours, 360 mL are remaining; describe your next action.	
Time remaining:	_____ hr
Recalculated flow rate:	_____ mL/hr
Recalculated flow rate:	_____ gtt/min
Variation:	_____ %
Action:	_____

Flow Rates for Electronic Regulation

Intravenous fluids may be monitored electronically by an infusion device, which is known as a controller or pump. The indication of an electronic infusion device is determined by the need to strictly control the IV. Manufacturers provide special volumetric tubing that must be used with their infusion devices. This volumetric tubing ensures accurate, consistent IV infusions. Each device may be set for a specific flow rate and will set off an alarm if this rate is interrupted.

Controllers depend on gravity to maintain the desired flow rate by a compression and decompression mechanism that pinches the IV tubing, rather than forcing IV fluid into the system (**Figure 15-9**). They are often referred to as electronic flow clamps because they control the selected rate of infusion by either drop counting (drops per minute) or volumetric delivery (milliliters per hour).

Infusion pumps do not rely on gravity but maintain the flow by displacing fluid at the ordered rate. Resistance to flow within the system causes positive pressure in relation to the flow rate (**Figure 15-10**).

A syringe pump is a kind of electronic infusion pump. It is used to infuse fluids or medications directly from a syringe. It is most often used in pediatric patients when small volumes of medication are administered at very low rates. It is also used in anesthesia, labor and delivery, and in critical

Figure 15-9 Alaris® Dual Pump, a volumetric Infusion Controller/Pump.
Photo courtesy of Cardinal Health, 2008. All rights reserved.

Figure 15-10 Infusion pump.
Photo courtesy of Cardinal Health, 2008. All rights reserved.

care when the drug cannot be mixed with other solutions or medications (**Figure 15-11**).

When an electronic infusion regulator is used, the IV volume is ordered by the physician and programmed into the device by the nurse. These devices are controlled in mL/hr. Usually, the prescriber orders the IV volume to be delivered in mL/hr. If not, it must be calculated. To regulate an IV volume by

Figure 15-11 Syringe pump.
Courtesy of Smiths Medical.

electronic infusion pump or controller calibrated in mL/hr, you should use the following formula:

$$\frac{\text{Total mL ordered}}{\text{Total hr ordered}} = \text{mL/hr}$$

■ **EXAMPLE 16:**

Ordered: D₅W 250 mL IV over the next 2

hours by infusion pump

Use the formula:

$$\frac{\text{Total mL ordered}}{\text{Total hr ordered}} = \text{mL/hr}$$

$$\frac{250 \text{ mL}}{2 \text{ hr}} = 125 \text{ mL/1 hr}$$

Stop and Review

Calculate the flow rate that you will program the electronic infusion regulator for the following IV orders.

1. Ordered:	380 mL D₅ 0.45% NaCl in 9 hr by infusion pump
Flow rate:	_____ mL/hr
2. Ordered:	150 mL antibiotic in D₅W IV in 2 hr by infusion pump
Flow rate:	_____ mL/hr
3. Ordered:	100 mL NS IV PB in 30 min by infusion pump
Flow rate:	_____ mL/hr

4. Ordered:	750 mL D$_5$W IV in 5 hr by infusion pump
Flow rate:	_____ mL/hr
5. Ordered:	3 L NS IV in 24 hr by controller
Flow rate:	_____ mL/hr
6. Ordered:	1800 mL Normal Saline IV to infuse in 15 hr by controller
Flow rate:	_____ mL/hr
7. Ordered:	1.5 L D$_5$ NS IV in 12 hr by controller
Flow rate:	_____ mL/hr
8. Ordered:	2000 mL D$_5$W IV in 24 hr by controller
Flow rate:	_____ mL/hr

HEPARIN INTRAVENOUS CALCULATIONS

Heparin is commonly available in the 1000 unit (2 units per mL) strength shown in **Figure 15-12**, as well as other sizes. This label shows the drug name and its dosage strength clearly printed in blue.

When a specific strength of heparin is not available, it must be prepared from a variety of available dosage strengths. The following examples refer to **Figure 15-13**, which shows four different heparin labels.

■ **EXAMPLE 1:**

Using **Figure 15-13a**, determine how many mL are needed to add 20,000 units to an IV solution. Answer: _____

■ **EXAMPLE 2:**

Using **Figure 15-13b**, determine how many mL are needed to add 20,000 units to an IV solution. Answer: _____

Figure 15-12 Heparin Sodium 1000 units.
© Cengage Learning 2013

(a)   (b)

(c)   (d)

Figure 15-13
© Cengage Learning 2013

■ EXAMPLE 3:

Using **Figure 15-13c**, determine how many mL are needed to add 12,000 units to an IV solution. Answer: _____

■ EXAMPLE 4:

Using **Figure 15-13d**, determine how many mL are needed to add 10,000 units to an IV solution. Answer: _____

> ⬤⬤⬤ **Remember**
>
> The mL/hr flow rate for an EID is identical to the gtt/min flow rate for a microdrip.

Calculating IV Flow Rate from Units Per Hour Ordered

Heparin is usually ordered in units per hour to be administered via an electronic infusion device (EID). Therefore, calculating the flow rate in milliliters per hour (mL/hr) is usually required.

■ EXAMPLE 5:

Heparin is ordered at 800 units/hr. It is on hand as 20,000 units in 1000 mL D5W. What is the mL/hr flow rate?

$$\frac{mL}{hr} = \frac{1000\ mL}{20,000\ units}$$

Enter the next ratio, 800 units/hr, using units to match the denominator.

$$\frac{mL}{hr} = \frac{1000\ mL}{20,000\ units} \times \frac{800\ units}{1\ hr}$$

Cancel units to double-check, and do the math.

$$\frac{mL}{hr} = \frac{1000\ mL}{20,000} \times \frac{800}{1\ hr} = 40\ mL/hr$$

A rate of 40 mL/hr is needed to infuse 800 units/hr from a solution strength of 20,000 units in 1000 mL.

■ EXAMPLE 6:

Heparin is needed at 1100 units/hr from an available solution of 60,000 units in 1 L D5W. What is the flow rate in mL/hr?

$$\frac{mL}{hr} = \frac{1000\ mL}{60,000\ units} \times \frac{1100\ units}{1\ hr}$$

$$\frac{mL}{hr} = \frac{1000\ mL}{60,000} \times \frac{1100}{1\ hr} = 18.33\ \text{(which is rounded to 18 mL/hr)}$$

Therefore, a rate of 18 mL/hr is needed to infuse 1100 units per hour from a 60,000 units in 1 L solution.

■ EXAMPLE 7:

Heparin must be infused at 1000 units/hr from a solution of 10,000 units in 250 mL D5W. What is the flow rate in mL/hr?

Enter the mL/hr being calculated, and then locate the ratio containing mL (the 10,000 units/250 mL strength). This should be entered as the starting ratio with mL as the numerator, matching the mL numerator of units being calculated. Therefore, 10,000 units becomes the denominator.

$$\frac{mL}{hr} = \frac{250\ mL}{10,000\ units}$$

In the next numerator, the starting ratio denominator (units) must be matched. The rate ordered (1000 units/hr) is entered, with units as the numerator.

$$\frac{mL}{hr} = \frac{250\ mL}{10,000\ units} \times \frac{1000\ units}{1\ hr}$$

You then cancel alternate denominator/numerator units, leaving only the mL and hr. Do the math.

$$\frac{mL}{hr} = \frac{250 \; mL}{10,000} \times \frac{1000}{1 \; hr} = 25 \; mL/hr$$

A rate of 25 mL/hr is needed to infuse 1000 units/hr from a solution strength of 10,000 units in 250 mL.

Stop and Review

Calculate the IV flow rate in mL/hr in the following scenarios.

1. The order is for 1500 units per hour of heparin from an available strength of 40,000 units in 1 L. _____

2. The order is for 50,000 units of heparin in 1 L D5W to infuse at a rate of 2000 units per hour. _____

3. The order is for 800 units of heparin per hour from an available solution strength of 25,000 units in 500 mL NS. _____

4. The order is for 1200 units per hour from a D5W solution of 15,000 units in 1000 mL. _____

5. The order is for 2500 units per hour. The solution strength is 50,000 units in 1 L D5W. _____

Calculating Units Per Hour Infusing from IV Flow Rate

Another type of heparin calculation involves units/hr infusing from the mL/hr flow rate. You must use the units/mL solution strength and mL/hr rate of infusion.

■ EXAMPLE 8:

A 500 mL IV containing 20,000 units of heparin is running at 30 mL/hr. How many units/hr are being infused?

$$\frac{units}{hr} = \frac{20,000 \; units}{500 \; mL} \times \frac{30 \; mL}{1 \; hr}$$

$$\frac{units}{hr} = \frac{20,000 \; units}{500 \; mL} \times \frac{30 \; mL}{1 \; hr} = 1200 \; units/hr$$

Therefore, a 500 mL solution containing 20,000 units heparin running at 30 mL/hr is being infused at 1200 units/hr.

■ EXAMPLE 9:

A 1 L solution of D5W with 15,000 units of heparin is running at 60 mL/hr. How many units/hr are being infused?

$$\frac{units}{hr} = \frac{15,000\ units}{1000\ mL} \times \frac{60\ mL}{1\ hr}$$

$$\frac{units}{hr} = \frac{15,000\ units}{1000\ mL} \times \frac{60\ mL}{1\ hr} = 900\ units/hr$$

Therefore, a 1 L (1000 mL) solution containing 15,000 units heparin running at 60 mL/hr is being infused at 900 units/hr.

■ EXAMPLE 10:

A 500 mL IV of D5W containing 5000 units of heparin is running at 30 mL/hr. How many units/hr are being infused?

$$\frac{units}{hr} = \frac{5000\ units}{500\ mL} \times \frac{30\ mL}{1\ hr}$$

$$\frac{units}{hr} = \frac{5000\ units}{500\ mL} \times \frac{30\ mL}{1\ hr} = 300\ units/hr$$

Therefore, a 500 mL solution containing 5000 units heparin running at 30 mL/hr is being infused at 300 units/hr.

Stop and Review

Determine the following calculations for intravenous heparin using the information that is given.

1. A physician ordered an IV of 750 mL containing 30,000 units of heparin running at 25 mL/hr. _____

2. A physician ordered a solution of 20,000 units in 500 mL running at 30 mL/hr. _____

3. A 1 L DNS IV is needed, containing 30,000 units of heparin running at 40 mL/hr. _____

4. A 1 L DNS IV is needed, containing 20,000 units of heparin running at 30 mL/hr. _____

5. 25,000 units of heparin in a 500 mL solution must run at 30 mL/hr.

   _____

6. An IV containing 40,000 units of heparin in 1000 mL must run at 25 mL/hr. _____

7. A 1000 mL solution with 25,000 units heparin is running at 20 mL/hr.

   _____

8. A 1 L solution with 35,000 units heparin is running at 25 mL/hr.

   _____

9. An IV of 1 L DNS containing 20,000 units heparin is running at 20 mL/hr. _____

10. An IV of 1000 mL containing 40,000 units heparin is running at 35 mL/hr. _____

INTERMITTENT INTRAVENOUS INJECTIONS

Intermittent intravenous infusions, such as IV piggyback and IV push, are used for IV administration of drugs and supplemental fluid. Intermittent peripheral infusion devices, also known as saline or heparin locks, are used to maintain venous access without continuous fluid infusion. In the case of a patient needing to get supplemental fluid therapy or IV medications, but not needing continuous replacement or maintenance IV fluid, intermittent IV infusion systems are generally used. These systems include IV piggyback, IV locks for IV push drugs, or volume control sets (such as Bureterol).

IV Piggybacks (IVPB)

A medication may be prescribed to be dissolved in a small amount of IV fluid, for example, 50 to 100 mL, and run "piggyback" to the regular IV fluids. Recall that the piggyback IV (or secondary IV) requires a secondary IV set.

■ EXAMPLE 1:

Ordered: Kefzol 500 mg in 100 mL D_5W IV PB to run over 30 min

Drop factor: 20 gtt/mL

Determine the flow rate in gtt/min.

$$\frac{V}{T} \times C = \frac{100 \text{ mL}}{30 \text{ min}} \times 20 \text{ gtt/mL} = \frac{200 \text{ gtt}}{3}$$

$$= 66.7 \text{ gtt/min} \_ 67 \text{ gtt/min}$$

Saline and Heparin IV Locks for IV Push Drugs

IV locks are attached to the hub of the IV catheter that is situated in the vein. The lock is called a **saline lock**, meaning that saline is used to flush or maintain the IV catheter patency, or a **heparin lock** if heparin is used to maintain the IV catheter patency. Sometimes a more general term, such as **intermittent peripheral infusion device**, may be used. Medications can be given IV push, meaning that a syringe is attached to the lock and medication is pushed in. An **IV bolus**, usually a quantity of IV fluid, can be run in over a specified period of time through an IV setup that is attached to the lock.

In the majority of cases, it is easy to calculate mL/hr by dividing the total mL by the total hr. However, an IV with medication added or a piggyback IV may be prescribed to be injected in less than 1 hour by an electronic infusion device, but the pump or controller must still be set in mL /hr.

In this situation, the following formula can be used:

$$\frac{\text{Total mL ordered}}{\text{Total min ordered}} \times 60 \text{ min/hr} = \text{mL/hr}$$

■ EXAMPLE 2:

Ordered: Amoxicillin 500 mg IV in 50 mL D$_5$ $\frac{1}{2}$ NS in 30 min by controller. Use the following formula:

$$\frac{\text{Total mL ordered}}{\text{Total min ordered}} \times 60 \text{ min/hr} = \text{mL/hr}$$

$$\frac{50 \text{ mL}}{30 \text{ min}} \times \frac{60 \text{ min}}{1 \text{ h}} = 100 \text{ mL/h}$$

Test Your Knowledge

For the following questions, use the drop factor to calculate the flow rate in gtt/min.

1. Ordered:	*1000 mL of 0.45% NaCl IV at 200 mL/hr*
Drop factor:	10 gtt/mL
Flow rate:	_____ gtt/min
2. Ordered:	*1000 mL of 0.45% NaCl IV at 200 mL/hr*
Drop factor:	15 gtt/mL
Flow rate:	_____ gtt/min
3. Ordered:	*1000 mL of 0.45% NaCl IV at 200 mL/hr*
Drop factor:	20 gtt/mL
Flow rate:	_____ gtt/min

4. Ordered:	*1000 mL of 0.45% NaCl IV at 200 mL/hr*
Drop factor:	10 gtt/mL
Flow rate:	_____ gtt/min
5. Ordered:	*1000 mL of 0.45% NaCl IV at 200 mL/hr*
Drop factor:	15 gtt/mL
Flow rate:	_____ gtt/min
6. Ordered:	*1000 mL of 0.45% NaCl IV at 200 mL/hr*
Drop factor:	20 gtt/mL
Flow rate:	_____ gtt/min
7. Ordered:	*1000 mL of 0.45% NaCl IV at 200 mL/hr*
Drop factor:	60 gtt/mL
Flow rate:	_____ gtt/min
8. Ordered:	*1 L hyperalimentation solution IV to infuse in 12 hr*
Drop factor:	60 gtt/mL
Flow rate:	_____ gtt/min
9. Ordered:	*1 L hyperalimentation solution IV to infuse in 12 hr*
Drop factor:	15 gtt/mL
Flow rate:	_____ gtt/min
10. Ordered:	*1 L hyperalimentation solution IV to infuse in 12 hr*
Drop factor:	10 gtt/mL
Flow rate:	_____ gtt/min

11. Ordered:	*1 L hyperalimentation solution IV to infuse in 12 hr*
Drop factor:	20 gtt/mL
Flow rate:	_____ gtt/min
12. Ordered:	*2 L D$_5$ NS IV to infuse in 20 hr*
Drop factor:	20 gtt/mL
Flow rate:	_____ gtt/min
13. Ordered:	*2 L D$_5$ NS IV to infuse in 20 hr*
Drop factor:	60 gtt/mL
Flow rate:	_____ gtt/min
14. Ordered:	*2 L D$_5$ NS IV to infuse in 20 hr*
Drop factor:	10 gtt/mL
Flow rate:	_____ gtt/min
15. Ordered:	*2 L D$_5$ NS IV to infuse in 20 hr*
Drop factor:	15 gtt/mL
Flow rate:	_____ gtt/min

Complete the flow rate in drops per minute or milliliters per hour as requested. For these situations, hospital policy permits recalculating IVs when off schedule with a maximum variation in rate of 25%.

16. Ordered:	*1L D$_{10}$ W IV to run from 1000 to 1800*
Drop factor:	*On electronic infusion pump*
Flow rate:	_____ mL/hr

17. Ordered:	*1000 mL D₅W IV per 24 hr*
Drop factor:	60 gtt/mL
Flow rate:	_____ gtt/min
18. Ordered:	*1000 mL D₅W IV for 6 hr*
Drop factor:	15 gtt/mL
After 2 hours, 800 mL remain. Explain your next action. _____	
19. Ordered:	*2.5 L NS IV to infuse at 125 mL/hr*
Drop factor:	20 gtt/mL
Flow rate:	_____ gtt/min
20. Ordered:	*1500 mL D₅ LR IV to run for 12 hr*
Drop factor:	20 gtt/mL
Flow rate:	_____ gtt/min

The IV tubing package in the following figure is the IV system available in your stock for manually regulated, straight gravity flow IV administration with macrodrop. The patient has an order for 500 mL D₅W IV q4h written at 1515, and you start the IV at 1530. Questions 21 through 30 refer to this situation.

Primary I.V. Set.
Photography courtesy of Abbott Laboratories

21. How much IV fluid will the patient receive in 24 hours? _____

22. Who is the manufacturer of the IV infusion set tubing? _____

23. What is the drop factor calibration for the IV infusion set tubing? _____

24. What is the drop factor constant for the IV infusion set tubing? _____

25. Using the shortcut (drop factor constant) method, calculate the flow rate of the IV as ordered. Show your work.

    Shortcut method calculation: _____

    Flow rate: _____ gtt/min

26. Using the formula method, calculate the flow rate of the IV as ordered. Show your work.

    Formula method calculation: _____

    Flow rate: _____ gtt/min

27. At what time should you anticipate the first IV bag of 500 mL D_5W will be completely infused?

    _____

    _____

28. How much IV fluid should be infused by 1730? _____ mL

29. At 1730, you notice that the IV has 210 mL remaining. After assessing your patient and confirming that his condition is stable, what should you do?

    _____

    _____

30. After consulting the physician, you decide to use an electronic controller to better regulate the flow rate. The physician orders that the controller be set to infuse 500 mL every 4 hours. You should set the controller for _____ mL/hr.

Answer the following questions.

31. 100 mL of ampicillin in NS is to run over 30 minutes. What is the flow rate?

    _____

    _____

32. 1600 mL of NS must be administered over 10 hours. How many mL/hour should be given?

    _____

    _____

33. 2 L of D5W must be administered over 24 hours. The drop factor is 10 gtt/mL. How many drops per minute should be given?

_____

_____

34. 450 mL of fluid must run over 90 minutes using a tubing set to deliver 60 gtt/mL. How many drops per minute should be given?

_____

35. 50 mL of an antibiotic must run over 30 minutes with tubing calibrated to deliver 45 gtt/mL. How many drops per minute should be given?

_____

_____

36. D5 ½ NS is prescribed to run at 35 mL/hour with a drop factor of 60 gtt/mL. How many drops per minute should be given?

_____

_____

37. An IVPB of 500 mg ampicillin in 50 mL of fluid is prescribed to run at 50 gtt/minute. The drop factor is 60 gtt/mL. How long will the infusion take?

_____

_____

38. 2 L of D5LR must infuse over 12 hours at 42 gtt/minute. After 6 hours, 850 mL of fluid remained. The drop factor is 30 gtt/mL. At what rate must the IV be set to complete the infusion in the original 12 hours?

_____

_____

39. A manually regulated IV is using a standard microdrop set (60 gtt/mL). How long will it take to infuse 150 mL of fluid to run at 30 gtt/minute?

_____

_____

40. 1 L of D5W was ordered to infuse over 6 hours by infusion pump. What is the flow rate?

_____

_____

41. 1600 mL of D5 $\frac{1}{2}$ NS was ordered to infuse over 24 hours. What is the flow rate?

_____

_____

42. 1500 mL of D5W was prescribed to be infused over 6 hours. With an IV set that delivers 10 gtt/mL, how many drops per minute should be infused?

_____

_____

43. 80 mL of an IVPB must run over 20 minutes with tubing calibrated to infuse 40 gtt/mL. How many drops per minute should be infused?

_____

_____

44. 600 mL of D5W must be given to a patient, running at 30 gtt/minute. The drop factor of the tubing is 60 gtt/mL. How long will the infusion take?

_____

_____

45. Lidocaine (2 grams) was prescribed in 500 mL of fluid at 2 mg/minute, to be administered via an infusion pump. What is the flow rate?

_____

_____

46. A physician ordered a medication (40 mg) in 500 mL of fluid at 1 mg/minute. What is the flow rate in milliliters per hour?

_____

_____

47. A prescriber ordered Pentids 600,000 units in 100 mL. IVPB is to infuse over 1 hour by infusion pump, to deliver 15 gtt/mL. Calculate the flow rate in drops per minute.

_____

_____

48. 1 L of NS must infuse over 6 hours using tubing calibrated to deliver 20 gtt/mL. How many drops per minute should be infused?

_____

_____

49. A physician ordered 150 mL of an antibiotic to infuse over 30 minutes by an infusion pump. Calculate the flow rate.

_____

_____

50. D5W must run at 150 mL/hour with a drop factor of 10 gtt/mL. Calculate how many drops per minute will be infused.

_____

_____

51. A 1000 mL solution containing 45,000 units of heparin must run at 25 mL/hr.

_____

CHAPTER 16

Pediatric Drug Administration

OBJECTIVES

Upon completion of this chapter, you should be able to:

1. Convert pounds to kilograms.
2. Use the two primary methods to calculate pediatric drug dosages.
3. Compare the ordered dosage with the recommended safe dosage.
4. Identify the steps in calculating body surface area from a pediatric nomogram and with the square root method.
5. Determine whether the ordered dosage is safe to administer.
6. Explain the dosage inaccuracies that can occur with pediatric drug formulas.

GLOSSARY

body surface area (BSA) – Calculated by using a graph that consists of weight and height variables called a nomogram. It is expressed as meters squared (m^2).

hypertonic solution – Used to maintain daily fluid needs; is generally a combination of saline, glucose, and potassium chloride.

nomogram – A quick reference graph for calculating pediatric doses.

safe-dosage range – Varying amounts of a drug that can be taken in a single dose and still have therapeutic value.

52. 25,000 units of heparin in a 1000 mL solution must run at 30 mL/hr.

_____

53. A 1 L solution containing 35,000 units of heparin must run at 45 mL/hr.

_____

54. A 500 mL solution containing 20,000 units of heparin must run at 20 mL/hr.

_____

55. A solution of 1 L containing 25,000 units of heparin must run at 30 mL/hr.

_____

56. A solution of 1 L of D5W containing 30,000 units of heparin must run at 50 mL/hr.

_____

57. Heparin 2000 units per hour is to be infused using a solution strength of 20,000 units in 500 mL.

_____

58. A solution of 35,000 units of heparin in 1 L D5W is to infuse via a volumetric pump at 1200 units/hour.

_____

Critical Thinking

An elderly patient who had pneumonia was prescribed Rocephin 1 g IV q12h by her physician. The medication, which utilized a new dispensing system, was delivered by the pharmacy technician to the hospital unit. 1 g of Rocephin was supplied as a powder attached to a 50 mL IV bag of 5% dextrose in water. The nurse hung the IV medication and infused the solution. Three days later, another nurse discovered that the Rocephin powder was still in the vial, and that the vial stopper had never been opened. The powder had not been mixed into the IV fluid during this entire period. The nurse who made the error had never worked with this new dispensing system and did not ask for instructions either from the pharmacy technician or another nurse. The pharmacy technician did not include the dispensing instructions or explain the dispensing procedure to the nurse.

1. As a result of this situation, what could possibly happen to the patient's pneumonia?

_____

2. What effects might this omission have on the patient's condition?

_____

OVERVIEW

Administration of medications to children requires special attention and care because of their size and the way they metabolize drugs. Pharmacy technicians must understand calculations used for pediatric dosages. Accuracy is essential in all calculations. The calculations performed by the pharmacy technician must be supervised by a pharmacist. Pharmacists have ultimate legal responsibility for all pediatric dosages.

Children of different ages respond to medications differently. For example, many organ systems in newborns, infants, and toddlers are varied. Metabolism of medications in these groups compared with an adult dose will be completely different. Therefore, variations for children are so significant that no foolproof formula exists to determine the dosage of medications that a child should receive.

CALCULATING PEDIATRIC DOSAGES

Pharmacists must be skillful in more advanced calculations for pediatric dosages. While pharmacy technicians must have an understanding of how this is done, pediatric dosing is actually regulated by law to pharmacists. The two main methods currently used for calculating safe pediatric dosages are body weight (such as mg/kg), and body surface area (BSA). The first method uses a specific number of milligrams, micrograms, or units for each kilogram of body weight. Usually, drug data for pediatric dosage (mg/kg) are supplied by manufacturers in a drug information insert. BSA, measured in square meters (m^2), is considered a more accurate method than body weight. BSA takes into consideration the relationship between basal metabolic rate and surface area. BSA has primarily been used to calculate the dosage of antineoplastic agents (which are used in chemotherapy). Manufacturers are beginning to include BSA parameters (mg/m^2, mcg/m^2, $units/m^2$) in drug information.

Body Weight Dosage Calculations

Standard adult dosages are determined by the drug manufacturer. Formulas must be provided for pediatric doses if the drug is intended to be given to children. Pediatric dose formulas are particularly important because dosage is usually recommended based on the requirements of an average-weight adult.

Dosages for newborns, infants, and children are based on their unique and changing body differences. Prescribers must consider the weight, height, body surface, age, and condition of the child as contributing factors to safe and effective drug dosages. The body weight method is more common in pediatric situations. Remember that both the body weight and BSA methods are also used for adults, especially in critical care situations, and the calculations are the same.

To calculate the amount of drug based on the child's body weight in kilograms, it is necessary to compare the child's ordered dosage to the recommended safe dosage from a reputable drug resource before administering the medication. During calculation and verification for safe pediatric dosages, follow these steps:

1. Convert the child's weight from pounds to kilograms.

2. Calculate the safe dosage in mg/kg or mcg/kg for a child of this weight, as recommended by a reputable drug reference: multiply mg/kg by the child's weight in kg (e.g., 1 kg = 2.2 lb or 1 g = 1000 mg).

3. Decide if the dosage is safe by comparing ordered and recommended dosages.

4. Calculate one dose.

5. Compare the prepared dosage to the ordered dosage and the recommended dosage, and have the pharmacist decide if the dosage is safe.

Note: The dosage per kg may be mg/kg, g/kg, mEq/kg, units/kg, milliunits/kg, and so forth.

■ EXAMPLE 1:

The physician orders morphine sulfate 1.8 mg IM stat. The child weighs 79 lb. Is this dosage safe? First, convert pounds to kilograms.

$$79 \text{ lb} = 79 = 2.2 \div 35.90 \text{ kg} = 35.9 \text{ kg}$$

Next, calculate the milligrams per kilogram as recommend by a reputable drug source. A reputable drug source indicates that the usual IM/SC dosage may be initiated at 0.05 mg/kg/dose.

Decide if the dosage ordered is safe. For this child's weight, 1.8 mg is the recommended dosage and 1.8 is the ordered dosage. This dosage is safe.

Calculate the dose.

Morphine 5mg/mL.
© Cengage Learning 2013

Ordered: *morphine sulfate 1.8 mg IM stat*

On hand: morphine sulfate 5 mg/mL

Administer:

$$\frac{D}{H} \times Q = \frac{1.8 \text{ mg}}{5 \text{ mg}} \times 1 \text{ mL} = 0.36 \text{ mL}$$

Or, apply the ratio and proportion method:

5 mg : X mL : : 1.8 mg : 1 mL

$$\frac{5\,mg}{1\,mL} = \frac{1.8\,mg}{X\,mL}$$

$$5X = 1.8$$

$$X = 0.36\,mL$$

This is a small child's dose. Measure 0.36 mL in a 1 mL syringe. Route is IM. The needle may need to be changed.

0.36 mL

© Cengage Learning 2013

Single-Dosage Ranges

Single-dosage drugs are intended to be given once or prn. Dosage ordered by the body weight method is based on mg/kg/dose and is calculated by multiplying the recommended mg by the patient's kg weight for each dose. Some single-dosage medications indicate a minimum and maximum range, or a *safe-dosage range*.

■ EXAMPLE 2:

The physician orders *Vistaril 20 mg IM q4–6h, p.r.n., nausea*. The child weighs 44 lb. Is this a safe dosage?

1. Convert lb to kg.

$$44\,lb = 44 \div 2.2 = 20\,kg$$

Vistaril 50 mg/mL.
Label reproduced with permisison of Pfizer, Inc.

Calculate the recommended dosage. A reputable drug resource indicates that the usual IM dosage is 0.5 mg to 1 mg/kg/dose every 4 to 6 hours as needed.

Calculate the minimum and maximum safe dosage range.

Minimum per dose: 0.5 mg/kg/dose × 20 mg = 10 mg/dose

Maximum per dose: 1 mg/kg/dose × 20 kg = 20 mg/dose

2. Decide if the ordered dosage is safe. The recommended dosage is 10 mg to 20 mg, and the ordered dosage of 20 mg is within this range. Yes, the ordered dosage is safe.

3. Calculate one dose. Apply the three steps of dosage calculation.

Ordered: *Vistaril 20 mg IM q4–6h p.r.n., nausea*

On hand: Vistaril 50 mg/mL

$$\frac{D}{H} \times Q \quad \frac{20\,mg}{50\,mg} \times 1\,mL = \frac{2}{5}\,ML = 0.4\,mL$$

Or, apply the ratio and proportion method.

$$\frac{50\,mg}{1\,mL} = \frac{20\,mg}{X\,mL}$$

$$50X = 20$$

$$\frac{50X}{50} = \frac{20}{50}$$

$$X = 0.4\,mL$$

This is a small child's dose. Measure it in a 1 mL syringe. Route is IM. The needle may need to be changed.

0.4 mL

© *Cengage Learning 2013*

Stop and Review
Calculate one safe pediatric dose.

1. Ordered:	*Keflex 125 mg p.o. q6h for a child who weighs 44 lb.* The recommended pediatric dosage of Keflex (cephalexin) is 25–50 mg/kg/day in 4 equally divided doses.	
Child's weight:	_____ kg	
Recommended minimum daily dosage for this child:	_____ mg/day	
Recommended minimum single dosage for this child:	_____ mg/dose	
Recommended maximum daily dosage for this child:	_____ mg/day	
Recommended maximum single dosage for this child:	_____ mg/dose	
Is the dosage in the recommended range for a healthy child?	_____	

2. Keflex is available in a suspension of 125 mg per 5 mL. If the dosage ordered in question 1a is safe, give _____ mL.

3. Ordered:	*Chloromycetin 55 mg IV q12h for an 8-day-old newborn who weighs 2200 g. The recommended dosage of Chloromycetin (chloramphenicol) for neonates less than 2 kg is 25 mg/kg once daily; and for neonates more than 2 kg and over 7 days of age, the recommended dosage is 50 mg/kg/day divided q12h.*
Child's weight:	_____ kg
Recommended daily dosage for this child:	_____ mg/day
Recommended single dosage for this child:	_____ mg/dose
Is the ordered dosage safe?	

4. Chloramphenicol is available as a solution for injection of 1 g per 10 mL. If the dosage ordered in question 1c is safe, how much should be given?

_____

5. Ordered:	*Suprax 120 mg p.o. q.d. for a child who weighs 33 lb.*
	The recommended dosage of Suprax (cefixime) for children under 50 kg is 8 mg/kg p.o. once daily or 4 mg/kg q12h.
Child's weight:	_____ kg
Recommended single dosage for this child:	_____ mg/dose
Is the ordered dosage safe?	_____

6. Suprax is available as a suspension of 100 mg per 5 mL in a 50 mL bottle. If the dosage ordered in question 1e is safe, give _____ mL.

How many doses are available in the bottle of Suprax? _____ dose(s)

The labels provided represent the drugs available to answer questions 7 through 13. Verify safe dosage, indicate the amount to give, and draw an arrow on the accompanying measuring device. Explain unsafe dosages and describe the appropriate action to take.

7. Ordered:	*Nebcin 8 mg IM q6h for an infant who weighs 5000 g. The recommended pediatric dosage of Nebcin (tobramycin) is 2–2.5 mg/kg q8h or 1.5–1.9 mg/kg q6h.*
Infant's weight:	_____ kg
Recommended minimum single dosage for this infant:	_____ mg/dose
Recommended maximum single dosage for this infant:	_____ mg/dose
Is the dosage ordered safe?	_____

NDC 00000-0000-00
2 mL VIAL
PEDIATRIC ℞
TOBRAMYCIN
INJECTION, USP
20 mg
per
2 mL
Multiple Dose
For I.M. or I.V. Use
Must dilute for I.V. use
Lot:
Exp. Date:
DCL DELMAR | Cengage Learning
For Educational Purposes Only
00000-0000-00

Nebcin Pediatric 20 mg.
© Cengage Learning 2013

8. If the dosage ordered in question 2a is safe, give _____ mL.

½   1   1½   ②   2½   3 mL

© Cengage Learning 2013

9. Ordered:	*gentamicin 40 mg IV q8h for a premature neonate who is 5 days old and weighs 1800 g.* The recommended dosage of gentamicin for children is 2–2.5 mg/kg q8h; for neonates, it is 2.5 mg/kg q8h; and for premature neonates less than 1 week of age, it is 2.5 mg/kg q12h.
Neonate's weight:	_____ kg
Recommended single dosage for this neonate:	_____ mg/dose
Is the dosage ordered safe?	_____

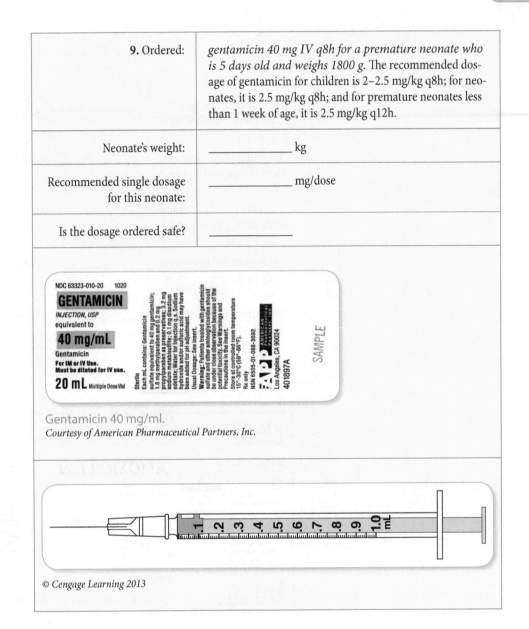

Gentamicin 40 mg/ml.
Courtesy of American Pharmaceutical Partners, Inc.

© Cengage Learning 2013

10. Ordered:	Amoxil oral suspension 100 mg p.o. q8h for a child who weighs 39 lb.
Recommended dosage: See the label. Child's weight:	_____ kg
Recommended minimum daily dosage for this child:	_____ mg/day
Recommended minimum single dosage for this child:	_____ mg/dose
Recommended maximum daily dosage for this child:	_____ mg/day
Recommended maximum single dosage for this child:	_____ mg/dose
Is the ordered dosage safe?	_____

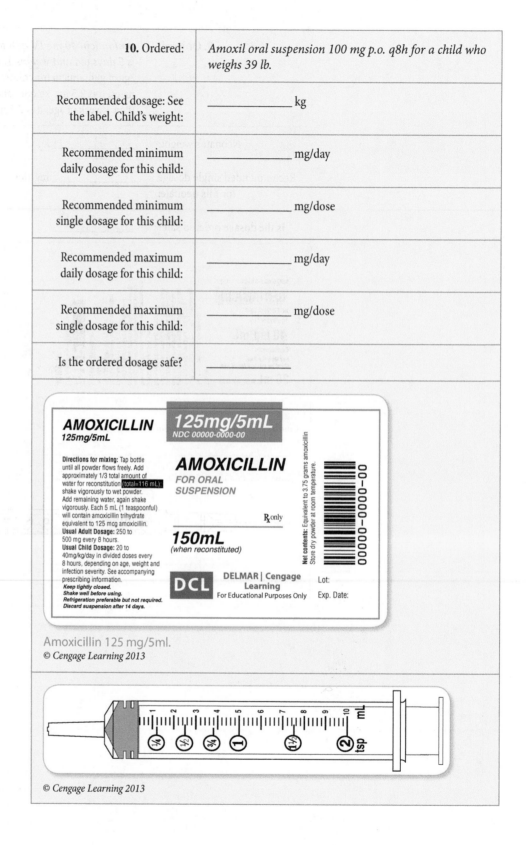

AMOXICILLIN
125mg/5mL

125mg/5mL
NDC 00000-0000-00

Directions for mixing: Tap bottle until all powder flows freely. Add approximately 1/3 total amount of water for reconstitution (total=116 mL): shake vigorously to wet powder. Add remaining water, again shake vigorously. Each 5 mL (1 teaspoonful) will contain amoxicillin trihydrate equivalent to 125 mcg amoxicillin.
Usual Adult Dosage: 250 to 500 mg every 8 hours.
Usual Child Dosage: 20 to 40mg/kg/day in divided doses every 8 hours, depending on age, weight and infection severity. See accompanying prescribing information.
Keep tightly closed.
Shake well before using.
Refrigeration preferable but not required.
Discard suspension after 14 days.

AMOXICILLIN
FOR ORAL
SUSPENSION

R only

150mL
(when reconstituted)

DCL   DELMAR | Cengage
Learning
For Educational Purposes Only

Lot:
Exp. Date:

Net contents: Equivalent to 3.75 grams amoxicillin Store dry powder at room temperature.

00000-0000-00

Amoxicillin 125 mg/5ml.
© Cengage Learning 2013

© Cengage Learning 2013

11. Ordered:	*Bactrim Pediatric Suspension 7.5 mL p.o. q12h for a child who weighs 15 kg and has a urinary tract infection. The recommended dosage of Bactrim (trimethoprim and sulfamethoxazole) for such infections in children is based on the trimethoprim at 8 mg/kg/day in 2 equal doses.*
Recommended daily trimethoprim dosage for this child:	_____ mg/day
Recommended single trimethoprim dosage for this child:	_____ mg/dose
Recommended single dose for this child:	_____ mL/dose
Is the ordered dose safe?	_____

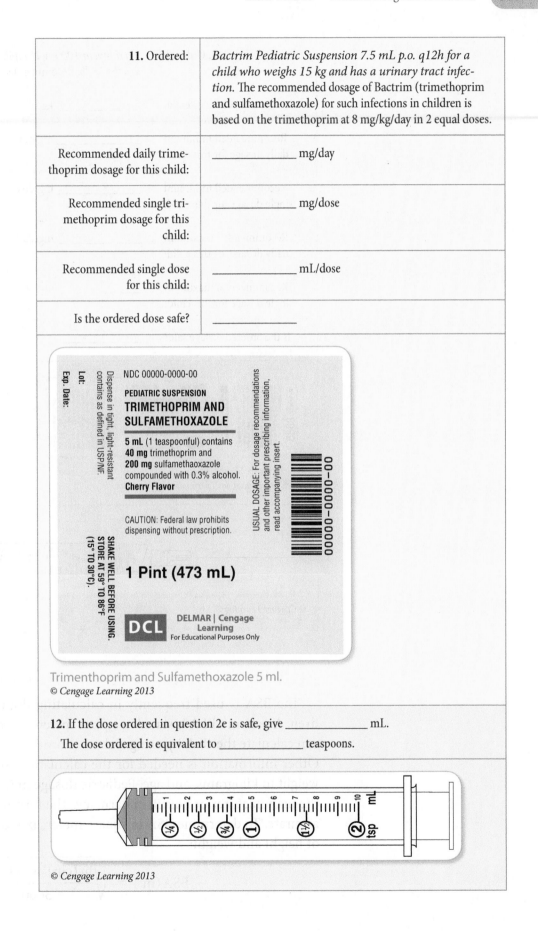

Trimenthoprim and Sulfamethoxazole 5 ml.
© Cengage Learning 2013

12. If the dose ordered in question 2e is safe, give _____ mL.

The dose ordered is equivalent to _____ teaspoons.

© Cengage Learning 2013

13. Ordered:	*Terramycin 100 mg IM q8h for a 9-year-old child who weighs 55 lb.* Recommended pediatric dosage: see the label.
Child's weight:	_____ kg
Recommended minimum daily dosage for this child:	_____ mg/day
Recommended minimum single dosage for this child:	_____ mg/dose
Recommended maximum daily dosage for this child:	_____ mg/day
Recommended maximum single dosage for this child:	_____ mg/dose
Is the ordered dosage safe?	_____

Terramycin 50 mg/ml.

Labels reproduced with permision of Pfizer, Inc.

© Cengage Learning 2013

Body Surface Area (BSA) Dosage Calculations

The BSA is used frequently in calculating dosages for infants and children. A patient's BSA is stated in square meters, or m². Pharmacy technicians can calculate the BSA by using a chart (nomogram) or formula calculation. Other information is needed for the calculation, such as the child's height, weight in kilograms, and age. Pediatric dosage in (square meters) is listed by the manufacturer or hospital pharmacy. The formula calculation is the most accurate. To determine BSA in square meters based on metric measurement of height and weight:

$$\text{BSA (m}^2) = \sqrt{\frac{\text{ht (cm)} \times \text{wt (kg)}}{3600}}$$

This formula may also be expressed as follows:

BSA = The square root of:

The patient's weight (in kilograms) multiplied by his or her height (in centimeters)

Divided by 3600

■ EXAMPLE 3:

Use the metric formula to determine the BSA for a child whose height is 85 cm and weight is 13.9 kg (note that square meters is signified by m^2):

$$BSA = \sqrt{\frac{85 \times 13.9}{3600}} \, m^2$$

$$\sqrt{\frac{1181.5}{3600}} \, m^2$$

$$= 0.573 \, m^2 = 0.57 \, m^2$$

■ EXAMPLE 4:

Calculate the BSA of a child who stands 98.4 cm and weighs 17.17 kg.

You need to find the square root of:

$$17.17 \times 98.4, \text{ divided by } 3600$$

Therefore,

$$\text{The square root of } 0.47 =$$

$$0.685 = 0.69 \, m^2 \text{ (rounded to hundredths)}$$

To calculate BSA in m^2 based on household measurement of height and weight:

$$BSA(m^2) = \sqrt{\frac{ht(in) \times wt(lb)}{3131}}$$

This formula may also be expressed as follows:

BSA = The square root of:

The patient's weight in pounds multiplied by his or her height in inches

Divided by 3131

■ EXAMPLE 5:

Calculate the BSA for a baby whose height is 24 in. and weight is 12.2 lb.

$$BSA = \sqrt{\frac{24 \times 12.2}{3131}} \, m^2$$

$$\sqrt{\frac{292.8}{3131}}\ m^2$$

$$= 0.306\ m^2 = 0.31\ m^2$$

■ **EXAMPLE 6:**

A child is 25 inches tall and weighs 35 pounds. What is his BSA?

You need to find the square root of:

35 pounds $\times$ 25 inches, divided by 3131

Therefore,

The square root of 0.28 =

0.529 = 0.53 m² (rounded to hundredths)

■ **EXAMPLE 7:**

A child weighs 95 lbs and stands 49 inches in height. What is her BSA?

You need to find the square root of:

95 $\times$ 49, divided by 3131

Therefore,

The square root of 1.49 =

1.220 = 1.22 m² (rounded to hundredths)

Nomogram

When practitioners use a chart to estimate the BSA by plotting the height and weight and then connect the dots with a straight line, it is called a nomogram (**Figure 16-1**). Use a nomogram for determining the BSA for a child who has a normal height and weight. For a child who is underweight or overweight, the surface area is indicated by a straight line connecting the height and weight, intersecting the surface area (SA) column. This chart can be used for both children and adults for heights up to 240 cm (95 in.) and weights up to 80 kg (180 lb).

West's nomogram uses a calculation of the body surface area of infants and young children to determine the pediatric dose. The nomogram is used as a quick reference for pediatric doses. To use the nomogram, you need a straightedge ruler. Place one end of the ruler on the patient's height (either centimeters or inches) and the other edge on the weight (either kilograms or pounds). Draw a line to connect these two points; the meter-squared number is where the line intersects on the line labeled meters squared (m²). Write this number down.

Figure 16-1 Nomogram for calculating body surface area.

From Nelson Texbook of Pediatrics *(16th ed.), by R.E. Behrman, R.M. Kliegman, and H.B. Jenson, 2000, Philadelphia: W.B. Saunders Company. Reprinted with permission.*

For pediatric doses, you can use the following formula:

$$\text{Pediatric dose} = \frac{\text{Body surface area (BSA) of child in m}^2}{1.7\,\text{m}^2\,\text{(average adult BSA)}} \times \text{Adult dose}$$

Stop and Review

Use the appropriate formula to determine the BSA.

1. A child's height is 88 cm and her weight is 13.2 kg.

   _____

2. A child measures 94 cm in height and weighs 18 kg.

   _____

3. A child measures 26 in. tall and weighs 21 lb.

   _____

4. A child measures 65 cm tall and weighs 15 kg.

   _____

5. A child measures 92 cm tall and weighs 24 kg.

   _____

6. A teenager measures 135 cm tall and weighs 46 kg.

   _____

7. A child measures 43 in. tall and weighs 35 lb.

   _____

Find the BSA on the West nomogram (see **Figure 16-1**) for children with the following height and weight.

8. 21 in. and 81 lb _____ m²

9. 106 cm and 25 kg _____ m²

10. 41 in. and 32 lb _____ m²

11. 80 cm and 11 kg _____ m²

12. 140 cm and 30 kg _____ m²

13. 34 in. and 28 lb _____ m²

14. 122 cm and 32 kg _____ m²

15. 38 in. and 31 lb _____ m²

Clark's Rule

The use of Clark's rule to calculate pediatric dosages is much more accurate than other pediatric methods. It is based on a child's weight and uses 150 lb (70 kg) as the average adult weight, while assuming that a child's dose is proportionately less. Calculate as follows:

$$\text{Pediatric dose} = \frac{\text{Child's weight in pounds}}{150 \text{ pounds}} \times \text{Adult dose}$$

■ EXAMPLE 8:

Find the dose of cortisone for a 45 lb infant (adult dose = 100 mg).

$$\frac{45}{150} \times 100 \text{ mg} = 30 \text{ mg}$$

NOTE: The use of Clark's rule, Young's rule, and Fried's rule has declined because of the use of nomograms and body surface area. However, it is still important for health professionals to understand the rules' concepts.

> **⫸ Remember**
>
> **Three steps are used to calculate pediatric drug dosages:**
>
> **Step 1: Convert pounds to kilograms, and then cross-multiply the ratio and round to the nearest whole number.**
>
> **Step 2: Calculate the drug dosage based on milligrams per kilogram of body weight and cross-multiply the ratio.**
>
> **Step 3: Calculate how much medication the patient would then receive based on the total amount allowed per day, divided into the proper amount of administrations per day.**

Young's Rule

Young's rule is used for children who are older than 1 year of age. Calculate as follows:

$$\text{Pediatric dose} = \frac{\text{Child's age in years} \times \text{adult dose}}{\text{Child's age in years} + 12}$$

■ EXAMPLE 9:

How much acetaminophen is the acceptable dosage for a 5-year-old child if the adult dose normally equals 1000 mg?

$$\frac{5 \text{ (years)} \times 1000}{5 \text{ (years)} + 12} = \frac{5000}{17} = 294 \text{ mg}$$

Young's rule is not valid for children who are older than 12 years of age. If a child over 12 is still small enough in size to require a reduced dose, Clark's rule should be used to calculate the proper amount.

Fried's Rule

Fried's rule helps to estimate correct medication dosages for infants who are younger than 1 year of age. Calculate as follows:

$$\frac{\text{Age in months}}{150} \times \text{average adult dose} = \text{child's dose}$$

■ **EXAMPLE 10:**

Find the dose of phenobarbital for an 11-month-old infant if the adult dose = 400 mg.

$$\frac{11}{150} \times 400\,mg = 29\,mg$$

INTRAMUSCULAR DRUGS

The amount of medication to be administered in pediatric patients requires the pharmacy technician to consider the age and the size of the child. To be precise in calculating injection amounts, round the amount of the drug calculation to the nearest hundredth. When a pharmacy technician calculates dosages for pediatric injections, he or she uses the same method used for adults. The maximum volume of "intramuscular injections" for infants is 0.5–1 mL and for children more than 1 year old, it is 1 mL. For preschoolers and elementary school-age children, the amount is 1–1.5 mL.

■ **EXAMPLE 1:**

Ordered: *Zinacef 50 mg/kg/day IM q6h*

On hand: Zinacef 750 mg for injection

Find the amount to administer.

According to the package insert, Zinacef may be administered to pediatric patients above 3 months of age at the rate of 50–100 mg/kg/day in divided doses every 6 to 8 hours.

$$1\,kg : 2.2\,lb : : ?\,kg : 44\,lb$$

$$\frac{1\,kg}{2.2\,lb} = \frac{X\,kg}{44\,lb}$$

$$44 = 2.2X$$

$$X = 20\,kg$$

Now, find the daily dosage.

$$\frac{50\,mg}{1\,kg} \times 20\,kg = \frac{50}{1} \times 20 = 1000\,mg$$

$$1000 \div 4 = 250\,mg\ \text{each dose}$$

After reconstitution, the Zinacef has a dosage strength of 220 mg/mL. To find the amount to administer for each dose:

$$250\,mg \times \frac{1\,mL}{220\,mg} = 250 \times \frac{1}{220} = 1.14\,mL$$

INTRAVENOUS DRUGS

According to the size and age of children, the amount of medication to administer for intravenous drugs compared with adults is smaller. Volume control sets (**Figure 16-2**) are most commonly used to administer hourly fluids and intermittent IV medications to children. The fluid chamber will hold 100 mL to 150 mL of fluid to be infused in a specified time period as ordered, for example, for 60 minutes or less. The medication is added to the IV fluid in the chamber for a prescribed dilution volume. The IV bag acts only as a reservoir to hold future fluid infusions and the nurse can fill the chamber for 1 to 2 hours. If more fluid infusions are needed, then the nurse can add to the amount. Only small, ordered quantities of fluid can be added, and the clamp above the chamber is fully closed.

Figure 16-2 Volume control set.
© *Cengage Learning 2013*

Intermittent IV Drug Infusion Using a Volume Control Set

In place of a continuous IV infusion, children receiving IVs may receive them via means of a saline or heparin lock. Medication is injected into the volume control set chamber, and then an appropriate volume of IV fluid (to dilute the drug) is added. Then the IV tubing is attached to the child's IV lock to infuse over a specified amount of time. Once the chamber is empty and all the medication is infused, a flush of IV fluid is used to make sure that all the medication has cleared out of the tubing. Once the chamber empties, remember that some medication remains in the drip chamber, IV tubing, and the IV lock (all above the height of the child's vein). Peripheral or central IV lines are not flushed with any standard amount of fluid. Manufacturers of IV tubing all have slight differences in their products, so the flush can vary from 15 mL to 50 mL, according to the tubing's overall length and any extra extensions added. It is necessary to verify hospital policy as to the correct volume to flush central and peripheral IV lines in children. For the examples in this text, 15 mL is used as the volume to flush a peripheral IV line unless otherwise specified.

In calculating the IV flow rate for the volume control set, consider the total fluid volume of the medication, the IV fluid used for diluting, and the volume of IV flush fluid. Volume control sets are microdrip sets that use a drop factor of 60 gtt/mL. Note that, usually, nurses are responsible for calculating flow rates or setting up equipment.

■ **EXAMPLE 1:**

Ordered: *Claforan 250 mg IV q6h in 50 mL D5 $\frac{1}{4}$ NS to infuse in 30 min followed by a 15 mL flush. Child has a saline lock.*

On hand: See the label.

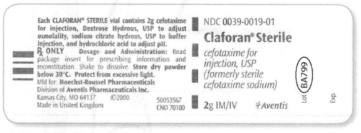

Claforan® Sterile.
Courtesy of Aventis Pharmaceuticals, Inc.

Instructions from the package insert for IV use are the following: Add 10 mL diluent for a total volume of 11 mL with a concentration of 180 mg/mL.

Step 1   Calculate the total volume of the intermittent IV flush: 50 mL + 15 mL = 65 mL

Step 2   Calculate the flow rate of the IV medication and the IV flush. Remember: The drop factor is 60 gtt/mL.

$$\frac{V}{T} \times C = \frac{65\,mL}{30\,min} \times 60\,gtt/mL$$

$$= \frac{65\,mL}{1\,min} \times \frac{2\,gtt}{1\,mL} = 130\,gtt/min$$

Step 3   Calculate the volume of the medication to be administered.

$$\frac{D}{H} \times Q = \frac{250\,mg}{180\,mg} \times 1\,mL = 1.39\,mL = 1.4\,mL$$

Step 4   Add 1.4 mL Claforan 2 g to the chamber and fill with IV fluid to a volume of 50 mL. This provides the prescribed total volume of 50 mL in the chamber.

Step 5   Set the flow rate of the 50 mL of intermittent IV medication for 130 gtt/min. Follow with the 15 mL flush also set at 130 gtt/min. When complete, detach the IV tubing and follow the saline lock policy.

■ EXAMPLE 2:

Ordered: *D5NS IV at 30 mL/hr for continuous infusion and gentamicin 30 mg IV q8h over 30 min*

On hand: See the label.

An infusion controller is in use with the volume control set.

Gentamicin 40 mg/ml.
Courtesy of American Pharmaceutical Partners, Inc.

Step 1   Calculate the dilution volume required to administer the gentamicin at the prescribed continuous flow rate of 30 mL/hr.

Calculate   Use ratio and proportion to verify your estimate.

$$\frac{30\,mL}{60\,min} = \frac{X\,mL}{30\,min}$$

$$60X = 900$$

$$\frac{60X}{60} = \frac{900}{60}$$

$$X = 15\,mL\ in\ 30\,min$$

Therefore, the IV fluid dilution volume required to administer 30 mg of gentamicin in 30 minutes is 15 mL to maintain the prescribed, continuous infusion rate of 30 mL/hr.

Step 2   Determine the volume of gentamicin and IV fluid to add to the volume control chamber.

$$\frac{D}{H} \times Q = \frac{30\,mg}{40\,mg} \times 1\,mL = \frac{3}{4}\,mL = 0.75\,mL$$

Add 0.75 mL gentamicin and fill the chamber with D5 NS to the total volume of 15 mL.

Step 3   Set the controller to 30 mL/hr to deliver 15 mL of intermittent IV gentamicin solution in 30 minutes. Resume the regular IV, which will also flush out the tubing. The continuous flow rate will remain at 30 mL/hr.

Stop and Review

Calculate the amount of IV fluid to be added to the volume control chamber.

1. Ordered:	*D5 0.33% NaCl IV at 66 mL/hr with Fortaz 720 mg IV q8h to be infused over 40 min by volume control set*
On hand:	Fortaz 1 g/10 mL
Add _____ mL medication and _____ mL IV fluid to the chamber.	
2. Ordered:	*D5W at 30 mL/hr for continuous infusion with medication × 60 mg q6h to be infused over 20 min by volume control set*
On hand:	Medication × 60 mg/2 mL
Add _____ mL medication and _____ mL IV fluid to the chamber.	
3. Ordered:	*D5 0.45% NaCl IV at 48 mL/hr with Vibramycin 75 mg IV q12h to be infused over 2 hr volume control set*
On hand:	Vibramycin 100 mg/10 mL
Add _____ mL medication and _____ mL IV fluid to the chamber.	

4. Ordered:	0.9% NaCl at 50 mL/hr for continuous infusion with Ancef 250 mg IV q8h to be infused over 30 min by volume control set
On hand:	Ancef 125 mg/mL
Add _____ mL medication and _____ mL IV fluid to the chamber.	

Calculate the IV flow rate to administer the following IV medications by using a volume control set, and determine the amount of IV fluid and medication to be added to the chamber. The ordered time includes the flush volume.

5. Ordered:	Antibiotic Z 15 mg IV b.i.d. in 25 mL 0.9% NaCl over 20 min. Flush with 15 mL.
On hand:	Antibiotic Z 15 mg 3 mL
Flow rate:	_____ gtt/min
Add _____ mL medication and _____ mL IV fluid to the chamber.	

6. Ordered:	Antibiotic Y 60 mg IV q8h in 50 mL D5 $\frac{1}{3}$ NS over 45 min. Flush with 15 mL.
On hand:	Antibiotic Y 60 mg/2 mL
Flow rate:	_____ gtt/min
Add _____ mL medication and _____ mL IV fluid to the chamber.	

7. Ordered:	Ancef 0.6 g IV q12h in 50 mL D5 NS over 60 min or an infusion pump. Flush with 30 mL.
On hand:	Ancef 1 g/10 mL
Flow rate:	_____ mL/hr
Add _____ mL medication and _____ mL IV fluid to the chamber.	

8. Ordered:	*Medication X 75 mg IV q6h in 60 mL D5 $\frac{1}{4}$ NS over 60 min. Flush with 15 mL.*
On hand:	Medication X 75 mg/3 mL
Flow rate:	_____ gtt/min
Add _____ mL medication and _____ mL IV fluid to the chamber.	

DAILY MAINTENANCE FLUID NEEDS

Pharmacy technicians should also be familiar with calculating 24-hour maintenance IV fluids for pediatric patients. They must use the following formula for calculations:

- 100 mL/kg/day for the first 10 kg of body weight
- 50 mL/kg/day for the next 10 kg of body weight
- 20 mL/kg/day for each kg above 20 kg of body weight

This formula uses the child's weight in kilograms to estimate the 24-hour total fluid need, including oral intake.

These types of IV solutions usually contain a combination of saline, glucose, and potassium chloride and are known as hypertonic solutions (**Figure 16-3**).

Figure 16-3 Dextrose Injection 5% USP.
© *Cengage Learning 2013*

Sodium chloride is usually concentrated between 0.225% and 0.9% ($\frac{1}{4}$ NS up to NS). Dextrose (glucose) for energy is usually concentrated between 5% and 12% for peripheral infusions. Plus, 20 mEq per liter of potassium chloride (20 mEq KCl/L) are added to continuous pediatric infusions.

■ EXAMPLE 1:

Child who weighs 26 kg: 100 mL/kg/day × 10 kg = 1000 mL/day (for the first 10 kg)

50 mL/kg/day × 10 kg = 500 mL/day (for the next 10 kg)

20 mL/kg/day × 6 kg = 120 mL/day (for the next 6 kg)

Total: 1000 mL/day + 500 mL/day + 120 mL/day = 1620 mL/day, or per 24 hour

$$\frac{1620 \text{ mL}}{24 \text{ hr}} = 67.5 \text{ mL/hr} = 68 \text{ mL/hr}$$

■ EXAMPLE 2:

Child who weighs 14 kg: 100 mL/kg/day × 10 kg = 1000 mL/day (for the first 10 kg)

50 mL/kg/day × 4 kg = 200 mL/day (for the remaining 4 kg)

Total: 1000 mL/day + 200 mL/day = 1200 mL/day or 24 hours

$$\frac{1200 \text{ mL}}{24 \text{ hr}} = 50 \text{ mL/hr}$$

■ EXAMPLE 3:

Child who weighs 8 kg: 100 mL/kg/day × 8 kg = 800 mL/day or per 24 hours

$$\frac{800 \text{ mL}}{24 \text{ hr}} = 33.3 \text{ mL/hr} = 33 \text{ mL/hr}$$

Stop and Review

Calculate the daily maintenance fluids for pediatric patients.

1. Calculate the total volume and hourly IV flow rate for a 3500 g infant receiving maintenance fluids. Infuse _____ mL at _____ mL/hr.

2. Calculate the total volume and hourly IV flow rate for a 13 kg child receiving maintenance IV fluids. Infuse _____ mL at _____ mL/hr.

3. Calculate the total volume and hourly IV flow rate for a 77 lb child receiving maintenance fluids. Infuse _____ mL at _____ mL/hr.

4. Calculate the total volume and hourly IV flow rate for a 25 kg child receiving maintenance IV fluids. Infuse _____ mL at _____ mL/hr.

5. Calculate the total volume and hourly IV flow rate for a 17.6 lb newborn receiving maintenance IV fluids. Infuse _____ mL at _____ mL/hr.

6. Calculate the total volume and hourly IV flow rate for an 8800 g child receiving maintenance IV fluids. Infuse _____ mL at _____ mL/hr.

7. Calculate the child's daily maintenance fluid needs for the following weights.

    a. 68.2 lb = _____ mL

    b. 13.3 lb = _____ mL

    c. 12 kg = _____ mL

    d. 43 kg = _____ mL

Test Your Knowledge

For Questions 1 through 7, verify the safety of the following pediatric dosages ordered. If the dosage is safe, calculate one dose and the IV volume to infuse one dose.

Ordered for a child weighing 15 kg:

D5 0.45% NaCl IV at 53 mL/h with ampicillin 275 mg IV q4h infused over 40 min by volume control set

Recommended dosage: ampicillin 100–125 mg/kg/day in 6 divided doses

On hand: ampicillin 1 g/10 mL

1. Safe daily dosage range for this child: _____ mg/day to _____ mg/day
   Safe single dosage range for this child: _____ mg/dose to _____ mg/dose. Is the ordered dosage safe? _____ If safe, give _____ mL/dose.

2. IV fluid volume to be infused in 40 min: _____ mL. Add _____ mL ampicillin and _____ mL D5 0.45% NaCl to the chamber.

Ordered for a child who weighs 55 lbs:

D5 NS at 60 mL/hr with penicillin G potassium 525,000 units q4h to be infused over 20 min by control set

Recommended dosage: penicillin G potassium 100,000–250,000 units/kg/day in 6 divided doses q 4 hr.

On hand: penicillin G potassium 200,000 units/mL

3. Child's weight: _____ kg

    Safe daily dosage for this child: _____ units/day to _____ units/day

    Safe single dosage for this child: _____ units/dose to _____ units/dose

4. Is the ordered dosage safe? _____

5. IV fluid volume to be infused in 20 min: _____ mL. Add _____ mL penicillin G potassium and _____ mL D5 NS to the chamber.

Ordered for a child who weighs 22 kg:

D5 0.225% NaCl IV at 50 mL/hr with Amikin 165 mg IV q8h to be infused over 30 min by volume control set

Recommended dosage: Amikin 15–22.5 mg/kg/day in 3 divided doses q 8 hr

On hand: Amikin 100 mg/2 mL

6. Safe daily dosage range for this child: _____ mg/day to _____ mg/day. Safe single dosage range for this child: _____ mg/dose to _____ mg/dose.

7. IV fluid volume to be infused in 30 min: _____ mL. Add _____ mL Amikin and _____ mL D5 0.225% NaCl to the chamber.

For questions 8 through 15, use the BSA formulas to calculate the BSA value.

8. Height: 4 ft Weight: 80 lb BSA: _____ m^2

9. Height: 5 ft 6 in. Weight: 136 lb BSA: _____ m^2

10. Height: 68 in. Weight: 170 lb BSA: _____ m^2

11. Height: 64 in. Weight: 63 kg BSA: _____ m^2

12. Height: 164 cm Weight: 58 kg BSA: _____ m^2

13. Height: 100 cm Weight: 17 kg BSA: _____ m^2

14. Height: 60 cm Weight: 6 kg BSA: _____ m^2

15. Height: 85 cm Weight: 11.5 kg BSA: _____ m^2

For questions 16 through 18, calculate the ordered medication for each of the following IV bags to achieve the ordered concentration. On hand is KCl 2 mEq/mL.

16. Ordered: *Add 30 mEq KCl per L of IV fluid.*

    On hand: 360 mL IV solution

    Add: _____ mEq; _____ mL

17. Ordered: *Add 20 mEq KCl per L of IV fluid.*

    On hand: 700 mL IV solution

    Add: _____ mEq; _____ mL

18. Ordered: *Add 15 mEq KCl per L of IV fluid.*

    On hand: 250 mL IV solution

    Add: _____ mEq; _____ mL

To calculate the daily volume of pediatric maintenance IV fluids to answer questions 19 through 22, allow the following:

100 mL/kg/day for the first 10 kg of body weight

50 mL/kg/day for the next 10 kg of body weight

20 mL/kg/day for each kg of body weight above 20 kg

19. Calculate the total volume and hourly IV flow rate for a 78 lb child receiving maintenance fluids.

    Infuse _____ mL at _____ mL/hr.

20. Calculate the total volume IV flow rate for a 21 kg child receiving maintenance fluids.

    Infuse _____ mL at _____ mL/hr.

21. Calculate the total volume and hourly IV flow rate for a 2400 g infant receiving maintenance fluids.

    Infuse _____ mL at _____ mL/hr.

22. Calculate the total volume and hourly IV flow rate for a 33 lb child receiving maintenance fluids.

    Infuse _____ mL at _____ mL/hr.

Calculate the volume for one dose of safe dosages. Refer to the BSA formulas or the West nomogram, as needed, to answer questions 23 through 32.

23. A child is 140 cm tall and weighs 43.5 kg. The recommended IV dosage of Adriamycin is 20 mg/m^2. Use the BSA formula to calculate the safe IV dosage of Adriamycin for this child. BSA: _____ m^2

    Safe dosage: _____ mg

24. Calculate the dose amount of Adriamycin for the child in Question 23.

    On hand: Adriamycin 2 mg/mL

    Give: _____ mL.

25. Use the BSA nomogram to determine the safe IM dosage of Oncaspar for a child who is 42 in. tall and weighs 45 lb. The recommended IM dosage is 2500 units/m^2/dose.

    BSA: _____ m^2. Safe dosage: _____ units.

26. Oncaspar is reconstituted to 750 units per 1 mL. Calculate one dose for the child in question 25. Give: _____ mL.

27. Should the Oncaspar in question 26 be given in one injection?

    _____

28. Ordered: Vincristine 2 mg direct IV stat for a child who weighs 85 lb and is 50 in. tall. Recommended dosage of vincristine for children: 1.5–2 mg/m^2 – 1 time/week; inject slowly over a period of 1 minute.

    On hand: vincristine 1 mg/mL

    BSA (per formula) of this child: _____ m^2

    Recommended dosage range for this child: _____ mg to
    _____ mg

29. Use the BSA nomogram to calculate the safe oral dosage and amount to give of amoxicillin for a child of normal proportions who weighs 25 lb.

    Recommended dosage: 80 mg/m^2/day once daily p.o.

    On hand: amoxicillin 50 mg/mL

    BSA: _____ m^2

    Safe dosage: _____ mg

    Give: _____ mL.

30. Use the BSA nomogram to calculate the safe IV dosage of sargramostim for a 1-year-old infant who is 25 in. tall and weighs 20 lb.

    Recommended dosage: 250 mcg/m^2/day once daily IV

    BSA: _____ m^2

    Safe dosage: _____ mcg

31. Sargramostim is available in a solution strength of 500 mcg/10 mL. Calculate one dose for the child in question 30. Give: _____ mL.

32. Ordered: *D5 0.45% NaCl IV at 66 mL/hr with Fortaz 620 mg IV q8h to be infused over 40 min*

    Use a volume control set and flush with 15 mL.

    On hand: Fortaz 0.5 g/5 mL

    Add _____ mL Fortaz and _____ mL D5 0.45% NaCl to the chamber.

Critical Thinking

1.   A pharmacy technician received an order to dispense Halotex®
     (antifungal) for topical use for a 4-year-old child. Fortunately, the tech-
     nician read the dosage and administration section of the package insert.
     He finds a warning that Halotex should not be administered to patients
     younger than 5 years of age. This patient should not receive Halotex.
     Whom should the pharmacy technician alert about his finding?

PHARMACY OPERATIONS

Business Math

OBJECTIVES

Upon completion of this chapter, you should be able to:

1. Define *gross* and *net profit*.
2. Explain inventory turnover.
3. Compute discounts.
4. Describe what markup is.
5. List familiar unit costs used in pharmacy.

GLOSSARY

average wholesale price – The national average cost of a drug product to a pharmacy; however, in practice, this is simply a "benchmark" price set by manufacturers.

copayment – A specific amount required to be paid by a patient for a prescription.

expenses – Costs associated with the operation of a pharmacy, which are often called "overhead"; expenses include salaries, wages, rent, utilities, telephone, insurance, legal and accounting fees, advertising, and depreciation.

gross profit – The marginal difference between actual cost and total reimbursement; it is also known as "gross margin."

inventory – A list of merchandise, itemized by various types, and its costs.

inventory control – The process of managing inventory in order to meet customer demand at the lowest possible cost, with a minimum of investment in inventory; average inventory is calculated by adding beginning and ending inventory, and dividing by two.

inventory turnover – A measure of how many times a year a pharmacy's average inventory "turns," or is sold; cost of goods sold divided by average inventory gives the inventory turnover rate.

markup – The difference between the purchase price and the selling price of an item, often expressed as a percentage; markup percentage is calculated by subtracting the purchase price from the selling price, and then dividing by the purchase price.

markup method – The cost of a medication based on price and dollar margin on the ingredient cost of the dispensed product.

net profit – The net amount of money left after all operating or overhead expenses have been subtracted from the gross margin; this amount may be a profit or a loss.

return on investment – A measure of the percentage of net profit as related to net worth; net profit divided by net worth, multiplied by 100, gives this percentage.

sales – The revenue generated by the sale of the pharmacy's inventory (or goods) and services.

third-party payer – A company that pays part of the cost of an invoice between a health-care provider and a patient.

turnover – A measure of time that a product remains in stock and is not used by a pharmacy.

OVERVIEW

Pharmacy practice has changed dramatically over the last several years. Pharmacists are more likely to be employees rather than owners and instead work for large organizations, such as hospitals, chain pharmacies, and managed care pharmacies, rather than in small, independently owned pharmacies. These changes have been associated with a dramatic decline in the number of pharmacists who own their businesses; they have not affected the number of pharmacists who are managers. However, most states require pharmacy managers to actually be pharmacists. In fact, the need for pharmacy managers has increased. Managers are responsible for planning, organizing, and controlling resources so that the organizations in which they are employed meet their goals. The most important concerns of pharmaceutical organizations are productivity, quality, service, and price. The pharmacy manager is responsible and accountable for the finances of the pharmacy. Without establishing the pharmacy's ability to make a regular profit, pharmacy managers will not be able to achieve the pharmacy's ultimate goal of serving the community.

INVENTORY

Inventory may be defined as a list of merchandise, itemized by various types, and their costs. The goal of sound inventory management in today's environment is a reasonable turnover of products combined with rapid billing and receiving and minimal waste. The objective is to purchase an adequate supply of often-used pharmaceuticals. Today's highly competitive market demands optimal cost management for the pharmacy to operate efficiently and productively.

Depending on the nature of the pharmacy, most institutional pharmacies do not operate under the profit-margin system. Hospitals, nursing homes, and other "closed" pharmacies must maintain cost efficiency but are not required, by their nature, to generate a significant profit.

Retail pharmacy establishments answer to private, corporate, or public investors, that is, stock shareholders, and must maintain a level of pharmacy profit dictated by the business. The cost of goods along with overhead costs, including professional labor, clerical support, utilities, capital investment, and government fees, must be considered in developing the actual margin of profit. The actual profit generated is known as net profit. This is the reported profit a pharmacy generates when all costs of the business are considered.

■ EXAMPLE 1:

Assume that Family Drug Mart has the following annual overhead **expenses**:

Pharmacist's Salary	$ 70,000
Technician's Salary	$ 23,250
Rent	$ 16,000
Utilities	$ 7,300
Liability Insurance	$ 3,400
Business Insurance	$ 4,000
Supplies and Drug Purchases	$1,691,000
Total Overhead	$1,814,950

When the Family Drug Mart has an annual income of $2,087,192.50, it will be making a 15% profit. If a 15% profit is desired, what amount of income has to be received to meet this goal?

$$\text{Overhead} \times 0.15 = \text{Profit}$$

$$\$1,814,950 \times 0.15 = \$272,242.50$$

Because profit is equal to incoming receipts minus overhead:

$$\text{Overhead} + \text{Profit} = \text{Income}$$

$$\$1,814,950 + \$272,242.50 = \$2,087,192.50$$

Because net profit is usually reported annually or semiannually, the retail pharmacy department may frequently measure the cost of goods as compared to the revenue generated by the sale of those goods. This reported margin of profit is known as **gross profit**. Gross profit is the marginal difference between actual cost and total reimbursement and is also known as "gross margin." The insurance reimbursement or private pay customer's service charge most dramatically influences the "gross profit" margin.

■ EXAMPLE 2:

(**sales** – acquisition cost = gross profit)

If a pharmacy has sales totaling $1,000,000 and the cost of the items sold is $750,000, then the *gross profit* is $250,000.

A well-managed inventory program will include waste control. In institutional settings, the amount and size of injectable pharmaceuticals is often analyzed to reduce costs through minimizing waste. In the retail pharmacy department, timely return for credit of a near-expired product may be considered a controllable cost-effective tool for inventory management. The technician should become familiar with his or her pharmacy's policies and procedures on inventory management in an effort to prevent product depreciation and improve turnover.

Turnover

Turnover is a measure of time that the product remains in stock and is not used by the pharmacy. For higher-cost pharmaceuticals, this value may be used to prevent excessive expenditures by the pharmacy. Select drugs that have short expiration dating or limited need would be required to have a very high turnover rate to prevent excessive waste and financial loss. An **inventory turnover** rate is a specific time period over which the total inventory is sold. The more often this occurs, the higher the turnover rate.

■ EXAMPLE 3:

During the past year, a pharmacy spent $900,000 on the items in its inventory. The average inventory value during the past year was determined to be $150,000.

What was the *turnover rate* of the inventory? Turnover rate = total purchases divided by average inventory

So, $900,000 divided by $150,000 = 6 times

PROFIT

The pharmacy, like other businesses, must make a profit. It must have more receipts than expenses to continue providing customer services. The pharmacy technician is also involved in this effort to help ensure that receipts are greater than expenses. The technician must understand the importance of cost, overhead, **markup**, discount, and **inventory control** as they relate to profit. The overall cost for the pharmacy may include the cost of drug purchases, salaries, operating expenses, utilities, and insurance (business and liability). The net profit for each drug sold is calculated as the difference between the overall cost and the selling price. The overall cost is made up of the cost to dispense added to the purchase price. The net profit amount can be calculated by multiplying the overall cost by the desired percent of profit.

■ EXAMPLE 1:

A liquid drug for oral administration costs $20/pint. The pharmacy technician calculates that it costs $5 (including pharmacy supplies, shipping, supply maintenance, pharmacist consultation, and personnel time) to dispense one bottle's entire contents. If a 15% profit is desired, what selling price is required for the pint bottle?

Purchase price	+ dispensing cost	= overall cost
$20	+ $5	= $25
Overall cost	× 0.15	= net profit
$25	× 0.15	= $3.75
Overall cost	+ net profit	= selling price
$25	+ $3.75	= $28.75

SELLING PRICES

When a manufacturer or a supplier offers an item at a lower price to a pharmacy, this lower price is considered to be "discounted." A discount is, simply put, a deduction from what is normally charged. Discounts provided by suppliers may be based on quantity buying and/or payment of invoices within a specified time period. These discounts provide the pharmacy with a means of increasing the gross profit on selected merchandise. Discounts are offered as incentives to purchase the products being discounted. They are calculated as follows:

$$DISCOUNT = Discount\ rate \times total\ purchase\ price$$

$$Purchase\ price - discount = DISCOUNTED\ PRICE$$

■ EXAMPLE 1:

Ten cases of ointment are purchased at $180 per case. If the account is fully paid within 15 days, the manufacturer offers a discount of 12%. What is the total discounted purchase price?

First, you must calculate the full purchase price: 10 cases × $180 per case = $1800

Next, calculate the discount if paid for within 15 days:

(DISCOUNT = Discount rate × total purchase price)

$$(12\%) \times (\$1800)$$

The DISCOUNT is equal to $216.

Finally, to obtain the discounted price, you would subtract the discount from the original total purchase price.

Total purchase price − discount = discounted purchase price

$$\$1,800 - \$216 = \$1584$$

Prescription pricing is designed so that the pharmacy receives a fair **return on investment** and costs. It gives the pharmacy the ability to provide the services that its community needs in a uniform and consistent manner. The following sections explain the most common methods of prescription pricing.

Markup

The term *markup* refers to the difference between the cost of merchandise and its selling price. Markup is sometimes called "margin of profit" or "gross profit." For example, if a pharmacist buys an item for $2.75 and sells it for $3.75, the markup is $1.00. The **markup method** bases price and dollar margin on the ingredient cost of the dispensed product. Consequently, as ingredient cost increases, both price and margin increase proportionally. The markup may be calculated as a percentage, which refers to the markup divided by the selling price. The percent of markup may be somewhat ambiguous because it may be based on either the cost or the selling price of merchandise. As of this writing, the percentage is based on selling price, and the term *markup percent* means a percentage of the selling price.

Calculating the merchandise's selling price to yield a certain percent of gross profit involves the following:

■ **EXAMPLE 2:**

The cost of 100 antihistamine tablets is $1.98. What should the selling price be for 100 tablets to yield a 66% gross profit on the cost?

$$\text{Cost} \times \% \text{ of gross profit} = \text{Gross profit}$$

$$\$1.98 \times 66\% = \$1.30$$

$$\text{Cost} + \text{Gross profit} = \text{Selling price}$$

$$\$1.98 + \$1.30 = \$3.28$$

A markup system automatically adjusts prices to accommodate changes in ingredient costs. A disadvantage of the markup system is that it subsidizes low-cost products with high-cost ones. For example, if prescription prices are calculated using a markup, low-cost products have lower markups because consumers are more likely to recognize and react to higher prices on expensive drugs than to lower prices on inexpensive ones.

You can also calculate the markup rate by using this formula:

$$\text{Markup rate} = \frac{\text{Markup}}{\text{Cost}} \times 100\%$$

■ **EXAMPLE 3:**

If Zocor® 10 mg in a 30-pack costs the pharmacy $98.64 and the price is $147.96, what is the markup rate?

The markup is $147.96 − $98.64 = $49.32

The markup rate is calculated via the formula given previously:

$$\text{Markup rate} = \frac{49.32}{98.64} \times 100\% = 50\%$$

Percent Markup

In this type of prescription pricing, the cost of the ingredients of a prescription is added to the cost of ingredients multiplied by the desired percentage of markup.

$$\text{Cost of ingredients} + (\text{cost of ingredients} \times \% \text{ of markup})$$
$$= \text{Prescription price}$$

Percentages vary but, in general, lower-priced items are marked up with a higher percentage, and higher-priced items are marked up with a lower percentage.

■ **EXAMPLE 4:**

What would be the prescription price in the following situation?

A package of a certain drug product costs $5. The pharmacist applies a 50% markup on cost.

$$\$5 + (\$5 \times 50\%) = \$5 + \$2.50 = \$7.50$$

Percent Markup Plus a Professional Fee

Utilizing this method, both a percent markup *and* a professional fee are added to the ingredient's cost. In this type of prescription pricing, the percent markup is usually a bit lower than in the preceding *percent markup* example. A minimum professional fee is added to help recover the costs of professional services, labeling, containers, and overhead.

Cost of ingredients + (cost of ingredients × % of markup) + professional fee = Prescription price

■ EXAMPLE 5:

If the package of a quantity of drug product costs $5 and the pharmacist applies a 50% markup on cost plus a professional fee of $3, what would the prescription price be?

$$\$5 + (\$5 \times 50\%) + \$3 = \$5 + \$2.50 + \$3 = \$10.50$$

Average Wholesale Price

The term average wholesale price (AWP) is used to describe the national average cost of a drug product to the pharmacy. This price usually represents the highest cost available for pharmaceuticals purchased from the most readily available vendor source. However, in practice, this is simply a "benchmark" price set by manufacturers.

While the drug product (cost of goods) represents the major cost in the business aspect of pharmacy, it is often the cost the pharmacy has least control over. Pharmacies use a variety of contracts and limited purchase agreements to reduce the cost of goods. The "laid-in" or actual cost of a drug product is the product cost after all contract discounts are applied. This often differs from the AWP.

Pharmacies may restrict multiple-source products to a select manufacturer or distributor as a means of reducing the cost of goods. For example, Cefazolin 1 g IV powder for injection is produced by a variety of manufacturers. The pharmacy may choose to contract with a specific manufacturer or distribution group to reduce the cost substantially. When a drug product is available generically, the cost of goods represents an opportunity for the pharmacy to control the cost of the product. For single-source or branded products protected by U.S. patent, the pharmacy has less of an opportunity to control the cost of goods unless the department maintains a pharmacy formulary and restricts therapy choices.

INSURANCE REIMBURSEMENTS

Average wholesale price (AWP) is often used by insurance carriers or third-party providers to determine a contract price. Third parties reimburse a pharmacy based on the AWP, less an established percentage, as the cost basis for the drug in reimbursement programs. The AWP is obtained from commercial listings. The reimbursed amount is calculated from a predetermined formula, for example, "AWP less 10% plus $3.50 professional fee." Many third-party programs have a copayment provision, which requires the patient to pay a portion of the charge for each prescription filled.

■ EXAMPLE 1:

If a **third-party payer** reimburses a pharmacy "AWP less 15%" plus a professional fee of $3.50, what would the total reimbursement be on a prescription written for 40 capsules having an AWP of $22 per 100 capsules?

AWP for 40 capsules $= \$5 - 15\% = \$7.50$

$$\$7.50 + \$3.50 = \$11$$

If the patient must pay a copayment of $2 for each prescription filled, how much would the third party reimburse the pharmacy in the preceding example?

$$\$11 - \$2 = \$9$$

Test Your Knowledge

Choose and circle the most correct answer from the choices provided.

1. Twice annually, your pharmacy department analyzes and reports the net profit of the business. When calculating net profit, which of the following statement are true?

   a. Net profit is the gross profit (difference between the cost of goods and services and the total reimbursement to the pharmacy for those goods and services) *minus* all overhead costs.

   b. Salaries and bonuses paid to all pharmacy employees must be calculated.

   c. Benefits paid for all pharmacy employees (i.e., health care, retirement account) must be calculated.

   d. All of the above

2. Product turnover is best described as

   a. the average amount of time your pharmacy retains a product before it is sold.

   b. the amount of time before a pharmaceutical expires.

   c. the amount of revenue a product generates by the time it is dispensed and sold.

   d. the interest charge that the pharmacy pays for inventory purchased and not used.

3. Sales minus cost equals gross profit. What is the gross profit for a pharmacy whose sales total $199,991 and whose costs total $19,191?

   a. $108,072

   b. $108,000

   c. $108,080

   d. $180,800

4. The manufacturer's average wholesale price is $1200 per unit of product. If the pharmacy purchases 24 units or more per year, the pharmacy will receive a 15% rebate. If the pharmacy purchases 12 units or more, the rebate is 10%. Calculate the product's actual cost if 15 units are purchased, and then choose the correct answer.

   a. $14,400

   b. $15,000

   c. $1200

   d. $1080

5. Using the actual cost calculated in question 4, calculate the gross profit percent of the prescription sold to a patient with an insurance program that pays the pharmacy as follows: average wholesale price (AWP) minus 6% plus a $2 dispensing fee. What is the correct answer?

   a. 4.4%

   b. 1.25%

   c. 6%

   d. 27%

6. Insurance company "A" will reimburse the pharmacy at AWP minus 8% with a further deduction of a $4.50 dispensing fee. Insurance company "B" will reimburse the pharmacy at AWP minus 10% plus a $6 dispensing fee. Using the example from question 5, which insurance will generate the greatest gross profit?

   a. Insurance company B

   b. Insurance company A

   c. Both insurance companies

   d. Neither insurance company

7. The pharmacy manager wants a comparison of gross profit dollars between insurance plan "A" and insurance "B" for 2012 for the product described in question 6. You are asked to examine the pharmacy purchase history to find the rebate your pharmacy received in 2012 so you can then calculate the correct actual cost. The purchase history from January 1 to December 31, 2012, shows 28 units purchased. Which insurance plan would reimburse more for the drug described in question 6, and by how many total dollars?

   a. Plan "A" by $22.50

   b. Plan "A" by $630

   c. Plan "B" by $66

   d. Plan "B" by $88.50

8. In questions 5 through 7, if the drug product expires and is returned to the vendor, the pharmacy receives 45% of AWP for credit. The pharmacy returned two units in 2012. How much credit did the pharmacy receive?

   a. $1300

   b. $1080

   c. $918

   d. $997

9. The pharmacy receives a 10% discount if a case of 12 ammonium lactate lotion, 365 mL, is ordered from the manufacturer. If the invoice is paid within 14 days, the pharmacy receives an additional 2% rebate. If the AWP unit cost of the lotion is $7.25, and the pharmacy pays the invoice in 10 days, what is the "laid-in" or actual acquisition cost of one bottle (365 mL) for the pharmacy?

   a. $7.25

   b. $6.53

   c. $6.38

   d. $6.66

10. The total operating cost for the pharmacy department is approximately $172,000 per month. The average monthly invoice total for all goods purchased is $164,000. The average monthly sales amount the pharmacy department generates is $358,000. What is the total profit from the pharmacy?

   a. $186,000

   b. $172,000

   c. $194,000

   d. $22,000

11. In the example from question 10, what is the approximate percent net profit generated?

   a. 20%

   b. 6%

   c. 54%

   d. 12%

Answer the following questions on the lines provided.

12. A drug prescribed to treat AIDS costs $300 per 60 tablets. Calculate the cost for a 6-month supply if the patient takes one tablet per day.

   _____

13. A treatment for an eye infection is priced at $50 per gallon, minus a limited-time discount of 25%. If the pharmacy purchases the solution and receives this discount, what would the net cost be of 32 ounces (1 quart) of the medication?

   _____

14. Antacid tablets cost $100 per 500 tablets, less a discount of 30%. What would 100 tablets cost if purchased at the discounted price?

   _____

15. Mouthwash sells for $2.50. A 25% profit had been added to its actual cost in order to reach the selling price. What was the actual cost of the mouthwash?

   _____

Critical Thinking

1. Each tablet in a bottle of 30 costs $4.60. The Pharmacy's cost (including: pharmacy supplies, shipping, pharmacist consult, and personnel time to dispense) is $1.40 per pill. If a 12% profit is desired, how much would the entire bottle cost?

   _____

Answers to Stop and Review Exercises

Chapter 1: Fundamentals of Math

Page 11

1. 2.5
2. 0.63
3. 1.6
4. 1.3
5. 0.5
6. 0.15
7. 0.85
8. 0.25
9. 5.5
10. 0.1

Page 12

1. 5 g
2. 200 ml
3. 0.5 L
4. 0.03 g
5. 400 mcg
6. 0.2 mg
7. 0.4 mg
8. 900 mcg
9. 10.3 mcg
10. 2.7 kg
11. 0.05 g
12. 6.4 kg

Page 12

1. mg
2. mm
3. g
4. mcg
5. kg
6. m
7. mL
8. L
9. cm
10. kl

Page 14

1. gr iii
2. dr $\frac{2}{3}$
3. ℥ viii
4. lb iv
5. gr $\frac{1}{200}$
6. dr $(\overline{ss})$

7. ʒ iii
8. lb ii
9. lb ii ʒ xi
10. gr $(\overline{ss})$

Page 16

1. 1
2. 3
3. 1.5
4. 32
5. 2.67

Chapter 2: Fractions and Decimals

Pages 35–37

1. 80
2. 5
3. 60
4. 25
5. 9
6. 82
7. c
8. a
9. 3
10. 1
11. $6\frac{1}{2}$
12. $1\frac{4}{5}$
13. $4\frac{13}{15}$
14. 25
15. 2
16. $10\frac{1}{3}$
17. $\frac{20}{3}$
18. $\frac{370}{19}$
19. $\frac{51}{10}$
20. $\frac{9}{4}$
21. $\frac{35}{9}$
22. $\frac{113}{2}$
23. $\frac{452}{3}$
24. $\frac{578}{3}$

Page 39

1. 12
2. 6
3. 60
4. 20
5. 16
6. 12
7. 24
8. 16
9. 8
10. 4
11. $\frac{1}{2}$
12. $\frac{2}{3}$

13. $\frac{3}{4}$
14. $\frac{1}{9}$
15. $\frac{1}{2}$
16. $\frac{1}{2}$
17. $\frac{1}{3}$
18. $\frac{7}{8}$
19. $\frac{3}{4}$
20. $\frac{7}{9}$

Pages 40–41

1. $\frac{13}{24}$
2. $\frac{71}{72}$
3. $4\frac{3}{5}$
4. $1\frac{17}{24}$
5. $\frac{2}{3}$
6. $\frac{2}{5}$
7. $3\frac{8}{11}$
8. $\frac{13}{42}$
9. $\frac{71}{105}$
10. $\frac{2}{3}$
11. $\frac{47}{60}$

12. $1\frac{11}{18}$
13. $2\frac{7}{10}$
14. $\frac{13}{15}$
15. 6
16. $3\frac{1}{5}$
17. $\frac{1}{5}$
18. $3\frac{1}{3}$
19. $5\frac{1}{2}$
20. $\frac{4}{5}$
21. $6\frac{4}{7}$
22. $\frac{3}{7}$

23. $\frac{7}{12}$
24. $5\frac{1}{8}$
25. $2\frac{1}{8}$
26. $11\frac{2}{5}$

27. $13\frac{4}{7}$
28. $4\frac{5}{6}$
29. $7\frac{2}{9}$
30. $\frac{7}{12}$

Pages 41–42

1. $\frac{1}{15}$
2. $\frac{8}{35}$
3. $\frac{3}{10}$
4. $1\frac{1}{3}$
5. $\frac{2}{9}$
6. $4\frac{1}{2}$
7. $\frac{25}{72}$
8. $\frac{1}{6}$
9. $1\frac{1}{3}$
10. $\frac{14}{15}$

11. 2
12. $14\frac{3}{10}$
13. $27\frac{1}{12}$
14. $1\frac{1}{2}$
15. $\frac{21}{128}$
16. $\frac{48}{125}$
17. $\frac{49}{108}$
18. $\frac{5}{6}$
19. $1\frac{17}{88}$
20. $\frac{35}{96}$

Pages 42–43

1. $\frac{3}{4}$
2. $\frac{20}{33}$
3. $\frac{8}{9}$
4. $\frac{4}{15}$
5. $2\frac{1}{7}$
6. $1\frac{5}{9}$

7. $1\frac{1}{2}$
8. $\frac{90}{161}$
9. $2\frac{1}{7}$
10. $\frac{5}{14}$
11. $2\frac{106}{171}$
12. $4\frac{5}{7}$

13. $\dfrac{4}{42}$

14. 16

15. $1\dfrac{1}{8}$

16. $\dfrac{16}{21}$

Pages 45–46

1. 0.5

2. 0.4

3. 0.17 (rounded)

4. 0.625

5. 0.13 (rounded)

6. 0.006 (rounded)

7. 0.015

8. 0.83 (rounded)

9. 0.002

10. 0.0003 (rounded)

11. $\dfrac{1}{200}$

12. $\dfrac{9}{1000}$

13. $\dfrac{33}{10,000}$

14. $\dfrac{1}{20}$

15. $\dfrac{1}{4}$

16. $\dfrac{1}{5000}$

17. $\dfrac{3}{40}$

18. $\dfrac{3}{20}$

19. $\dfrac{21}{25}$

20. $2\dfrac{3}{4}$

Pages 47–48

1. 14.24

2. 186.09

3. 17.469

4. 77.224

5. 4.86

6. 5.459

7. 0.705

8. 8.033

9. 53.55

10. 17.135

11. 7.8

12. 15.6

13. 4.62

14. 12.023

15. 8.977

16. 16.93

Page 49

1. 83.42

2. 3.43

3. 20.724

4. 0.5648

5. 0.539

6. 0.0492

7. 0.00027

8. 0.2125

9. 90.72

10. 1.36

11. 0.0591

12. 0.38535

Pages 50–51

1. 4.43

2. 61.33

3. 47

4. 2

5. 3

6. 1.55

7. 4

8. 7.3

9. 100

10. 0.1

11. 0.3906

12. 0.004

13. 2222.2

14. 20705

15. 0.06313

16. 18.295

17. 60

18. 23.5454

19. 0.00089

20. 2.7308

Chapter 3:
Ratios, Proportions, and Percents

Pages 58–59

1. 1 : 4

2. 1 : 5

3. 2 : 3

4. 3 : 4

5. 1 : 3

6. 1 : 8

7. 1 : 20

8. 1 : 20

9. 1 : 3

10. 1 : 2

11. 2 : 5

12. 1 : 10

13. 1 : 20

14. 2 : 25

15. 1 : 200

16. 1 : 20

17. 1 : 4

18. 1 : 5

19. 1 : 4

20. 1 : 10

Pages 60–61

1. 75

2. 15

3. 12

4. 50

5. 135

6. 16

7. 45

8. 40

9. 3

10. 640

11. 125

12. 50

Pages 63–64

1. 12

2. 500

3. 0.02

4. 10

5. 250

6. 7.5

7. 8

8. 187.5

9. 3

10. 35

11. 10.8

12. 250

13. 1.25

14. 60

15. 30

Chapter 4:
Celsius and Fahrenheit Temperature Conversions

Page 70

1.	98.6°F	9.	42.8°C
2.	33.9°C	10.	71.6°F
3.	16.7°C	11.	37°C
4.	40°C	12.	31.1°C
5.	108.9°F	13.	39.3°C
6.	86.7°C	14.	42.8°C
7.	212°F	15.	101.3°F
8.	188.6°F		

Chapter 5:
Ratio and Proportion Method

Pages 79–81

1.	0.16	8.	32.4	15.	True	22.	2.4 mL
2.	38.1	9.	8.1	16.	2.9 mL	23.	2.7 mL
3.	0.46	10.	0.25	17.	1.9 mL	24.	0.5 mL
4.	0.625	11.	True	18.	0.4 mL	25.	2 mL
5.	1.89	12.	True	19.	1.3 mL		
6.	32,000	13.	True	20.	0.6 mL		
7.	7.28	14.	Not True	21.	1.5 mL		

Pages 82–83

1.	True	4.	Not true
2.	True	5.	True
3.	True		

Pages 84–85

1.	0.8 mL	3.	1.1 mL
2.	1.1 mL	4.	2.2 mL

5.	1.3 mL	7.	2.7 mL
6.	15 mL		

Chapter 6:
Dimensional Analysis

Page 97

1.	0.06 mL	4.	15 mL
2.	2.7 mL	5.	1.1 mL
3.	1.3 mL		

Chapter 7:
Formula Method

Pages 114–115

1.	1.5 mL	3.	1.2 mL
2.	0.9 mL	4.	0.55 mL

Page 116

1.	0.9 mL	3.	1.2 mL
2.	4.5 mL	4.	1 mL

Pages 117–118

1.	1.9 mL	3.	5 mL
2.	0.6 mL	4.	1.9 mL

Chapter 8:
Interpretation of Prescriptions and Drug Labels

Pages 126–127

1. Twice a day

2. 1 capsule

3. The prescriber's address and phone number, the patient's address, the Rx symbol

4. 28 capsules

5. None (zero)

6. 20 milligrams

7. Three times a day

8. 90

9. 360

10. The prescriber's address and phone number, the patient's address, the Rx symbol

11. The prescriber's address and phone number, the patient's address, the date, the Rx symbol

12. 90 tablets

13. Three times per day

14. 1 tablet

15. Five

Pages 128–130

1. Demerol	5. Once		8. Oral and intravenous
2. Six doses or 3900 mg	6. Lasix		9. 10:00 p.m.
3. SC	7. Milliequivalent		10. Oral
4. Before breakfast			

Pages 138–141

1. IM

2. *Film sealed tablet*

3. 2 tablets

4. 0.5 mg

5. All of the labels

6. Roche Pharmaceuticals, Inc.

7. Zeneca

8. F

9. B

10. E

11. A

12. C

13. D

14. Pfizerpen

15. Penicillin G potassium

16. 5,000,000 units per vial; reconstituted to 250,000 units/mL, 500,000 units/mL, or 1,000,000 units/mL

17. IM or IV

18. 0049-0520-83

19. Pfizer-Roerig

20. 10 mg per mL

21. 1%

22. 1 g, 100 mL

Pages 142–144

1. Receiving the prescription; reading and checking it; numbering, dating, and putting information into the computer; labeling

2. The technician *must* request the pharmacist to counsel the patient.

3. Because filling a prescription with accuracy and precision can reduce medication errors

4. Computer systems allow the entering and keeping of all information about patients, prescribers, and medication in order to prevent medication errors.

5. Labeling of medications gives information such as brand name, generic name, dosage strength, route of administration, frequency that the drug should be used, refilling, expiration date, and so on.

6. Instill 2 drops of 1% atropine sulfate in both eyes every 15 minutes for 4 applications.

7. Give 250 mg of Biaxin orally 2 times a day.

8. Give 20 mg of Lasix intramuscularly before breakfast.

9. Give $\frac{1}{400}$ grain of nitroglycerin sublingually immediately.

10. Give 10 mg of Solu-Medrol intramuscularly every 6 hours.

11. Give 20 mg of meperidine subcutaneously every 3–4 hours, as needed, for pain.

12. Give 750 units of heparin subcutaneously immediately.

13. Give 0.3 mg of Narcan intramuscularly immediately.

14. Give 40 mg of Benadryl orally immediately.

15. Give 3.5 mg of Valium intramuscularly every 6 hours, as needed, for anxiety.

16. Give 150 mcg of Synthroid orally each day.

17. Give 90 mg of tobramycin sulfate intramuscularly every 8 hours.

18. Instill 2 drops of Cortisporin otic suspension in left ear 3 times a day.

19. Give 250 mg of Fortax intravenously every 12 hours.

20. Give 0.24 g of Elixophyllin orally immediately.

Page 147

1a. Rechecks calculations

1b. Verifies drug orders

1c. Checks for allergy history

1d. Identifies the patient

2. Bar coding will require changes in label designs, production process, and size of packages, all of which combine to reduce medication errors.

3. Elixir "sulfanilamide" in 1937

4. They maintain accurate patient records and drug information.

Chapter 9:
Percentage of Error Due to Equipment
Page 166

1. 6%

4. 10%

2. 1.4%

5. 75 mg

3. 0.5 g or 500 mg

Chapter 10
Dilutions and Solutions
Page 174

1. water; saline

6. 800

2. solvents

7. 1500

3. total

8. 40

4. stock

9. 3; 7

5. 1; 7

10. 1; 10

Page 178

1. 129 g of 10% and 321 g of 3%

2. 400 mL of 30% and 100 mL of 20%

3. 231 mL of 23.4% and 5,769 mL of water

4. 167 mL of 60% and 83 mL of water

5. 366 mL of NaCl and 633 mL of water

6. 1 L of 31% and 1 L of 27%

7. 1000 mL of 42% and 500 mL of 18%; 86 mL of stock solution and 34 mL of water

Chapter 11:
Concentrations
Page 188

1. 180 g

2. 6 g

3. 1800 mL of stock solution and 1200 mL of water

Page 189

1. 0.95%

Page 190

1. 700 mL

2. 270 mL

3. 240 mL

4. $166\frac{2}{3}$ mL

5. 157 mL

Page 193

1. 0.03 mL concentrate; 1.97 mL diluent

2. 5 mL concentrate; 20 mL diluent

3. 500 mg; 18 mL diluent

4. 17.5 mL diluent

5. 4 mL concentrate

6. 0.05 mL concentrate

7. 1 mL concentrate

8. 3.57 mL concentrate

Chapter 12:
Oral Medication Labels and Dosage Calculation
Pages 206–212

1. 2 tablets   400X = 800

2. 2 tablets   10X = 20

3. 1 tablet   60:1::X mg:5 gr

4. 4 tablets   15X = 60 = 4

5. 2 tablets   0.4 mg:1 tab::X mg:2 tab X = 0.4 × 2 = 0.8 mg (which, in practice, would be 1 tablet)

6. 3 tablets $= \dfrac{600}{200} = 3$

7. 1.5 tablets $= x = \dfrac{7.5}{5} = 1.5$

8. 2 tablets $= x = \dfrac{250}{125} = 2$

9. 1 tablet

10. $2\dfrac{1}{2}$ tablets

11. B, 1 caplet

12. I, 2 tablets

13. F, 1 tablet

14. H, 2 tablets

15. C, 1 tablet

16. E, 2 tablets

17. D, 2 tablets

18. G, 2 tablets

19. A, 1 tablet

Pages 214–219

1. 10 mL		12. 20 mL	
2. 7.5 mL		13. 2.5 mL	
3. 2.5 mL		14. 8 mL	
4. 4 mL		15. 10 mL	
5. 10 mL		16. 2 mL	
6. 10 mL		17. 2 mL	
7. 7.5 mL		18. 5 mL	
8. 3 mL		19. 0.75 mL	
9. 6 mL		20. 10 mL	
10. 5 mL		21. 3 mL	
11. 2.5 mL			

Chapter 13: Reconstitution of Powdered Drugs

Pages 228–234

1. Sterile water for injection or bacteriostatic water for injection

2. 0.9 mL

3. 1.7 mL

4. 3.4 mL

5. 6.8 mL

6. 250 mg per 1 mL

7. 5 mL

8. Inject slowly over 3 to 5 minutes

9. Rapid administration may result in seizures

10. 250,000 units per mL

11. Yes

12. Expires June 8 at 2 p.m.

13. 20 million units

14. Your initials

15. Package insert

16. 10 mL

17. 20 mL

18. Sterile water for injection

19. 50 mg per mL

20. 14 days

21. Expires May 18 at 1350 hours

22. Your initials

23. 1 g

24. 2.1 mL

25. 350 mg/mL

26. 200 mcg; 0.2 mg

27. 5 mL

28. 0.9% sodium chloride

29. Must be used immediately

30. 40 mcg/mL

31. Package insert

32. 10 mL

33. Bacteriostatic Water for Injection with Benzyl Alcohol

34. 1 gram

35. 25°C (77°F)

36. 100 mg per mL

37. 48 hours

38. Expires February 16 at 0840 hours

39. 19 mL

40. Water for injection

41. 10 mg/mL

42. 200 mg

43. 29 mL

44. Distilled water

45. Shake the bottle to loosen granules, add half (15 mL) of the distilled water, shake vigorously to dissolve the granules, and then add the balance of the water and shake vigorously.

46. 100 mg/5 mL

47. 14 days

48. 500 mg

49. Bacteriostatic Water with Benzyl Alcohol

50. 10 mL

51. 50 mg per mL

52. 48 hours

Chapter 14: Parenteral Medication Labels and Dosage Calculation

Pages 246–251

1. Insulin Brand Name: Humulin R Regular
Action Time: Rapid-Acting

2. Insulin Brand Name: Novolin N
Action Time: Intermediate-Acting

3. Insulin Brand Name: Humulin U
Action Time: Long-Acting

4. Insulin Brand Name: Humalog
Action Time: Rapid-Acting

5. Insulin Brand Name: Humulin L
Action Time: Intermediate-Acting

6. Standard, dual-scale 100 unit/mL U-100 syringe;
Lo-dose, 50 unit/0.5 mL U-100 syringe;
Lo-dose, 30 unit/0.3 mL U-100 syringe

7. Lo-dose, 30 unit U-100 syringe

8. Lo-dose, 50 unit U-100 syringe

9. 0.6

10. 0.25

11. Standard dual-scale 100 unit U-100 syringe

12. False

13. 68

14. 15

15. 23

16. 57

17.

80 units

18.

15 units

19.

66 units

20.

16 units

21.

32 units

22.

15 units   21 units   Total = 36 units
NPH   Regular
            (drawn first)

23.

42 units

16 units
Regular
(drawn first)

Total = 58 units

24.

40 units
NPH

32 units
Regular
(drawn first)

Total = 72 units

25.

12 units 8 units
NPH Regular
(drawn first)

Total = 20 units

Pages 252–253

1. 30 mEq; 15 mL
2. 2 mEq/mL
3. 7.5 mL
4. 2 mEq/mL
5. 20 mL
6. 10 mL
7. 1 mEq/mL
8. 50 mL/50 mEq; 1 mEq/mL
9. 4.2 g/mL
10. 10 mL

Chapter 15: Intravenous Flow Rate Calculations

Pages 269–271

1. 0.6 mL; 2.4; 144
2. 167
3. 1.5; 0.19
4. 120
5. 50
6. 25
7. 133
8. 200
9. 3; 3
10. 2; 18; 2.5

Page 274

	Letter of Matching Illustration	Components and Strength	Osmolarity (mOsm/L)
1.	C	sodium chloride 0.9%, 0.9 g/100 mL	308 mOsm/L
2.	E	dextrose 5%, 5 g/100 mL	252 mOsm/L
3.	G	dextrose 5%, 5 g/100 mL sodium chloride 0.9 g/100 mL	560 mOsm/L
4.	D	dextrose 5%, 5 g/100 mL sodium chloride 0.45 g/100 mL	406 mOsm/L
5.	A	dextrose 5%, 5 g/100 mL sodium chloride 0.225%, 0.225 g/100 mL	329 mOsm/L
6.	H	dextrose 5%, 5 g/100 mL sodium lactate 0.31 g/100 mL, NaCl 0.6 g/100 mL; KCl 0.03 g/100 mL; CaCl 0.02 g/100 mL	525 mOsm/L
7.	B	dextrose 5%, 5 g/100 mL sodium chloride 0.45%; 0.45g/100 mL; potassium chloride 20 mEq per liter	447 mOsm/L
8.	F	sodium chloride 0.45% 0.45 g/100 mL	154 mOsm/L

Pages 278–279

1. 2.25
2. 150; 27
3. 25; 1.65
4. 25
5. 50; 9
6. 6.75
7. 3.375
8. 36; 2.7
9. 25; 2.25
10. 50; 1.125

Pages 282–283

1. 15
2. 10
3. 60
4. 60
5. 10

Page 285

1. 28		**4.** 42	
2. 42		**5.** 49	
3. 16		**6.** 42	

Page 287

1. 26		**4.** 31	
2. 23		**5.** 42	
3. 28		**6.** 23	

Pages 288–290

1. 50		**5.** 20	
2. 40		**6.** 55	
3. 80		**7.** 33	
4. 50		**8.** 83	

Pages 290–291

1. 11		**5.** 25	
2. 28		**6.** 50	
3. 31		**7.** 60	
4. 8		**8.** 28	

Pages 293–297

1.
Original flow rate:	31
Solution remaining:	1350
Time remaining:	10
Recalculated flow rate:	135
Recalculated flow rate:	34
Variation:	10%
Action:	reset to 34 gtt/min (10% increase is acceptable).

2.
Original flow rate:	100
Time remaining:	5
Recalculated flow rate:	100
Recalculated flow rate:	100
Variation:	0%
Action:	IV is on time, so no adjustment is needed.

3.
Original flow rate:	21
Time remaining:	4
Recalculated flow rate:	188
Recalculated flow rate:	31
Variation:	48% (48% increase is unacceptable).
Action:	Consult the physician.

4.
Original flow rate:	33
Time remaining:	3
Recalculated flow rate:	83
Recalculated flow rate:	28
Variation:	−15% (−15% slower is acceptable)
Action:	IV is ahead of schedule. Slow rate to 28 gtt/min, and observe the patient's condition.

5.
Original flow rate:	42
Time remaining:	6
Recalculated flow rate:	142
Recalculated flow rate:	47
Variation:	12%
Action:	reset to 47 gtt/min (12% increase is acceptable).

6. Original flow rate: 42

Time remaining: 4

Recalculated flow rate: 200

Recalculated flow rate: 67

Variation: 60%

Action: recalculated rate 67 gtt/min (60% increase is unacceptable). Consult the physician.

7. Original flow rate: 13

Time remaining: 10

Recalculated flow rate: 60

Recalculated flow rate: 15

Variation: 15%

Action: reset to 15 gtt/min (15% increase is acceptable).

8. Original flow rate: 42

Time remaining: 2

Recalculated flow rate: 180

Recalculated flow rate: 45

Variation: 7%

Action: reset to 45 gtt/min (7% increase is acceptable).

Pages 299–300

1. 42	**5.** 125
2. 75	**6.** 120
3. 200	**7.** 125
4. 150	**8.** 83

Page 303

1. 38 mL/hr	**4.** 80 mL/hr
2. 40 mL/hr	**5.** 50 mL/hr
3. 16 mL/hr	

Pages 304–305

1. 1000 units/hr	**6.** 1000 units/hr
2. 1200 units/hr	**7.** 500 units/hr
3. 1200 units/hr	**8.** 875 units/hr
4. 600 units/hr	**9.** 400 units/hr
5. 1500 units/hr	**10.** 1400 units/hr

Chapter 16: Pediatric Drug Administration

Pages 318–324

1. 20; 500; 125; 1000; 250; yes

2. 5

3. 2.2; 110; 55; yes

4. 0.55

5. 15; 120; yes

6. 8

7. 5; 7.5; 12.5; yes

8. 0.8

9. 1.8; 4.5; no

10. 17.7; 354; 118; 708; 236; no

11. 120; 60; 7.5; yes

12. 7.5; $1\frac{1}{2}$

13. 25; 375; 125; 625; 208; no

Page 328

1. 0.57 m^2	**7.** 0.69 m^2
2. 0.69 m^2	**8.** 0.29 m^2
3. 0.42 m^2	**9.** 0.88 m^2
4. 0.52 m^2	**10.** 0.64 m^2
5. 0.78 m^2	**11.** 0.5 m^2
6. 1.40 m^2	**12.** 1.08 m^2

13. 0.34 m²   **15.** 0.38 m²

14. 1.08 m²

Pages 334–336

1. 7.2; 36.8

2. 2; 8

3. 7.5; 88.5

4. 2; 23

5. 120; 3; 22

6. 87; 2; 48

7. 80; 6; 44

8. 75; 3; 57

Pages 337–338

1. 350; 14.6

2. 1150; 48

3. 1800; 75

4. 1600; 67

5. 800; 33

6. 880; 35

7a. 1720

7b. 600

7c. 1100

7d. 1960

Chapter 1: Fundamentals of Math

1. V
2. XVIII
3. IX
4. XVI
5. XIX
6. XXII
7. XXIV
8. XXVII
9. XXIX
10. XXX
11. XLV
12. LXXXIX
13. CXII
14. CLV
15. CXCVIII
16. CCII
17. DVI
18. DXXXIV
19. M
20. MXXV
21. 4
22. 7
23. 9
24. 13
25. 14

26. 18
27. 19
28. 24
29. 27
30. 29
31. 18
32. 12
33. 11
34. 31
35. 21
36. 6
37. 18
38. 10
39. 9
40. 3
41. ɱ
42. pt
43. gr
44. fl oz
45. dr
46. gtt
47. fl dr
48. qt
49. kg
50. L

51. mg
52. g
53. mL
54. mcg
55. m
56. cm
57. T or tbsp
58. c
59. t or tsp
60. gal
61. oz
62. 0.04 g
63. 17.5 kg
64. 3.5 kg
65. 5.3 mL
66. 10.4 mcg
67. 200 mcg
68. 15.2 mcg
69. 0.6 L
70. 8 g
71. 0.4 mL
72. 0.09 mg
73. gr v
74. $\frac{1}{2}$ t or $\frac{1}{2}$ tsp
75. 9 oz
76. $7\frac{1}{2}$ oz
77. gr xvi

78. gr $\overline{ss}$
79. dr iv
80. 25 mEq
81. 10,000 units
82. $\frac{1}{2}$ T or $\frac{1}{2}$ tbsp
83. $3\frac{1}{2}$ oz
84. $\frac{1}{2}$ oz
85. 15
86. 6
87. 32
88. 40
89. 60 gtt
90. 3
91. 1.5t
92. 2
93. meter
94. dram
95. minim
96. grain
97. quart
98. ounce
99. ounce
100. $\frac{1}{2}$
101. millimeter
102. gram
103. gtt

104. gr

105. t or tsp

106. ℳ

107. T or tbsp

108. dr

109. mEq

110. pt

111. oz

112. length

113. volume

114. weight

115. 1000

116. 1

117. 10

118. 1000

119. 10

120. 1000

121. 0.1

122. 10 mg

123. 4.5 mL

124. 7 kg

125. 2.5 mm

126. 8.5 mcg

Critical Thinking

1a. The patient should use a tablespoon to administer the medication.

1b. The patient should take one tablespoon three times a day.

1c. 45 mL per day × 10 days equals 450 mL total. Because 450 mL is equivalent to 0.95 of a pint, the patient needs 2 half-pint bottles to contain enough medication for the 10-day period.

2. The pharmacy technician should ask the pharmacist or check a Web site to understand what the "L" stands for in the Roman numeral system.

Chapter 2: Fractions and Decimals

1. $2\frac{1}{3}$

2. 2

3. $\frac{13}{25}$

4. $9\frac{3}{8}$

5. $1\frac{1}{3}$

6. $\frac{1}{20}$

7. $3\frac{5}{8}$

8. $2\frac{5}{7}$

9. $\frac{2}{3}$

10. $\frac{3}{14}$

11. 12

12. $8\frac{1}{4}$

13. $\frac{3}{8}$

14. $24\frac{16}{39}$

15. $8\frac{5}{8}$

16. $\frac{1}{5}$

17. $\frac{9}{7}$

18. $\frac{171}{8}$

19. $\frac{43}{5}$

20. $\frac{13}{2}$

21. $\frac{9}{2}$

22. $\frac{34}{3}$

23. $\frac{1}{4}$

24. $\frac{33}{46}$

25. 6

26. $11\frac{1}{2}$

27. $1\frac{25}{31}$

28. 2

29. 10 and $\frac{6}{10}$; 1 and $\frac{1}{10}$

30. $\frac{9}{18}$ and $\frac{8}{18}$; $\frac{17}{18}$

31. $\frac{56}{60}, \frac{15}{60},$ and $\frac{40}{60}$; 1 and $\frac{37}{60}$

32. $\frac{18}{30}, \frac{45}{30}, \frac{5}{30}$; 2 and $\frac{4}{15}$

33. 4.6

34. 7.8

35. 9

36. 0.1

37. 8.09

38. 0.44

39. 64

40. 9.88

41. 20

42. 7

43. 1

44. 13

45. 0.901

46. 21.56

47. 5.39

48. 17.308

49. 5.08

50. 2.95

51. −0.206

52. 18.373

53. 41.87

54. 0.00268

55. 8.928

56. 12.19881

57. 23.1524 (rounded)

58. 2.0464 (rounded)

59. 40

60. 20

61. 0.15

62. 0.073

63. False

64. False

65. True

Critical Thinking

1. The instruments should be arranged as follows (smallest to largest):

$$\frac{1}{16}, \frac{3}{16}, \frac{1}{4}, \frac{5}{16}, \frac{7}{16}, \frac{1}{2}$$

2. Yes, the missing instrument sizes in the sequence are the following:

$$\frac{1}{8} \text{ and } \frac{3}{8}$$

Chapter 3:
Ratios, Proportions, and Percents

1. 0.06	20. 1:300
2. 0.35	21. 4
3. 0.003	22. 1
4. 0.0001	23. 2
5. 0.00004	24. $\frac{1}{3}$
6. $\frac{1}{20}$	25. 500
7. $\frac{1}{5}$	26. 4
	27. 0.375
8. $\frac{3}{1000}$	28. 0.5
	29. 9
9. $\frac{1}{400}$	30. $\frac{2}{3}$
10. $\frac{1}{2000}$	31. T
11. 1:3	32. T
12. 1:500	33. F
13. 8:9	34. T
14. 1:75	35. F
15. 2:1	36. F
16. 1:100	37. F
17. 1:2	38. F
18. 1:8	39. T
19. 1:400	40. F

Critical Thinking

1. No, the technician made a mistake during calculation.

2. The pharmacy technician should use the ratio formula as follows:

$$\frac{250 \text{ mcg}}{1 \text{ tablet}} = \frac{125 \text{ mcg}}{X \text{ tablets}}$$

By cross-multiplying, the answer reveals that one-half of a tablet contains 125 micrograms of medication. Therefore, the patient must take only one-half of a tablet per dose.

Chapter 4:
Celsius and Fahrenheit Temperature Conversions

1. 17.44°C	13. 32°F
2. 37.5°C	14. 44.2°F
3. 30.7°C	15. 36.3°F
4. 81.1°C	16. 99.3°F
5. 55.6°C	17. 212°F
6. 0°C	18. 110.5°F
7. 44.4°C	19. 89.6°F
8. 100°C	20. 47.1°F
9. 6.7°C	21. 131°F
10. 36.6°C	22. 62.6°F
11. 73.3°C	23. 32.2°F
12. 8.9°C	24. 80.6°F

Critical Thinking

1. 38.33°C

2. 46.4°F

Chapter 5:
Ratio and Proportion Method

1. 0.8 mL	4. 5 mL
2. 1.5 mL	5. 0.9 mL
3. 0.4 mL	6. 1.5 mL

7. 0.38 mL

8. 0.8 mL

9. 2.4 mL

10. 0.8 mL

11. 8 mL

12. 2 mL

13. 1.5 mL

14. 0.45 mL

15. 2 mL

16. 1.8 mL

17. 15 mL

18. 0.8 mL

19. 1.7 mL

20. 2.5 mL

21. 8 mL

22. 1.6 mL

23. 1.5 mL

24. 1.6 mL

25. 1.5 mL

26. 0.8 mL

27. 1.3 mL

28. 2.4 mL

29. 0.9 mL

30. 0.7 mL

Chapter 6:
Dimensional Analysis

1. $2\frac{1}{2}$ tablets

2. 1.3 mL

3. 0.5 mL

4. 2.5 mL

5. 2.3 mL

6. 2.6 mL

7. 3 mL

8. 1.5 mL

9. 7 mL

10. 3 mL

11. 0.8 mL

12. 1.4 mL

13. 3 mL

14. 0.9 mL

15. 1.5 mL

16. 0.38 mL

17. 0.8 mL

18. 1.2 mL

19. 1.5 mL

20. 0.45 mL

21. 1.6 mL

22. 2 mL

23. 2.3 mL

24. 2.4 mL

25. 15 mL

26. 1.5 mL

27. 0.8 mL

28. 1.6 mL

29. 2.5 mL

30. 3 mL

31. 8 mL

32. 1.2 mL

33. 1.6 mL

34. 0.6 mL

35. 1.5 mL

36. 1.6 mL

37. 1.3 mL

38. 1.5 mL

39. 1.5 mL

40. 2.5 mL

41. 1.7 mL

42. 2 mL

43. 0.9 mL

44. 1.4 mL

45. 10 mL

46. 1.8 mL

47. 0.8 mL

48. 2 mL

49. 0.8 mL

Chapter 7:
Formula Method

1. 1.3 mL

2. 0.8 mL

3. 1.5 mL

4. 1.6 mL

5. 1.4 mL

6. 1.2 mL

7. 1.2 mL

8. 2.4 mL

9. 0.7 mL

10. 0.8 mL

11. 2 mL

12. 12 mL

13. 3 mL

14. 4 mL

15. 2.6 mL

16. 4 mL

17. 1.4 mL

18. 20 mL

19. 1.6 mL

20. 0.8 mL

21. 1.5 mL

22. 30 mL

23. 1.5 mL

24. 0.8 mL

25. 2.5 mL

26. 1.6 mL

27. 0.8 mL

28. 1.6 mL

29. 2.5 mL

30. 20 mL

31. 0.7 mL

32. 0.8 mL

33. 1.3 mL

34. 25 mL

35. 1.2 mL

36. 0.8 mL

37. 30 mL

38. 1.3 mL

39. 2.5 mL

40. 35 mL

Chapter 8: Interpretation of Prescriptions and Drug Labels

1. The components of a prescription include all of the following: name, address, and phone number of the prescriber's office; name and address of the patient; date; medication prescribed (inscription); Rx symbol (superscription); dispensing directions to the pharmacist (subscription); directions for the patient (signa), refill and special labeling; prescriber's signature; and license number or Drug Enforcement Administration (DEA) number (on controlled substances only).

2. A "stat" order means *immediately*. These orders are used on prescriptions and other medical orders.

3. Controlled substances only

4. Inscription; signa; subscription; superscription

5. Two

6. Five

7. 30 tablets

8. One

9. 100 mg

10. 1 every 4 hours

11. One drop twice a day in affected eye

12. 0.5%

13. Two

14. Three

15. One tablet

16. 180

17. Every four hours, as needed

18. Two

19. None

20. Ointment

21. Every

22. Verbal order

23. Amount

24. Before meals

25. Write on label

26. After meals

27. At bedtime ("hour of sleep")

28. Water

29. As needed

30. Drop

31. Without

32. Immediately

33. With

34. 50 mEq/50 mL or 1 mEq/mL

35. 84 mg/mL

36. 63323-006-50

37. IV (injection)

38. cefpodoxime proxetil

39. Shake bottle to loosen granules. Add approximately one-half the total amount of distilled water required for constitution (total water = 29 milliunits). Shake vigorously to wet the granules. Add remaining water and shake vigorously.

40. Pharmacia and Upjohn

41. 0009-3615-03

42. 250 mg (25 mg/mL)

43. 10 mL

44. 1 mL

45. tobramycin

46. Nebcin®

47. 40 mg

48. 30 mL

49. Intramuscular solution

50. Intramuscular (injection)

51. 10 mL

52. Store below 86 degrees Fahrenheit (30 degrees Celsius); protect from freezing.

53. Pfizer/Roerig

54. propranolol hydrochloride

55. Tablets

56. Ayerst Laboratories Inc.

57. 0046-0422-81

58. 40 mEq (2 mEq per mL)

59. 12/2007 (Dec 2007)

60. Give 30 mg of Apresoline intravenously every 6 hours.

61. Give 0.5 mg of neostigmine by intramuscular injection three times a day.

62. Give 25 units of Novolin N NPH U-100 insulin subcutaneously before breakfast.

63. Give 50 mg of Demerol by intramuscular injection every 3 to 4 hours as needed for pain.

64. Give 0.25 mg of Lanoxin orally every day.

65. Give 5 mL of Maalox orally 1 hour before meals, 1 hour after meals, and at bedtime.

66. Give 600 mg of Motrin orally twice a day.

67. Give 50 mg of Cytoxan orally every day.

68. Give 0.5 g of Cephalexin orally 4 times a day.

69. Give 16 mEq of potassium chloride orally every day.

70. Give 60 mg of Toradol intramuscularly immediately and every 6 hours.

71. Give 4 mg of Decadron intravenously twice a day.

72. Not listed

73. Label H

74. Label I

75. Schedule III

76. PO, since the drug is in tablet form

77. Label H

78. 2 mL

79. 2%

80. 20

Critical Thinking

1. A pharmacy technician should always ask for assistance when a prescription is not clear due to handwriting. The prescription should never be filled until it is accurately understood.

2. Metadate is commonly prescribed for ADHD, while methadone is strong synthetic opioid usually prescribed for withdrawal from morphine, as well as for pain.

Chapter 9: Percentage of Error Due to Equipment

1. 6.67%

2. 1%

3. 69%

4. 6.6%

5. 5.5%

6. 7.14%

7. 247.5 mg would have actually been weighed because of the 10% overage.

8. 1.25%

9. 60 mg

10. The smallest weight would be 0.08 g, and an aliquot could be made to get the desired amount of weight.

Critical Thinking

1. This spoon is not calibrated identically to a conventional teaspoon.

2. The child is still sick because she is not receiving enough medication per spoonful because the spoon being used is not equivalent to a full teaspoon.

Chapter 10: Dilutions and Solutions

1. $3\frac{1}{3}$ mg

2. 15 mg

3. $6\frac{2}{3}$ mg

4. 100 g

5. $\frac{2}{5}$; $\frac{2}{7}$

6. $\frac{3}{7}$; $\frac{7}{10}$

7. $\frac{4}{11}$; $\frac{11}{15}$

8. $\frac{5}{7}$; $\frac{7}{12}$

9. $\frac{1}{7}$; $\frac{1}{7}$

10. $\frac{3}{14}$; 3; 14

11. $\frac{2}{17}$; $\frac{2}{17}$

12. $\frac{5}{23}$; $\frac{5}{23}$

13. $\frac{2}{5}$

14. $\frac{5}{13}$

15. $\frac{1}{11}$

16. $\frac{3}{13}$

17. Take 162 mL urine and add it to 108 mL water.

18. Take 40 mL urine and add it to 60 mL water.

19. Take 50 mL urine and add it to 30 mL water.

20. $\frac{3}{12} = \frac{1}{4}$

21. $\frac{2}{14}$ or $\frac{1}{7}$

22. $\frac{2}{7}$

23. 15 microliters serum and 105 microliters diluent are needed.

24. 18 mL total solution; 14 mL diluent are needed

25. 10 microliters serum and 140 microliters diluent are needed.

26. 12 mL total solution; 9 mL diluent are needed

27. Take 300 mL concentrate and add it to 200 mL diluent.

28. Take 160 mL concentrate and add it to 240 mL diluent.

29. 12.5 microliters

30. Take 125 mL concentrate and add it to 125 mL diluent.

31. 2 microliters

32. 12.5 mL

33. 20 g of 20% ichthammol ointment and 40 g of 15% ichthammol ointment

34. 20 g of 20% zinc oxide ointment and 40 g of 5% zinc oxide ointment

35. 60 g of 10% coal tar and 100 g of 2% coal tar

36. 45 g of benzocaine 10% ointment and 75 g of benzocaine 2% ointment

37. 19 g of 10% hydrocortisone cream and 71 g of 2.5% hydrocortisone cream.

38. 250 mL of 90% alcohol and 1750 mL of 10% alcohol

39. 9 bottles

40. Combine 750 mL of D10W and 250 mL of SWFI.

41. 15 g of petrolatum

42. 180 mL of 1:10 solution and 300 mL of 1:50 solution

Critical Thinking

1. 400 mL ÷ 8 = 50 mL

2. 350 mL of water are needed.

Chapter 11: Concentrations

1. 1.5%

2. 0.8%

3. 5%

4. 25%

5. 1.5%

6. $\frac{1}{5}$

7. $\frac{1}{2}$

8. $\frac{1}{4}$

9. $\frac{1}{3}$

10. 0.2%

11. 1%

12. 10%

13. 4.8%

14. 7.5%

15. 90 mL

16. 87.5 mL

17. 125 mL

18. 96 mL

19. 1.25%

20. 0.5%

21. 1.75%

22. 0.75%

23. 0.4%

24. 400 mL

25. approx 171 mL

26. approx 233 mL

27. 700 mL

28. Need 22.5 g

29. Need 37.5 g

30. Need 6.75 g

31. 90 g

32. Add 45 mL isopropyl alcohol to 205 mL water.

33. Add 40 mL isopropyl alcohol to 160 mL water.

34. Add 22.5 mL isopropyl alcohol to 202.5 mL water.

35. Add 49 mL isopropyl alcohol to 21 mL water.

36. Dissolve 37.5 g NaCl in 150 mL diluent.

37. Dissolve 12 g ampicillin in 200 mL diluent.

38. Dissolve 1 g NaCl in 50 mL diluent.

39. Dissolve 15 g cephapirin in 125 mL diluent.

40. Dissolve 21 g cephapirin in 150 mL diluent.

41. 150 g

42. 1350 g

43. 2 g

44. 20 g

45. 600 mL

46. 1000 mL = 1 L

47. Approx 583 mL

48. 250 mL

49. 3%

50. 8%

51. 6%

52. Approx 8.3%

53. 20%

54. 18.75%

Chapter 12:
Oral Medication Labels and Dosage Calculation

1. 2 capsules

2. 2 tablets

3. 1 tablet

4. 1 tablet

5. $\frac{1}{2}$ tablet

6. 2 capsules

7. 4 tablets

8. 4 tablets

9. 1 capsule

10. 1 tablet

11. 2 tablets

12. 2 tablets

13. 1 tablet

14. 2 tablets

15. 2 tablets

16. 2 tablets

17. 4 tablets

18. 2 tablets

19. 4 tablets

20. 1 tablet

21. 10 mL

22. 1.5 mL at bedtime

23. 5 mL

24. 12.5 mL

25. 7.5 mL

26. 1.9 mL

27. 0.5 mL

28. 1 oz per dose

29. 6 mL

30. 5 mL

31. 2.5 mL

32. 2.5 mL

33. 5 mL

34. 20 mL

35. 5.5 mL

36. 3.3 mL

37. 3 oz per dose

38. 3.3 mL

39. 2.5 mL

40. 20 mL

Critical Thinking

1. 480 mg; no, the correct dosage is 120 mg per day, or six 20 mg tablets.

Chapter 13:
Reconstitution of Powdered Drugs

1. Sterile Water for Injection

2. 10 mL

3. 500 mg

4. Within 12 hours

5. 2 g

6. 20 mL

7. Bacteriostatic Water for Injection USP with Benzyl Alcohol

8. 100 mg/mL

9. 48 hours

10. One million units

11. 10 mL

12. 1.8 mL

13. 20 mL

14. Package insert

15. Refrigerate

16. Expires at 1:10 a.m. on Dec. 25

17. Your initials

18. Space considerations; handwriting is difficult to read

19. azithromycin

20. 500 mg

21. Sterile Water for Injection

22. 4.8 mL

23. 100 mg per mL

Chapter 14:
Parenteral Medication Labels and Dosage Calculation

1. 0.3

2. 1.6

3. 0.4

4. 2.5

5. 1.2

6. 22

7. 0.8

8. 0.6

9. 1.4

10. 0.75

11. 86

12. 46

13. 0.7; 1 mL or 3 mL, with 1 mL being best

14. 0.8; 1 mL or 3 mL

15. 1; 1 mL or 3 mL

16. 0.7; 1 mL or 3 mL

17. 6; 10 mL

18. 0.7; 1 mL or 3 mL, with 1 mL being best

19. 0.75; 1 mL or 3 mL, with 1 mL being best

20. 2.5; 3 mL

21. 1.5; 3 mL

22. 2; 3 mL

23. 0.5; 1 mL or 3 mL

24. 0.6; 1 mL or 3 mL, with 1 mL being best

25. 1; 1 mL or 3 mL

26. 0.4; 1 mL

27. 0.7; 1 mL or 3 mL, with 1 mL being best

28. 0.4; 1 mL

29. 0.25; 1 mL

30. 2.5; 3 mL

31. 0.24; 1 mL

32. 0.75; 1 mL

Critical Thinking

1. Compazine would be injected intramuscularly (IM). Therefore, it would be absorbed through the blood capillaries around the muscle injected.

2. There is a possibility of infection and nerve damage due to the patient's lack of knowledge of properly self-injecting.

Chapter 15: Intravenous Flow Rate Calculations

1. 33

2. 50

3. 67

4. 8

5. 11

6. 15

7. 45

8. 83

9. 21

10. 14

11. 28

12. 33

13. 100

14. 17

15. 25

16. 125

17. 42

18. Assess the patient. If stable, recalculate and reset to 50 gtt/min; observe the patient closely.

19. 42

20. 42

21. 3000 mL

22. Abbott Laboratories

23. 15 gtt/mL

24. 4

25.

$$\text{mL/hr} = \frac{500 \text{ mL}}{4 \text{ hrs}} = 125 \text{ mL/hr}$$

$$\frac{\text{mL/hr}}{\text{Drop factor constant}} = \text{gtt/min}$$

$$\frac{125 \text{ mL/hr}}{4} = 31.2 \text{ gtt/min} = 31 \text{ gtt/min}$$

26.

$$\frac{V}{T} \times C = \frac{125 \text{ mL}}{60 \text{ min}} \times 15 \text{ gtt/mL}$$

$$= \frac{125 \text{ gtt}}{4 \text{ min}} = 31.3 \text{ gtt/min or } 31 \text{ gtt/min}$$

27. 1930 (or 7:30 PM)

28. 250

29. Recalculate 210 mL to infuse over the remaining 2 hours. Reset the IV to 26 gtt/min and observe the patient closely.

30. 125

31. 200 mL/hour

32. 160 mL/hour

33. 14 gtt/min

34. 233 gtt/min

35. 75 gtt/min

36. 35 gtt/min

37. 60 minutes

38. 70.8 or 71 gtt/min

39. 30 gtt/min over 300 minutes (5 hours)

40. 125 mL/hour

41. 66.6 or 67 mL/hour

42. 41.6 or 42 gtt/min

43. 160 gtt/min

44. 30 gtt/min over 1200 minutes (20 hours)

45. 0.5 mL

46. 750 mL/hour

47. 25 gtt/min

48. 55.5 gtt/min

49. 300 mL/hour

50. 25 gtt/min

51. 1125 units/hr

52. 750 units/hr

53. 1575 units/hr

54. 800 units/hr

55. 750 units/hr

56. 1500 units/hr

57. 50 mL/hr

58. 34 mL/hr

Critical Thinking

1. The patient's pneumonia could worsen.
2. As a result, the patient may die.

Chapter 16: Pediatric Drug Administration

1. 1500–1875; 250–312.5; Yes; 2.8
2. 35; 2.8; 32.2
3. 25; 2,500,000–6,250,000; 416,667–1,041,667
4. Yes
5. 20; 2.6; 17.4
6. 330–495; 110–165
7. 25; 3.3; 21.7
8. 1.11
9. 1.69
10. 1.92
11. 1.68
12. 1.63
13. 0.69
14. 0.32
15. 0.52
16. 10.8; 5.4
17. 14; 7
18. 3.8; 1.9
19. 1809; 75
20. 1520; 63
21. 240; 10
22. 1250; 52
23. 1.3; 26
24. 13
25. 0.8; 2000
26. 2.7
27. No
28. 1.17; 1.8–2.3

29. 0.52; 42; 0.84 **31.** 2.2

30. 0.43; 108 **32.** 6.2; 37.8

Critical Thinking

1. The pharmacy technician should alert the pharmacist.

Chapter 17:
Business Math

1. d **3.** d

2. a **4.** d

5. a **11.** b

6. b **12.** $900

7. b **13.** $9.38

8. b **14.** $14.00

9. c **15.** $2.00

10. d

Critical Thinking

1. $4.60 + ($4.60 × 12%) + $1.40 = $6.55

$6.55 × 30 = $196.50

Case Studies with Answers

1. The physician prescribes dopamine 400 mg in 250 mL D_5W to start at 5 mcg/kg/min in a 55-year-old man weighing 178 lb. The nurse would set the infusion pump to how many milliliters per hour?

   A. 12.8
   B. 15.1
   C. 17.5
   D. 21.1

2. A 60-year-old woman is brought to the hospital because of her hypertensive condition. Her weight is 165 pounds, and her physician prescribed Nipride 3 mcg/kg/min. IV. Nipride 50 mg is added to a 250 mL solution of D_5W. What would be the concentration of Nipride in this solution?

   A. 120 mcg/mL
   B. 150 mcg/mL
   C. 200 mcg/mL
   D. 250 mcg/mL

3. In question 2, by using an infusion pump, the nurse would set the flow rate at how many milliliters per hour?

   A. 47–48
   B. 57–58
   C. 67–68
   D. 97–98

4. A pediatrician ordered Benadryl® for a 9-year-old to relieve itching from chickenpox. Benadryl® comes in an elixir of 12.5 mg/5 mL. The normal adult dose is 25 mg every 12 hours as needed. Which of the following doses would you give?

   A. 5 mg in 2 mL
   B. 5 mg in 4 mL
   C. 7.5 mg in 2 mL
   D. 10 mg in 4 mL

5. A family practitioner prescribed 1.0 mg IM of leucovorin calcium to be administered once a day for the treatment of megaloblastic anemia. The medication is available as a powder in a 50 mg vial. The nurse reconstitutes it with 5.0 mL of sterile water for injection and shakes it well. Solution concentration will yield 10 mg/mL and fluid volume

will equal 5.0 mL. How much would the nurse give once a day?

   A. 0.1 mL
   B. 0.3 mL
   C. 0.5 mL
   D. 0.9 mL

6. A pediatrician ordered 100 mg of Augmentin every 8 hours for a 4-year-old. These antibiotics come in a powder for an oral suspension with a concentration of 200 mg/5 mL. The nurse would administer ____ mL for each dose. The child would receive ____ mg and ____ mL in 24 hours.

7. The physician prescribed 0.4 mg of atropine sulfate to be administered intramuscularly. The medication was labeled in grains/mL. The pharmacy technician knew to look for an ampule labeled ____ grains/mL.

8. The physician ordered 120 mg of furosemide to administer intramuscularly every 8 hours for 2 days. The medication is available for injection as 10 mg/mL. How much should the nurse give every 8 hours?

   A. 2 mL
   B. 4 mL
   C. 6 mL
   D. 10 mL

9. A cardiologist prescribes a continuous labetalol infusion to control hypertension. The label indicates that you should remove 90 mL from a 250 mL NSS bag, and add 200 mg of labetalol. The labetalol vial has 5 mg/mL. You would add ____ mL of labetalol to the IV bag. The concentration of labetalol would be ____ mg/mL (remember to include the volume of labetalol in the calculation of the total volume). In order to administer 1 mg/min, you would set the infusion pump at ____ mL/hr.

10. A child was prescribed 1 fluidram of cough syrup, four times a day, as needed. The child's mother wants to know how many teaspoon(s) should be given.

    A. 1
    B. $1\frac{1}{2}$
    C. 2
    D. $2\frac{1}{2}$

11. A physician prescribed 300 mg of Tagamet four times a day. The nurse would administer ____ tablet(s) for each dose. The patient would receive ____ mg of Tagamet in 24 hours.

12. A patient is to receive Nitrostat 20 mcg/min IV. Nitrostat is available in a 10 mL vial labeled 5 mg/mL. To prepare a 200 mcg/mL solution with a concentration of 50 mg in 250 mL, the nurse would add ____ mL of Nitrostat to 250 mL of D_5W, and set the infusion pump flow rate at ____ mL/hr to deliver 20 mcg/min.

13. The usual adult dose for Celebrex is 100 mg twice daily for a total dose of 200 mg/day. How much should a child weighing 52 lb receive per dose?

   A. 49.34
   B. 59.34
   C. 69.34
   D. 82.26

14. A 4-year-old child is to receive 250 mg of Ceclor three times daily. The medicine is available in oral suspension, 250 mg per 5 mL. The nurse would give how many teaspoons?

   A. 1 / 2
   B. 1
   C. 1 1 / 2
   D. 2

15. The physician prescribed an IV of Ringer's lactate at 75 mL/hr. There is a drop factor of 15. How much would the nurse administer to the patient?

   A. 13 gtt/min
   B. 19 gtt/min
   C. 22 gtt/min
   D. 27 gtt/min

16. The nurse increases a lidocaine infusion of 2 g in 250 mL D_5W to 30 mL/hr to control the patient's dysrhythmia. She should document that the patient is now receiving how many milligrams per minute?

   A. 2
   B. 3
   C. 4
   D. 5

17. Mrs. Brown goes to her participating HMO provider for a checkup and a flu shot. The allowed charge for a checkup is $65, and the physician's usual fee is $70. The allowed charge for the flu shot is $40, and the physician's usual fee is $25. How much is Mrs. Brown charged for the visit?

   A. $7   C. $18
   B. $12   D. Nothing

18. A pharmacy technician has been given 100 mL of a 10% acetic acid solution. The pharmacist asks the technician to dilute the solution to 500 mL with sterile water and to label the solution. What percentage should appear on the label?

   A. 1.5%
   B. 2.0%
   C. 2.5%
   D. 3.0%

19. A drug is available in the following strengths and dosage forms: 125 mg tablets, 250 mg capsules, and 125 mg/5 mL liquid. A child weighs 55 lb and the recommended dose is 10 mg/kg/24 hr (to be given in 6- or 12-hour intervals). Determine which of the following would not be an appropriate dosage regimen using the information provided.

   A. One-half of a 125 mg tablet every 6 hours
   B. 5 mL of 125 mg/5 mL liquid every 12 hours
   C. One 250 mg capsule every 12 hours
   D. One 125 mg tablet every 12 hours

20. The cost of 250 tablets of furosemide 80 mg is $246.84. If your pharmacy marks up the cost by 13% and adds a $2.35 dispensing fee, what would be the retail charge for 60 tablets?

   A. $54.51
   B. $62.43
   C. $69.29
   D. $76.64

21. The pediatrician ordered ampicillin 75 mg/kg/24 hr to be given in divided doses every 8 hours for days. The child weighs 44 lb. The pharmacy has a 150 mL bottle that contains 250 mg/5 mL. What is the patient's weight in kg?

   A. 10 kg
   B. 20 kg
   C. 25 kg
   D. 32 kg

22. A nurse received an order to administer 5 mEq of potassium acetate per hour. The bag of IV fluid contains 30 mEq/L. How many drops per minute would be needed to provide the prescribed dose using a set that delivers 15 gtt/mL?

   A. 26
   B. 42
   C. 51
   D. 64

23. The recommended dose of Demerol® is 6 mg/kg/24 hr for pain. It is given in divided doses every 4 to 6 hours. How many milliliters of Demerol® injection (50 mg/mL) should be administered to a 33 lb child as a single dose every 6 hours?

    A. 0.45 mL
    B. 0.65 mL
    C. 0.85 mL
    D. 1.25 mL

24. A pharmacy technician receives a prescription that orders 12.5% dextrose solution. There are 20% dextrose and 5% dextrose solutions available in stock. If the technician wants to mix these stock solutions, which of the following ratios would be correct?

    A. 1 : 1
    B. 1 : 2
    C. 1 : 3
    D. 2 : 1

25. A patient is to receive cefamandole (Mandol®) 500 mg IM by injection. The vial of powdered medication on hand is labeled Mandol® 1 gram. The directions state: For IM solution, add 3 mL of sterile diluent to provide an approximate volume of 3.5 mL = 1 gram. How many milliliters should the nurse inject?

    A. 1.25
    B. 1.50
    C. 1.75
    D. 2.25

26. The physician prescribed Aldomet 125 mg IV stat for Mrs. Johnston to be added into 100 mL NSS and hung as an intermittent infusion. The medication is available as 250 mg/5 mL. The nurse should prepare how many milliliters?

    A. 1.5
    B. 2.5
    C. 3.5
    D. 4.5

27. A pediatrician ordered Benadryl® 25 mg orally every 8 hours for a 2-year-old child who weighs 16 kg. Pediatric dosage range is 5 mg/kg/day. If this drug is available as 12.5 mg/5 mL, how many milliliters would you give?

    A. 2.5 mL
    B. 5.0 mL
    C. 7.5 mL
    D. 10 mL

28. The physician has prescribed tobramycin sulfate injection (Nebcin®) 70 mg in 100 mL of D_5W via IVPB to be infused in 75 minutes. Nebcin® 80 mg in 2 mL is available. The drop factor of the infusion set is 60. How much Nebcin® should be added to the 100 mL bag of D_5W? ____ mL

    How many drops per minute should be infused to deliver Nebcin® 70 mg in 75 minutes? ____ gtt/min

    If an electronic infusion device is used, the nurse should set the hourly rate at ____ mL/hr.

29. A child is brought to the emergency department with an asthma attack. His weight is 64 lb, and he requires aminophylline IV at 1 mg/kg/hr. The solution is prepared using premixed aminophylline 400 mg in 500 cc D_5W. Which of the following will be the correct rate?

    A. 22.32 mL/hr
    B. 32.46 mL/hr
    C. 64.64 mL/hr
    D. 94.94 mL/hr

30. A pregnant woman was prescribed 60 mg of Fergon® daily. Her cumulative monthly dose (30 days) would be approximately how many grams?

    A. 0.8 g
    B. 1.8 g
    C. 2.8 g
    D. 4.8 g

Answer Key

1. B	16. C
2. C	17. D
3. C	18. B
4. D	19. C
5. A	20. C
6. 2.5; 300; 7.5	21. B
7. 1/150	22. B
8. B	23. A
9. 40; 1; 60	24. A
10. C	25. C
11. 1; 1,200	26. B
12. 10; 6	27. D
13. C	28. 1.75 or 1.8; 82; 82
14. B	29. C
15. B	30. B

Generic Name	Brand Name	Manufacturer
hydrocodone w/apap	(generic only)	Watson
atorvastatin	Lipitor	Pfizer
hydrocodone w/apap	(generic only)	Mallinckrodt
levothyroxine sodium	(generic only)	Mylan
lisinopril	(generic only)	Lupin
amoxicillin	Augmentin	Teva
esomeprazole	Nexium	AstraZeneca
clopidogrel bisulfate	Plavix	Bristol-Myers Squibb/ sanofi-aventis
metoprolol tartrate	(generic only)	Mylan
montelukast sodium	Singulair	Merck/Schering-Plough
escitalopram oxalate	Lexapro	Forest
levothyroxine sodium	Synthroid	Abbott
albuterol sulfate	ProAir HFA	Teva
simvastatin	(generic only)	Teva
amlodipine besylate	(generic only)	Mylan
azithromycin	(generic only)	Greenstone/Pfizer
metformin hydrochloride	(generic only)	Teva
levothyroxine sodium	(generic only)	Lannett
metoprolol succinate	(generic only)	Par
simvastatin	(generic only)	Lupin
hydrochlorothiazide	(generic only)	Teva
rosuvastatin calcium	Crestor	AstraZeneca
furosemide	(generic only)	Mylan
warfarin sodium	(generic only)	Teva
fluticasone/salmeterol	Advair Diskus	GlaxoSmithKline
simvastatin	(generic only)	Dr. Reddy's
ibuprofen	Ibuprofen (Rx)	Amneal
sertraline hydrochloride	(generic only)	Greenstone/Pfizer
azithromycin	(generic only)	Teva
valsartan	Diovan	Novartis
zolpidem tartrate	(generic only)	Teva
lisinopril	(generic only)	Teva
oxycodone/apap	(generic only)	Mallinckrodt
duloxetine hydrochloride	Cymbalta	Lilly
quetiapine fumarate	Seroquel	AstraZeneca
venlafaxine hydrochloride	Effexor XR	Pfizer
tamsulosin hydrochloride	Flomax	Boehringer Ingelheim
amlodipine besylate	(generic only)	Greenstone/Pfizer
alprazolam	(generic only)	Actavis
valsartan and hydrochlorothiazide	Diovan HCT	Novartis
trazodone hydrochloride	(generic only)	Teva
pioglitazone hydrochloride	Actos	Takeda
alendronate sodium	(generic only)	Teva
sulfamethoxazole/trimethoprim	(generic only)	Amneal
lansoprazole	Prevacid	Takeda
clonazepam	(generic only)	Teva
tramadol hydrochloride	(generic only)	Amneal
levofloxacin	Levaquin	Johnson & Johnson
fluoxetine hydrochloride	(generic only)	Teva
prednisone	(generic only)	Watson

Generic Name	Brand Name	Manufacturer
omeprazole	(generic only)	Sandoz/Novartis
hydrochlorothiazide	(generic only)	Qualitest
atenolol	(generic only)	Mylan
insluin glargine	Lantus	sanofi-aventis
omeprazole	(generic only)	Mylan
amoxicillin trihydrate/potassium clavulanate	(generic only)	Sandoz/Novartis
oxycodone/apap	(generic only)	Watson
alprazolam	(generic only)	Greenstone/Pfizer
fenofibrate	Tricor	Abbott
celecoxib	Celebrex	Pfizer
donepezil hydrochloride	Aricept	Eisai
ezetimibe/simvastatin	Vytorin	Merck/Schering-Plough
cephalexin	(generic only)	Teva
mometasone furoate monohydrate	Nasonex	Merck/Schering-Plough
drospirenone/ethinyl estradiol	Yaz-28	Bayer
hydrocodone/apap	(generic only)	Qualitest
ergocaliferol (vitamin d)	Vit D	Teva
ezetimibe	Zetia	Merck/Schering-Plough
simvastatin	(generic only)	Aurobindo
gabapentin	(generic only)	Greenstone/Pfizer
pregabalin	Lyrica	Pfizer
sildenafil citrate	Viagra	Pfizer
apap/codeine	(generic only)	Teva
lisinopril	(generic only)	Mylan
fluconazole	(generic only)	Teva
fluticazone propionate	(generic only)	Roxane/Boehringer Ingelheim
omeprazole	(generic only)	Apotex
losartan potassium	Cozaar	Merck/Schering-Plough
warfarin sodium	(generic only)	Taro
lisinopril	(generic only)	Sandoz/Novartis
valacyclovir hydrochloride	Valtrex	GlaxoSmithKline
alprazolam	(generic only)	Sandoz/Novartis
albuterol sulfate	Ventolin HFA	GlaxoSmithKline
atenolol	(generic only)	Sandoz/Novartis
lorazepam	(generic only)	Actavis
metformin hydrochloride	(generic only)	Zydus
metoprolol succinate	Toprol-XL	AstraZeneca
pantoprazole sodium	(generic only)	Greenstone/Pfizer
amlodipine besylate/benazepril	(generic only)	Teva
amoxicillin trihydrate/potassium clavulanate	(generic only)	Teva
conjugated estrogens	Premarin	Pfizer
oseltamivir phosphate	Tamiflu	Roche
tiotropium bromide	Spiriva Handihaler	Boehringer Ingelheim
aripiprazole	Abilify	Otsuka
furosemide	(generic only)	Teva
methylphenidate hydrochloride	Concerta	Johnson & Johnson
azithromycin	(generic only)	Wockhardt
digoxin	(generic only)	Lannett
fluticasone propionate	(generic only)	Apotex

(Based on information found at **www.pharmacytimes.com**)

The Most Common Poisonous Substances and Their Antidotes

Drug	Antidote
Acetaminophen	Acetylcystein
Anticholinesterases	Atropine, pralidoxime (cholinergics)
Antidepressants	Phentolamine (MAO inhibitors and tyramine-containing foods)
Benzodiazepines	Flumazenil
Cyanide	Amyl nitrite, sodium nitrite, sodium thiosulfate
Digoxin, digitoxin	Digoxin immune Fab (Digibind)
Fluorouracil (5FU)	Leucovorin calcium
Heparin	Protamine sulfate
Ifosfamide	Mesna
Iron	Deferoxamine
Lead	Edentate calcium disodium, dimercaprol, succimer
Methotrexate	Leucovorin calcium
Opioid analgesics, heroin	Nalmefene, naloxone
Thrombolytic agents	Aminocaproic acid (Amicar)
Tricyclic antidepressants	Physostigmine
Warfarin (Coumadin)	Phytonadione (vitamin K)

Glossary

A

alligation A mathematical process that allows for calculation of amounts of substances based on their different percentage strengths. (Ch. 10)

apothecary system A system of measurement that was used in pharmacies until the early twentieth century; it has been replaced by the metric system. (Ch. 1)

Arabic numbers The numerical system commonly used, based on the digits 0, 1, 2, 3, 4, 5, 6, 7, 8, and 9. (Ch. 1)

average wholesale price The national average cost of a drug product to a pharmacy; however, in practice, this is simply a "benchmark" price set by manufacturers. (Ch. 17)

B

bar coding A system of marking products with printed horizontal bars and spaces (and sometimes numerals) that uniquely reference information; they are read via scanners attached to computers and offer improved timeliness and accuracy in recordkeeping and dispensing of medical products. (Ch. 8)

body surface area (BSA) Calculated by using a graph that consists of weight and height variables called a nomogram. It is expressed as meters squared (m^2). (Ch. 16)

C

capsules Solid oral dosage forms in which a medication is enclosed in a hard or soft soluble container, usually made of gelatin. (Ch. 12)

Celsius scale A temperature measurement scale wherein water freezes at 0 degrees and boils at 100 degrees; Celsius was the last name of the scale's inventor. (Ch. 4)

centigrade Identical to the Celsius scale and used interchangeably. (Ch. 4)

class A prescription balances One- or two-pan balances that are commonly used by pharmacists; they may be electronic or torsion balances. (Ch. 9)

clinical ratios Common fractions used in dimensional analysis calculations. (Ch. 6)

common fraction A fraction in which both the numerator and denominator are whole numbers as opposed to fractions themselves. (Ch. 2, 5)

complex fraction A fraction in which the numerator or the denominator, or both, may be a whole number, proper fraction, or mixed number. (Ch. 2)

concentrate A highly condensed drug product that is diluted prior to administration. (Ch. 11)

concentration The amount of a particular substance in a given volume. (Ch. 11)

conical graduates Cone-shaped containers with graduated markings for measuring liquids; their slanted sides may make estimations of quantity difficult. (Ch. 9)

continuous IV infusion Replaces or maintains fluids and electrolytes and serves as a vehicle for medication administration. (Ch. 15)

controllers Devices that are often referred to as electronic flow clamps because they control infusion rate by either drop counting or volumetric delivery, using gravity to maintain desired flow rates. (Ch. 15)

copayment A specific amount required to be paid by a patient for a prescription. (Ch. 17)

cylindrical graduates Cylinder-shaped containers with graduated markings for measuring liquids. (Ch. 9)

D

D_5W (Dextrose 5% in water) In this mixture, the solute is dextrose, and the solvent is water. (Ch. 15)

decimal fraction A fraction with a denominator of 10, 100, 1000, or any multiple or power of 10; also known as a decimal. (Ch. 2)

denominator The number the whole is divided into. (Ch. 2)

desired dosage The amount of a medication that is needed for administration. (Ch. 7)

diluents Substances used to dilute another substance, solvents, used to prepare solutions; when added, they decrease concentrations. (Ch. 10)

dilutions Parts of concentrate in total volume; they make a mixture weaker in concentration. (Ch. 10)

dispensing The preparation and distribution of prescription medications. (Ch. 8)

dividend The number that is being divided. (Ch. 2)

divisor The number performing the division. (Ch. 2)

dosage ordered The amount of a medication in milligrams, grams, and so forth from a prescriber for a patient. (Ch. 7)

dosage strength available The amount of medication on hand in milligrams, grams, and so forth. (Ch. 7)

E

electronic balances Scales that use electronic components and digital readouts to calibrate the weighing of different substances. (Ch. 9)

expenses Costs associated with the operation of a pharmacy, which are often called "overhead"; expenses include salaries, wages, rent, utilities, telephone, insurance, legal and accounting fees, advertising, and depreciation. (Ch. 17)

expiration date A specific date when it is determined that a drug product will have lost a significant amount of potency. (Ch. 8)

exponent A method of expressing a number that is multiplied by itself. (Ch. 1)

extremes The two outside terms in a ratio. (Ch. 3)

F

Fahrenheit scale A temperature measurement scale wherein water freezes at 32 degrees and boils at 212 degrees; Fahrenheit was the last name of the scale's inventor. (Ch. 4)

fraction An expression of division with a number that is the portion or part of a whole. (Ch. 2)

G

gram The basic unit of weight in the metric system. (Ch. 1)

gross profit The marginal difference between actual cost and total reimbursement; it is also known as "gross margin." (Ch. 17)

H

heparin lock A device attached to the hub of the IV catheter that allows access to the vein for IV push medications; also known as a saline lock or an intermittent peripheral infusion device. (Ch. 15)

household system A system of measurement primarily used by patients at home; it is less accurate than the metric system. Its most common units of measure include drops, teaspoons, and tablespoons. (Ch. 1)

hypertonic solution Used to maintain daily fluid needs; is generally a combination of saline, glucose, and potassium chloride. (Ch. 16)

I

improper fraction A fraction with the numerator larger than or equal to the denominator. (Ch. 2)

infusion pump A device that maintains flow by displacing fluid at an ordered rate, rather than relying on gravity. (Ch. 15)

inscription The part of a prescription that lists the names and quantities of the ingredients to be used. (Ch. 8)

intermittent intravenous infusion Medication administration as a single dose into a vein that has been maintained open with an IV catheter. (Ch. 15)

intermittent peripheral infusion device A device attached to the hub of the IV catheter that allows access to the vein for IV push medications; also known as a heparin lock or a saline lock. (Ch. 15)

international unit A measurement used to describe potency of vitamins and chemicals. The quantity that measures biological activity, or effect, of substances, developed from the French "Système Internationale." (Ch. 1)

inventory A list of merchandise, itemized by various types, and its costs. (Ch. 17)

inventory control The process of managing inventory in order to meet customer demand at the lowest possible cost, with a minimum of investment in inventory; average inventory is calculated by adding beginning and ending inventory, and dividing by two. (Ch. 17)

inventory turnover A measure of how many times a year a pharmacy's average inventory "turns," or is sold; cost of goods sold divided by average inventory gives the inventory turnover rate. (Ch. 17)

IV bolus A quantity of IV fluid that can be run over a specified period of time through an IV setup attached to the lock. (Ch. 15)

IV push Drugs that are administered by the direct IV injection route. (Ch. 15)

L

liter The basic unit of volume in the metric system. (Ch. 1)

lot number A number printed by a drug manufacturer on each medicine bottle that identifies the batch that the medication came from. (Ch. 8)

M

markup The difference between the purchase price and the selling price of an item, often expressed as a percentage; markup percentage is calculated by subtracting the purchase price from the selling price, and then dividing by the purchase price. (Ch. 17)

markup method The cost of a medication based on price and dollar margin on the ingredient cost of the dispensed product. (Ch. 17)

means The two inside terms in a ratio. (Ch. 3)

meniscus The bottom portion of the concave surface of a liquid; used to measure the volume of a liquid in a container such as a graduate. (Ch. 9)

meter The basic unit of length in the metric system. (Ch. 1)

metric conversion A process of converting between different metric values, such as from milligrams to grams. (Ch. 6)

metric system The most commonly used system of measurement; it is simple to use because it is based on parts and multiples of 10. (Ch. 1)

milliequivalent One-thousandth of an equivalent, the mass of a chemical ion that will combine with 1 gram of hydrogen or 8 grams of oxygen. (Ch. 1)

milliunit One-thousandth of a unit. (Ch. 1)

mixed fraction A fraction consisting of a whole number and a proper fraction combined. (Ch. 2)

multiplicand A number to be multiplied by another. (Ch. 2)

multiplier A number by which another is multiplied. (Ch. 2)

N

National Formulary A part of the United States Pharmacopeia that contains public pharmacopeia standards. (Ch. 12)

net profit The net amount of money left after all operating or overhead expenses have been subtracted from the gross margin; this amount may be a profit or a loss. (Ch. 17)

nomogram A quick reference graph for calculating pediatric doses. (Ch. 16)

normal saline A general term referring to a sterile solution of sodium chloride in water. (Ch. 11)

numerator The portion of the whole being considered. (Ch. 2)

P

parenteral   Injectable; this term indicates medications that are administered other than by the oral (enteral) route. (Ch. 14)

percent   A fraction whose numerator is expressed and whose denominator is understood to be 100. (Ch. 3)

percentage solutions   Liquid mixtures that may be calculated with percentages pertaining to mass/mass, mass/volume, or volume/volume. (Ch. 14)

pipets   Graduated tubes used to transfer small volumes of liquids; also spelled *pipettes*. (Ch. 9)

proper fraction   A fraction with the numerator smaller than the denominator. (Ch. 2)

proportion   A statement of two equal ratios. (Ch. 3)

Q

quotient   The answer to a division problem. (Ch. 2)

R

ratio   A statement of the relation of one quantity to another. (Ch. 5)

ratio strength   A numerator expressing an active ingredient and a denominator expressing the number of parts of a whole preparation. (Ch. 11)

reconstitution   The return of a substance to its original liquid state. (Ch. 13)

return on investment   A measure of the percentage of net profit as related to net worth; net profit divided by net worth, multiplied by 100, gives this percentage. (Ch. 17)

Roman numerals   The numerical system in which symbols (letters) are used to represent Arabic numbers. (Ch. 1)

S

safe-dosage range   Varying amounts of a drug that can be taken in a single dose and still have therapeutic value. (Ch. 16)

sales   The revenue generated by the sale of the pharmacy's inventory (or goods) and services. (Ch. 17)

saline lock   A device attached to the hub of the IV catheter that allows access to the vein for IV push medications; also known as a heparin lock or an intermittent peripheral infusion device. (Ch. 15)

scientific notation   A shorthand method of expressing large numbers that are a product of a number between 1 and 10 and a power of 10. (Ch. 1)

scored   Manufactured with a groove or indentation so that it may be easily broken; scored tablets are designed to be broken into one or more pieces so that lower dosages can be administered. (Ch. 12)

signa   A Latin term that means "mark" or "label." The signa is the portion of a prescription where the prescriber writes the directions for use. (Ch. 8)

solute   The substance being dissolved in a solvent to form a solution. (Ch. 11)

solution   A liquid preparation of several soluble chemical substances, often dissolved in water. (Ch. 13)

solvents   Materials (usually fluids) that can dissolve other substances; common solvents include water, alcohol, and acetone; often referred to as "diluents." (Ch. 10)

stat   An abbreviation used on prescriptions and other medical orders; it means "immediately." (Ch. 8)

subscription   The part of a prescription that includes directions for compounding. Most physicians do not include this information anymore, and pharmacists prepare the compound based on accepted standards. (Ch. 8)

superscription   The area on a prescription form below the patient's name and address. The superscription usually is designated with the "Rx" symbol and is considered the "body of the prescription." (Ch. 8)

supply dosage   An amount of a drug's measured units per a specific quantity. (Ch. 8)

syringe pump   A kind of electronic infusion pump used to infuse fluids or medications directly from a syringe. (Ch. 15)

Système International (SI)   A complete metric system of measurement for scientists; it includes measurements for length, weight, electric current, temperature, matter, and luminous intensity. (Ch. 1)

T

tablets   Solid oral dosage forms containing a medication with or without a diluent. (Ch. 12)

temperature   The measure of heat associated with metabolism of the body, or from any heat source. (Ch. 4)

third-party payer   A company that pays part of the cost of an invoice between a health-care provider and a patient. (Ch. 17)

true proportion   A proportion in which the ratios have been proven to be equal by multiplying the means and extremes. (Ch. 5)

turnover   A measure of time that a product remains in stock and is not used by a pharmacy. (Ch. 17)

U

unit   A standard of measurement based on the biological activity of a drug rather than its weight; used to express measurement quantities of vitamins, some antibiotics, and certain biologics such as vaccines. (Ch. 1)

unit conversion   Dimensional analysis (also known as "units conversion"). This is the process of mathematically changing or converting units of measure. (Ch. 6)

United States Pharmacopeia (USP)   An organization that sets official public standards for all prescription and OTC medications, dietary supplements, and other health care products. (Ch. 12)

Index

A

abbreviations
    apothecary system, 14
    household system, 15
    IV, 272
    metric system, 9–10
    in prescriptions, 123–125
accounting. *See* pharmacy operation and
    business math
adding
    decimals, 46
    fractions, 30–31
adjusting IV flow rates, 292–293
alligation, 174–178
alligation alternate, 174
apothecary, 13
apothecary system, 13–14
Arabic system, 4
average wholesale price (AWP),
    350–351

B

balances, 160, 161
bar code symbols, 137
bar coding, 146–147
beef insulin, 241
beef-pork insulin mixture, 241
biosynthetic insulin, 241
body surface area (BSA), 324–327
    dosage calculations, 324–327
body weight of children, 315–318
bolus, IV, 305–306
brand name, 130, 131

BSA. *See* body surface area
business math. *See* pharmacy operation and
    business math

C

calibrated dropper, 163
calibrated spoon, 163
capsules, 201–212
Celsius scale, 68–71
centi-, 9
centigrade, 68
centiscale, 68
chart order, 127–129
children. *See* pediatric drug
    administration
Clark's rule, 329
Class A prescription balance, 160
clinical ratios, 95
combination drug, 137
complex fraction, 27
computers, 146
concentration, 185–188
conical graduates, 162
continuous IV infusion, 271–273
controller, 297, 298
converting/conversions
    decimals/fractions, 44–45
    fractions, 29–32
    percents/decimals, 61
    percents/fractions, 62
    Roman numeral/Arabic systems, 6–7
    temperature, 68–71
copayment, 351
cylindrical graduates, 162

Dedication

This book is dedicated to

my granddaughter, Laila Jade Mabry

Table of Contents

Part II   Dosage Calculations

Part III   Prescriptions, Drug Labels, and Percentage of Error

Part V   Pharmacy Operations

Appendices

Preface

Pharmaceutical Calculations for Pharmacy Technicians: A Worktext, Second Edition is primarily for undergraduate and postgraduate pharmacy technician students. It features a great amount of expansion on the original edition, including three new chapters, plus a thorough reworking of the book's organization. However, other health science students whose roles involve drug therapy (such as medical assistants and nurses) should also find much of the material relevant to their studies. Some pharmaceutical calculation texts have been strong on pharmacy technician considerations, yet relatively weak in organization of content and practice problems, or have lacked instructor resources and learning resources for students.

My goal in this book is to empower pharmacy technicians through an understanding of the fundamental skills of calculating drug dosages and converting them within the metric, apothecary, and household systems. Additional calculations in the book focus on pediatric dosages.

I believe that developing an understanding of basic math and becoming proficient in drug dosage calculation and conversion are critical skills for pharmacy technicians, in that they play an important role in preventing medication errors that occur all too frequently in the United States.

ORGANIZATION OF THE TEXT

The book is organized in a natural progression of information, allowing users to master the information in order, ranging from simple to more complex. It is divided into 5 parts and 17 chapters, followed by five appendices. Chapters 1 through 4 focus on basic math skills such as number systems, fractions, decimals, ratios, proportions, and temperature conversions. Chapters 5 through 7 focus on calculation methods, including ratio and proportion, dimensional analysis, and the formula method. Chapters 8 and 9 focus on prescriptions, drug labels, and percentage of error. Chapters 10 and 11 focus on dilutions, liquid measures, and concentrations. Chapters 12 through 16 focus on dosage calculations, including oral medications, reconstitution of powdered drugs, parenteral medications, intravenous flow rates, and pediatric drug administration. Chapter 17 features business math as used in pharmacy operations.

The first two appendices feature answers to the Stop and Review activities and the Test Your Knowledge questions. The third appendix features Case

Studies with answers. Appendix D notes the most commonly prescribed drugs in 2011, and Appendix E focuses on poisonous substances and antidotes.

This text is published in full color, which helps to illustrate key points and concepts. It highlights unique learning tools that will reinforce skills and competencies.

NEW TO THE SECOND EDITION

The following chapters are all new to this second edition:

- Chapter 5 – Ratio and Proportion Method
- Chapter 6 – Dimensional Analysis
- Chapter 7 – Formula Method
- Chapter 8 – Interpretation of Prescriptions and Drug Labels
- Chapter 9 – Percentage of Error Due to Equipment
- Chapter 10 – Dilutions and Solutions
- Chapter 11 – Concentrations
- Chapter 12 – Oral Medication Labels and Dosage Calculation
- Chapter 13 – Reconstitution of Powdered Drugs
- Chapter 14 – Parenteral Medication Labels and Dosage Calculation
- Chapter 15 – Intravenous Flow Rate Calculations

The following chapters have been revised in this second edition:

- Chapter 1 – Fundamentals of Math
- Chapter 2 – Fractions and Decimals
- Chapter 3 – Ratios, Proportions, and Percents
- Chapter 4 – Celsius and Fahrenheit Temperature Conversions
- Chapter 16 – Pediatric Drug Administration
- Chapter 17 – Business Math

TOOLS FOR INSTRUCTORS

This text is accompanied by an Instructor Companion Website that includes a testbank featuring over 1000 questions and case studies that correspond to all of the chapters and focus on key points and skills that students must master. Also found on the Website are in-depth PowerPoint presentations. The PowerPoint presentations follow the structure of each chapter to complement the learning experience of each chapter and reinforce key points and concepts. An instructor's manual is also included and can be downloaded by instructors. The instructor's manual features further insights into key concepts that students must grasp.

Reviewers of the Second Edition

Christy Bevins, BS
Pharmacy Technology Professor
Licensed Pharmacist
North Georgia Technical College
Clarkesville, Georgia

Brenda A. Ghigliotto
Pharmacy Technician Instructor
San Pablo, California

Christie E. Martin, ABD, MSM, CPhT
Pharmacy Program Coordinator
Northwest Vista College
San Antonio, Texas

Michelle Miller
Pharmacy Technician Instructor
Kirkwood Community College
Cedar Rapids, Iowa

Mary G. Nelson
Pharmacy Technician
Specialty Pharmacy Services, Inc.
Melbourne, Florida

Douglas Scribner, MEd, CPhT
Director of Pharmacy Technology
Central New Mexico Community College
Albuquerque, New Mexico

Bobbi Jane Steelman, CPT, BSEd, MAEd
Pharmacy Technician Program Director
Daymar Colleges Group
Bowling Green, Kentucky

Mohamad Tlass, BS, CPhT, PhTR
Pharmacy Technician Professor
Houston Community College
Houston, Texas

About the Author

Dr. Moini was assistant professor at Tehran University School of Medicine for nine years teaching medical and allied health students. Dr. Moini is a professor and former director (for 15 years) of allied health programs at Everest University (formerly Florida Metropolitan University). Dr. Moini established, for the first time, the associate degree program for pharmacy technicians in 2000 at Everest's Melbourne, Florida, campus. For five years, he was the director of the pharmacy technician program. He also established several other new allied health programs for Everest in his 22-year career with the university.

Dr. Moini is actively involved in teaching and helping students to prepare for service in various health professions, including the roles of pharmacy technicians, medical assistants, and nurses. He is retired from the Brevard County Health Department, where he was county epidemiologist and health educator consultant in 1990, offering continuing education courses and keeping nurses up-to-date on the latest developments related to pharmacology, medication errors, immunizations, and other important topics.

Dr. Moini is a published author of many allied health books since 1999, notably eight books related to pharmacy technology for Delmar Cengage Learning, including "Flash Cards for the Pharmacy Technician."